Bovine Tuberculosis and the Culling of Badgers

Table of Contents

Preface

Bovine tuberculosis is an infectious disease that affects cattle such as cows, bulls, oxen, calves, buffaloes, and some other farm animals. It is caused by a bacterial species named Mycobacterium bovis (M.bovis). This disease can also be transmitted to mammals including humans, cats, dogs and badgers. In the initial stages of infection, usually there are no visible signs and symptoms. Some common signs of bovine tuberculosis that develop with the gradual progression of disease include weight loss, lack of appetite, weakness, and a low-grade fever. Bovine tuberculosis can also spread from a badger's den called sett through excretions and exhalations of the infected animal. Badger culling is a method adopted to reduce the transmission of bovine tuberculosis. In this method, badgers are slaughtered to reduce the incidence and spread of this infection. This book analyzes the impact of badger culling on the spread of bovine tuberculosis in detail. Coherent flow of topics, student-friendly language, and extensive use of examples make this book an invaluable source of knowledge.

This book is a comprehensive compilation of works of different researchers from varied parts of the world. It includes valuable experiences of the researchers with the sole objective of providing the readers (learners) with a proper knowledge of the concerned field. This book will be beneficial in evoking inspiration and enhancing the knowledge of the interested readers.

In the end, I would like to extend my heartiest thanks to the authors who worked with great determination on their chapters. I also appreciate the publisher's support in the course of the book. I would also like to deeply acknowledge my family who stood by me as a source of inspiration during the project.

David Hill

PART I

Background

1

Bovine Tuberculosis and Badgers: An Introduction

1.1 Badgers, Cows, TB, Science and Policy: A Primer for the Perplexed

For over a generation, the vexed question of whether to cull wild badgers (*Meles meles*: a nocturnal, burrowing relative of weasels and otters) to control the spread of bovine tuberculosis (bTB) in British cattle herds has plagued politicians. Questions of *what is known*, *who knows*, *who cares*, *who to trust* and *what should be done* about connections between cows, badgers and the bacterium *M. bovis* have been the source of scientific, veterinary, policy and increasingly vociferous public debate. Over this time, the controversy has spread—from a local problem involving a handful of people, to a national debate attracting extensive media coverage, costing the country millions of pounds and occupying the time, care and attention of many thousands of ordinary people. Alongside the disease, controversy has spread from its original highly localised context, and has become more visible and significant, creating in recent years a deeply polarised dynamic—tightly focused on badger culling—between increasingly angry opposed sides. Culling advocates argue that tuberculous badgers form a 'reservoir' of bTB infection, which must be removed to prevent bTB from re-infecting cattle and spreading the disease further. They emphasise why bTB must be controlled in the first place: it is a zoonotic disease, meaning that people can also catch it. Until well into the twentieth century *M. bovis* was a significant cause of human TB, particularly in children who drank infected milk: while this public health risk is now well controlled in the

UK, it remains a problem elsewhere.[1] Opponents of culling argue that bTB is more likely to be spread between the cows themselves, particularly when stressed by modern farming techniques and as cattle are increasingly moved around the country. They also contend that badger culling disrupts the complex social groupings of these wild animals, causing the survivors to move around more, disrupting ecosystems and spreading bTB along the way. They argue that policy should instead focus on alternative solutions which may be more sustainable, such as vaccination (of cattle and badgers) and stricter regulatory controls on farming. Others have deep moral objections to killing badgers, wildlife or any animals under any circumstances.

It is estimated that bTB currently costs the British Government around £100 million each year; since culling was resumed in 2010, these have been worsened by policing costs, the political fallout of the controversy, and the emotional and psychological impacts of the disease on farmers and other affected parties.[2] There are important continuities between bTB and previous British animal health crises, most notably the 2001 foot and mouth disease (FMD) epidemic, and policy responses to the emergence of BSE. All three episodes have involved publicly contested scientific uncertainties; political disagreements over how government should act; conflicts between farmers, policymakers and publics, and the death of many millions of animals.[3] However, unlike its notorious predecessors, bTB is curiously invisible: sick badgers and cows are nowhere to be seen, while there are only about forty cases of bTB infecting humans each year, mostly in people working directly with animals.[4] Bovine TB is rarely depicted by the media as a public health issue. Instead, it is framed as two mutually exclusive stories: either a chronic agricultural problem affecting already embattled farmers and a long-suffering government; or an environmental risk and additional threat to fragile wildlife and ecosystems. In Britain at least, the zoonotic risks of bTB are controlled by a regulatory and healthcare system that tests cattle for disease, mostly prevents people from eating diseased meat, pasteurises most milk, and treats the rare human cases. People and animals elsewhere in the world, in countries with weaker, less well-resourced health systems are not so fortunate: however, public debates in the UK rarely acknowledge the global aspects of bTB. Paradoxically, the twenty-first-century controversy over badgers and bTB in Britain may be the consequence of a successful (but largely invisible) regulatory system, which displaces risks from medicine and biology into the more contestable domains of economic, political and moral risk.[5]

Tuberculosis (TB) is an old, familiar disease problem, also characterised by deep scientific uncertainties and problems still defying resolution in the face of twenty-first-century biomedicine. The clinical disease in humans and other animals is caused by microorganisms known as *mycobacteria*—a group which also includes the bacterium causing leprosy, and many non-pathogenic environmental bacteria. Those causing TB are referred to by biologists as the *M. tuberculosis* complex (MTBC): they mostly include microbes which infect a single species, such as *M. tuberculosis* (humans) or *M. suricattae* (meerkats). The most unusual member of this group is *M. bovis*, which infects a much wider range of mammal hosts, including humans, cattle, badgers, deer, llamas, wild boar and domestic cats and dogs. *M. bovis* is the causative agent of the disease known as bovine TB, increasingly being renamed 'zoonotic TB'.[6] Mycobacteria grow slowly and have thick, acid-resistant cell walls: this makes them notoriously difficult to culture and develop reliable laboratory tests for. This slowness and toughness makes TB a very counter-intuitive disease: a long time can pass between infection and the appearance of clinical symptoms, which appear and disappear as the bacteria are active or go dormant, forming cysts (tubercles) in multiple organs of the body (not just the lungs). Unlike, say, influenza, it is not immediately obvious that someone has contracted TB (and it may not be so for many years); testing and vaccination regimes are not fully reliable and use technologies over a century old: while treatments exist, they are neither cheap nor easy, and drug-resistant strains of TB are proliferating. Bovine TB is even more counter-intuitive: it expresses itself in different kinds of animals very differently, it is difficult to directly trace transmission routes, even harder to test for and is resistant to many standard antibiotic treatments.[7] For these reasons, veterinary disease control regimes tend to use surveillance, movement restriction and culling of sick individuals to stop the spread of infection, rarely turning to human public health tools such as vaccination and treatment. This rarely discussed contrast between human and animal public health lies at the core of today's controversy, as does the 'fundamental ontological uncertainty' (the difficulties of fully knowing) what *M. bovis* is up to as it passes between humans, livestock and wild animals.[8]

Over the near half-century that badgers and bovine TB (badger/bTB) have been debated in Britain, the issue has passed across several generations of scientists, veterinarians, farmers, policymakers and politicians. So far, it has been the responsibility of nine prime ministers, fifteen government administrations and twenty-one Cabinet Ministers. As of 2018, there will have been nine expert led reviews of the situation.[9] Badger/bTB has provided scientists with steadily increasing opportunities for investigation and advancement, with publications on the topic going from only one or two a year during the 1970s to between thirty and forty a year in the past decade.[10] While several studies and accounts from participants have discussed the recent history of badger/bTB in the UK, these have generally focused upon a single aspect of the issue, such as farming, animal health policy, animal protection or conservation.[11] In this book, I will bring these varying accounts together to analyse how the worlds of farming, animal health, field biology, natural history and animal advocacy have interacted to create the controversy we see today. The timeline in Fig. 1.1 is therefore designed to orient the reader in these intersecting stories, and how they have contributed to the ongoing development of the public controversy.

Bovine TB was first found in wild badgers in 1971, at a time when regulatory systems had brought levels of disease in humans and cattle to historic lows. Following a frantic period of investigation and legislative change, MAFF introduced a full-scale badger culling policy by 1975: however, it was rapidly mired in controversy. Following a review conducted in 1980 by Lord Solly Zuckerman, scientific investigations confirmed the reports of badger advocates that 'gassing' (pumping sodium cyanide powder into the animals' underground setts) was not working quickly enough to be 'humane', resulting in the withdrawal of the technique. Between 1982 and 1995, a range of alternative culling policies were tried; over the same period animal advocates won further legal protections for badgers. In 1996, senior scientist Prof. John Krebs was commissioned by government to review the situation once again. He concluded that while MAFF's existing research suggested that there was a link between bTB in badgers and cattle, the evidence was 'circumstantial', and that a 'proper experiment' was needed to directly test the effects of badger culling on bTB in cattle.[12] The incoming Labour government was convinced, suspending culling and commissioning the largest field experiment ever conducted in the UK, the Randomised Badger Culling Trial (RBCT) to do exactly that. After nearly ten years and approximately £49 million, the Independent Scientific Group (ISG) conducting the work concluded that—contrary to widespread expectations—culling had the potential to make things worse; that it 'cannot make a meaningful contribution to bTB control in cattle'.[13] This inflamed the controversy, with other scientists, farmers and veterinarians contesting their findings in

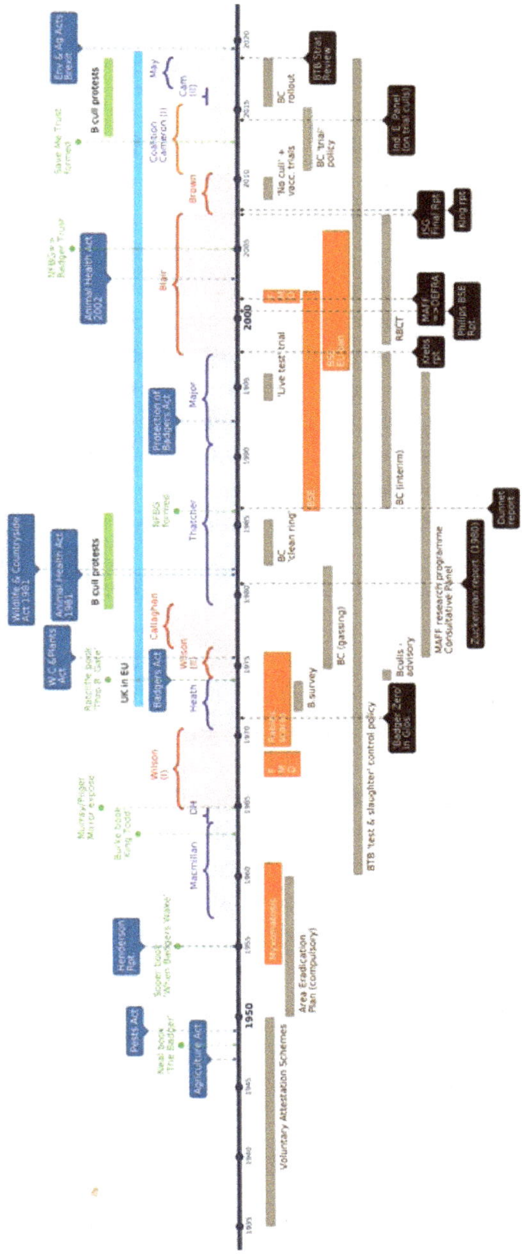

Fig. 1.1 Timeline of the badger/bTB controversy. Animal health events are shown below the line; political, legal and environmental events above. See https://time.graphics/line/83803 for an annotated online version

policy, Parliament and the wider public sphere. Following a change of government, the new minister reversed MAFF's (by then Defra) long-standing commitment to return to culling, taking the ISG's advice and making the (short-lived) decision to not cull, investing in vaccination as an alternative policy solution.[14]

In 2010, the incoming Coalition government declared its intention to return to badger culling, starting with two pilot culls using a new 'free shooting' technique—carried out by private consortia under licence, and paid for by industry.[15] As the policy was implemented, the badger/bTB debate moved from a specialist policy concern, mostly of interest to farmers, veterinarians, conservationists and animal advocates, into the political and media mainstream. The new policy was met by legal challenges and widespread protests (including marches, social media campaigning and local action directly disrupting culls), attracting more media coverage in more prominent places than ever before. Despite the concerns of another group of government-commissioned scientists about their 'effectiveness, safety and humaneness', and widespread criticism from scientists including Krebs, the culls continued. Since 2015, following the election of a Conservative majority government, Defra has started a 'rollout' of the policy, issuing licences in seven new areas. This was followed by further licences in 2017, and the 2018 announcement of licencing across the country, including in areas with low bTB rates in cattle.[16] This geographical extension has been accompanied by a gradual relaxation of the conditions attached to licencing culls—originally shaped by the ISG's findings.[17]

To move towards a deeper understanding of the controversy, we need to think about the development of badger/bTB debates in a broader context. To start with, how do these events relate to what the disease itself was doing? Figure 1.2 conveys a broad picture of how the incidence of bTB in British cattle herds has changed since the 1950s, when mandatory disease control measures were originally introduced.[19] By the late 1960s, this regime appeared to have been a resounding success, with rates of bTB in cattle dropping to unprecedentedly low levels: when badgers were first connected with bTB in the early 1970s these rates had levelled out, but there was little to hint at the problems to come. It is also worth noting the timing of the resurgence of bTB: the lowest point of incidence was in the early 1980s. While bTB was returning during the 1990s, it was not until after the FMD outbreak of 2001 that today's epidemic became fully apparent. From a socio-historical point of view, the lack of any clear correlation between disease incidence and episodes of public controversy (see Chap. 7,

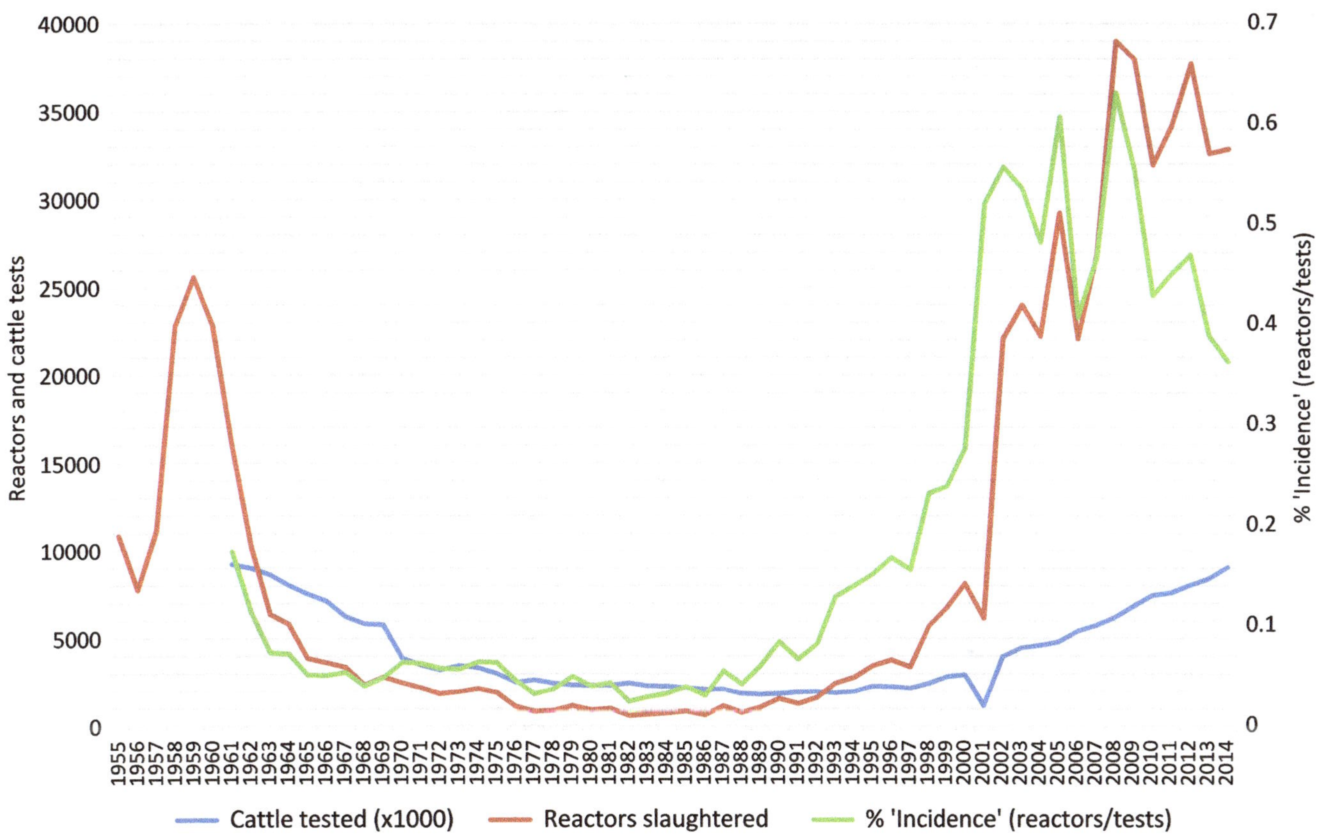

Fig. 1.2 Long-term indicators of UK bTB incidence [N.B. note multiple data sources]. Data sourced with thanks from Atkins (*A History of Uncertainty*, 301)[18]

Figs. 7.1 and 7.2) is particularly significant. Badger/bTB was already a notoriously difficult policy problem long before the resurgence of *M. bovis*, and whenever the issue hits the news, it's rarely for biological reasons.

The timeline in Fig. 1.2 therefore moves beyond animal health to introduce broader contexts of political, legal and environmental events and long-term trends since the middle of the last century. Beyond the swinging back and forth of power between Conservative and Labour governments, we have seen an underlying agenda of retreating and adjusting the role of the state, towards new models of shared governance across government, industry and civil society. The other most significant political and policy change has of course been the UK's entry to, increasing integration with and likely withdrawal from the European Union. Following the post-war boosting of agricultural productivity, we have seen further intensification of agriculture in general, particularly in livestock and the dairy industry, with herd size increasing alongside yields of milk and meat, while many farmers have struggled to turn a profit.[20] Agricultural intensification was a critical factor contributing to the rise of environmental, animal welfare and animal rights movements in the UK: concerns which have in turn precipitated widespread changes supporting sustainability and welfare in protective legislation, policy structures and industry practice.[21] Finally, we have seen two bouts of public crises over the governance of animal health, agriculture and the environment: first over myxomatosis, FMD and rabies between the 1950s and 1970s; and second over bovine spongiform encephalopathy (BSE), FMD, genetically modified foods and bTB since the 1990s.

These shifts in governance, agricultural and environmental politics in the UK have been accompanied by corresponding shifts in scientific understandings of *M. bovis*, badgers, cows, humans and the complex entanglements between these organisms. The 2018 Godfray report provides a detailed and reasonably balanced overview of the current situation, while several other recent review articles and reports provide a range of perspectives.[22] I refer the reader to these sources, but provide here my interpretation of the past and present state of scientific knowledge about relationships between *M. bovis*, cattle, badgers, farming and culling. At the start of our story (in the early 1970s) bTB was considered to be well understood following the success of eradication policies and was not a particularly active topic of research. BTB was also generally understood to be a livestock disease. While it was held as a primary example of zoonosis (human–animal transmission; hence regulatory structures) in the research literature, there was little consideration of the disease beyond veterinary and some public health publications, barring occasional reports of cases in other wild animals.[23] Badgers were also neglected, but for the opposite reason: beyond the writings of a few mammologists and naturalists, very little was known about them.[24] While the burgeoning field of disease ecology was exploring dynamics of infectious disease in wildlife via myxomatosis and plague, these scientists were dealing with rodents and rabbits.[25]

As this book will recount, encountering tuberculous badgers brought together previously unrelated policy, campaigning and scientific worlds. The various forms of badger culling deployed in England and Wales—both scientific trials and disease control policies—have taught us much more, but also uncovered further complexities and generated more questions along the way. This dynamic could be seen following the 1980 Zuckerman and 1996 Krebs reviews, both of which recommended that more scientific research should be conducted. In the former case the uncertainties were around how to cull badgers, while in the latter about the effects of culling on disease spread. Today there seems to be a broad consensus that both cattle and badgers get infected with *M. bovis*; that infection passes between the two populations; and that infection rates in badgers are much higher than in any other wild animals. However, these ideas were contested prior to the completion of the RBCT. While there may be 'a broad consensus among epidemiologists' that this poses a risk to cattle herds,[26] other scientists disagree. This is over whether infections in badgers are mostly a 'spill-over' from cattle (making cattle–cattle transmission the main problem), or are 'self-sustaining' within the badger population (making it more likely that badger–cattle transmission is a problem too).[27] Similarly, the effects and efficacy of badger culling on bTB rates in cattle are still contested. While the underlying theory of *perturbation*—human-induced disruption of ecosystems—is broadly accepted, the extent to which culling-induced perturbation exacerbates the spread of bTB is contested, particularly between ecologists and veterinarians. The picture becomes more complex once you consider what type of culling is involved (gassing, trapping, free shooting), who is doing the job (Ministry employees, private contractors, random people who don't like badgers), over what geographic- and time-scales, and whether it is done as a pre-emptive or post-infection intervention.[28] There are also significant issues around the accuracy of current regimes of bTB testing, and arguments over the risk factors for cattle, which may include broader factors such as herd size and infection history as well as the presence of bTB in local badger populations.[29]

Research and policy experiences from other countries paint a rather different picture. Across Europe, the countries experiencing the highest levels of infection are England, Wales, N. Ireland (not Scotland), the Republic of Ireland (RoI) and Spain. In the RoI (the only other country where badgers play a significant role), scientists are convinced that perturbation is not an issue and culling has brought their bTB rates down. That said, the RoI appear to be in the process of shifting bTB management policies away from badger culling and towards a vaccination-focused strategy, although its efficacy is not fully established.[30] In Spain, wild boar and deer are the main wildlife affected, both of which are culled for bTB control. Elsewhere in the world bTB wildlife 'hosts' include several species of deer, water buffalo, antelope and, in New Zealand, the brushtailed possum. While several of these countries have implemented wildlife culling policies with greater or lesser degrees of policy success (i.e. reductions in cattle bTB), perturbation and other ecological effects have been reported.[31] Furthermore, in the case of New Zealand, possums are a widely reviled invasive species and pest, while the governance situation has also been significantly different in that bTB regulation is controlled and paid for primarily by industry.[32] As we will explore through the rest of this book, the badger/bTB situation in Britain has been shaped by a unique set of ecological, epidemiological, agricultural, social, political and cultural factors for many decades. As such, any simple conclusions drawn by comparisons between other countries and the 'perfect storm'[33] experienced in Britain should be taken with a large dose of salt, as should any attempt at characterising 'the science' of this complex topic as fully in support of—or against—badger culling.

1.2 Knowing Animal Health in the Environment

This book will investigate what happened when the previously unconnected worlds of bTB and the badger were forcibly brought together—when Ministry veterinarians recorded and reported evidence of tuberculous badgers living and dying in a 'hotspot' of cattle TB infection in the early 1970s. It will explore controversies over the connections between *M. bovis*, badgers and cattle since that time, over which bTB went from a well-controlled disease, with policy primarily driven by public health agendas, to a resurgent, poorly understood epidemic, contested between animal health and conservation/animal welfare interests. While the key scientific and policy events have often been documented, they have rarely been explained, or addressed beyond the specific domain of animal health.[34] This book will perform such an analysis, with a central focus on the dynamics of debate amongst the various actors involved with *M. bovis*, badgers and cows in Britain over the past fifty years. This work is important not just as an intellectual exercise, but as a contribution to ongoing scientific, policy and public debates—about bTB itself, about how to control the disease, and about how to consider wildlife in policy decisions about (domestic) animal health, agriculture and the environment. The events of the recent past are often used as a resource by participants in today's controversy, who cite factors such as the introduction of badger protection; intensification of cattle farming and trading; changes in regulatory regimes; or culling itself as explanations for the current disease situation. However, these tend to be picked and used strategically and are often based on anecdotal rather than a critical historical evidence base. By collating this evidence and analysing it, this book can create better public and institutional memories of a notoriously 'intractable' policy problem.[35]

In this book, I combine social science and historical approaches to understanding how science, technology and medicine interact with policy and the public sphere. For a long-standing controversy like this, a historical perspective is essential in order to understand how the badger/bTB debate has developed over time, how it has shaped and been shaped by social and political changes since the 1960s, and also how past decisions led to present policy. I have also drawn upon the ideas of scholars working in fields such as environmental history and animal studies to help me understand how human–badger relationships have become entangled with animal health policy. I have used three key sets of ideas in this book: ideas about how knowledge is built through public controversies; ideas about care, caring practices and how they are built; and ideas about human–animal relationships, including how non-humans shape societal change.

Knowledge Controversies and Epistemic Communities. At its heart, this book is a study of what researchers in science and technology studies (STS) and the history of science call a 'knowledge controversy'—an academic and/or policy and/or public debate centred upon questions of scientific knowledge, expertise and evidence.[36] Controversies are key processes through which scientists build knowledge about the world, and therefore a key site of study for scholars like myself. The painstaking business of publishing a journal article—gathering, interpreting and analysing data; integrating it with theory and research questions; communicating persuasively that the findings mean something; and successfully passing through peer review—is only the beginning. Once an article—a knowledge claim—is published, the real work begins as other researchers working on the topic publish further articles supporting, reinterpreting or directly contesting that claim. This process, scaled up, creates the interwoven fabric of what sociologists and philosophers of science have described as 'normal science', or 'science in the making'.[37] Given the inherently social, collaborative and persuasive nature of this process, it should not be that surprising that once STS scholars started looking closely at how scientists do what they do, they found that everyday scientific practices involve the continual negotiation of uncertainty, personal rivalries and a deep interweaving with other social and political processes.[38]

Public knowledge controversies move out beyond the relatively closed worlds of academia, and start taking place in the wider public sphere, generally involving a wider range of people. In these situations, knowledge is not established within science, then 'popularised' in mass media—instead scientific communication is multidirectional, with information moving back and forth between 'popular' media, policy or campaigning contexts and 'specialist' academia.[39] Public knowledge controversies often involve multiple sources of knowledge and forms of expertise, including scientists, professionals (doctors, lawyers, farmers), non-professional specialists (naturalists, enthusiasts, fans), people with experiential knowledge (patients, parents) and members of relevant publics (local communities, campaigners).[40] Sometimes public knowledge controversies involve multiple disciplines: the need to communicate across disciplinary boundaries (and pursue disciplinary rivalries) is another factor which moves these disputes into the wider public sphere.[41] All these factors make public knowledge controversies even more complex than 'normal' scientific controversies, and more fiercely contested, as more people become invested in scientific debates over topics of deep concern to them. Such controversies often relate to questions of how people should act (politics), as well as what government should do (policy)—contemporary examples might include debates over climate change, artificial intelligence (AI) and gene editing. In these situations, scientific knowledge is still in the process of being built, meaning that what is 'known' about the issues can be highly uncertain and speculative or deeply contested, at times by specific political and economic interests. This further complicates how politicians and policymakers engage with—and formulate policy based upon—the evidence presented to them.[42]

But how and why do scientists come to disagree in the first place? Part of the answer lies in the sheer difficulty of gathering and interpreting data while integrating it with theory to find good explanations, but this is not the whole story. Scientific research is a social process, which breaks down enquiry into many specialist disciplines, each of which establishes their own methods, theories and modes of communication. When thinking about science and policy, another useful concept is that of the 'epistemic community'—a group of people 'concerned with producing and disseminating knowledge', who work together and have shared beliefs, working practices and criteria for assessing validity.[43] The difference between an epistemic community and an academic discipline or field is that the former has a shared *policy* focus, which can pull together specialists from multiple disciplines. Classically, epistemic communities are understood to be 'a network of professionals with recognised expertise' involved with policy problems:[44] policy research explores how such experts can (or can't) contribute to 'policy learning' over time. Indeed, some of this work has examined the increasingly strained relationships between scientists and policymakers over the management of bTB since the 1990s—a situation which has been described as a 'pathology of policy learning'.[45] I argue that public knowledge controversies often involve multiple epistemic communities, who therefore form different understandings of the situation. Other scholars have combined the idea of epistemic communities with that of 'communities of practice', when professional experts work alongside others with relevant knowledge. These epistemic communities have much fuzzier boundaries, which are constantly changing as they work together.[46] Given that the longer history of the badger/bTB controversy involves multiple, overlapping and distinctly fuzzy groupings, which change over time, it is this latter version of epistemic communities that I will use to understand this case.

Following the established practice of many STS researchers and historians of science, technology and medicine, I have taken what is known as a 'symmetrical' stance in relation to the controversy itself. This means that, as far as I am able, I have tried to understand and provide explanations of all sides in the debate, and what they know—explaining positions for and against badger culling, as well as everything in-between. As David Bloor famously argued, such an analysis must also be 'impartial with respect to truth and falsity, rationality or irrationality, success or failure'.[47] In effect, this means that the research deliberately sets aside questions of who is factually 'right' in the debate, and as far as possible investigates the perspectives of all those involved 'symmetrically' (with equal attention). While Bloor and his colleagues may have paid less attention to questions of moral or political normativity, I think these must be directly addressed in a charged debate like this, which taps into deeply held beliefs. For me, it seems a logical extension of the symmetrical approach to likewise set aside questions of who is morally 'right' in the badger/bTB controversy. This parallels debates in animal studies where, broadly speaking, some scholars argue that gaining a deep understanding of animals in society is, or should be, inextricably linked to a normative position advocating for their interests.[48] Others, such as the anthropologist Garry Marvin, who has studied many 'troubling' human–animal relationships (including bull-fighting and fox-hunting), argue that in order to fully understand such practices *from multiple points of view*, researchers need to have 'a shared commitment to no overarching political agenda'.[49] In neither Bloor nor Marvin's case does this imply full moral, ethical or epistemological objectivity nor relativism—I understand these positions as part of a *methodological stance*, making it possible to reach a deeper understanding of controversies.[50] While I am sceptical that anyone could provide a truly impartial analysis of a controversy like this, I think there is a lot to be gained by retaining this as a (possibly futile) goal.[51] In this research, I have done this by being as 'interested' (rather than disinterested) as possible in all sides of the controversy, while refusing to be drawn into any single agenda.[52] I hope that this strategy of reflexive engagement is aided by foregrounding my disciplinary and other backgrounds in the Preface of this book.[53] That said, I have drawn together my thoughts and suggestions on how the badger/bTB debate might move forward in my conclusions in Chap. 8.

Good Care, Good Work, Good Knowledge. The second set of ideas centres upon *care*—what it means to care, about what, and how caring practices are (like knowledge practices) formed by people as they work together. Human medicine is based on a series of core ethical principles, including respect for the autonomy and confidentiality of patients, and acting in their best interests—this generally implies a fierce commitment to the preservation of human *life*. The translation of these ethical principles into the working practices of doctors and nurses has been described by the anthropologist Anne-Marie Mol as the 'logic of care' in human medicine. Mol vividly articulates how this logic structures the day-to-day interactions between patients and healthcare workers in modern Dutch hospitals, down to the smallest details. She also describes how the logic of care interacts and conflicts with a contrasting 'logic of choice', based upon the decisions made by individual patients, about their own behaviour and as they navigate increasingly market-based health systems.[54] These interactions profoundly shape who makes medical decisions and what decisions are made. While Mol's logic of care is physical, practical, relational and able to deal with the inherent uncertainty and unpredictability of health and illness, it also tends towards a parental mode in which it can be difficult for patients to exercise much agency. By contrast, while the logic of choice creates 'the illusion of control',[55] playing on consumer desires in the marketing of medical devices, it also increases the possibilities for patients to exercise agency over decisions made about caring for their own bodies. This idea of 'logics'—or modes—of care has been taken up and used to understand other working practices, including those of farmers, veterinarians and scientists. This work has demonstrated that such tensions and negotiations over choice and agency are not unique to human healthcare and are central to caring relationships between humans and animals.[56]

While practicing and delivering good care is essential to understanding what it is to be a 'good' doctor, farmer, scientist or vet, this research has shown how these modes of care are highly variable, and at times come into conflict.[57] What 'good care' might mean in practice can look very different at different places and times, as well as who or what is or should be cared about, and how to care under varying economic circumstances. Like the knowledge of epistemic communities, modes of care are created as groups of people work together towards common goals. Care and epistemic communities have therefore been brought together to understand how caring and knowledge-building practices co-create each other—in the work of running a laboratory or a museum, in developing standards for what constitutes 'good science', or in caring for laboratory animals.[58] In this book, I draw upon recent research by Gail Davies and colleagues on the 'cultures of care' of laboratory research. I argue that the fuzzy and changing epistemic communities involved in badger/bTB have created correspondingly fuzzy 'cultures of care',[59] constantly renegotiated over the past half-century. When tuberculous badgers were found in the early 1970s, the separate epistemic communities around bTB and around badgers were forcibly brought together, sometimes mutually reshaping and at other times violently clashing with one another. I will discuss in turn the epistemic communities of farmers and veterinarians (trying to protect cows and humans from TB); of pest control scientists and field biologists (trying to protect human agriculture while also caring for wildlife); and of conservationists and animal advocates (trying to protect badgers and environments from harm). I will also explore how these differing cultures of care have also entailed differing expectations of agency—in 'experts', politicians, policy-makers, publics and the organisms involved (*M. bovis*, humans, badgers and cows)—expectations which have been repeatedly confounded over the years. These differences in care have in turn further driven the overall knowledge controversy.

Animal Roles and Traces. This third set of ideas was developed in collaboration with Abigail Woods and colleagues, as we researched the roles played by animals in the history of modern medicine.[60] It is part of a new body of scholarship documenting how animals, plants and environments have shaped a wide range of human activities, from obvious sites such as zoos and research laboratories, through human–animal working partnerships and the production of animals as human food, to the creation and manipulation of ecosystems and societies. Tools for decentring the human in social and historical research have been developed in the burgeoning fields of animal studies and animal history, where scholars have investigated how animal agency—their bodies, minds and actions—have shaped human knowledge, actions, societies and histories.[61] Historical researchers (and anyone working with texts) face a particular challenge: how to build better accounts of non-verbal non-humans when most records have been created by verbal, literate humans. We built upon the idea of using 'animal traces' (the indirect marks left by animals in historical records, such as photographs and accounts of animal actions).[62] Historians of biology and medicine can analyse primary sources deriving from physical traces made by and upon animal bodies, which the scientists of the past have examined, manipulated, interpreted and eventually recorded. These form multiple layers of animal 'traces' which gain meaning in relation to one another—from the immediate remains of animal bodies, through the images, statistics and interpretations made by scientists, out to the new knowledge practices, social relationships, institutions and even imaginaries of animals that are built in response. We drew upon well-established techniques for writing 'histories from below'—work which brings to the fore the experiences of powerless and/or illiterate people in the past. We argued that while such approaches have generally been used to explore the neglected histories of groups of people, these tools can be extended and applied to the challenges of animal history.

Finally, we explored the multiple *roles* that animals have played in medical research and practice since the nineteenth century. These include obvious, well-studied examples such as experimental subjects and models for human health in laboratory research; or disease victims, patients and transmitters of infection. However, our work also investigated no less important, but far less well-studied animal roles: as pathological specimens, shapers of and commodities in food systems, points of cross-species comparison, and vehicles for (human) personal and professional advancement. These are of course related to the wider roles and categories that human societies assign to animals, such as food, pets, workers, experimental subjects, charismatic wildlife and pests—and these roles change over time as society changes.[53] Understanding and exploring these multiple social roles—particularly beyond the immediately obvious ones—can reveal previously unexplored histories. It can also teach us a great deal about how scientific and medical knowledge has been and continues to be built in partnership with non-human animals. In this book I have further developed this approach, following veterinarians, scientists, conservationists and animal advocates as they have followed *M. bovis*, cows and badgers, documenting the traces left behind by these organisms as people sought to understand their complex interconnections.

Methods, Sources, Questions. The most succinct way of describing the methodology of this project would be a *bricolage*—a tinkered together set of techniques, which has grown and changed as my understanding has grown. Another way of describing this would be a 'mixed methods' research design, combining together quantitative and qualitative analyses of texts, with interviews with those involved in badger/bTB.[64] The variety of sources and methods employed has made it easier to conduct this research in an iterative way, with each stage of the work informing the next, feeding back into my research questions along the way.[65] I found material from a huge variety of sources: archives; mass media; policy documents and online materials; clippings and memories from friends and colleagues; and a profusion of images. I helped colleagues in oral history to organise a 'witness seminar' on the history of bTB in Britain, where people who had worked on bTB in the past shared their memories.[66] I have also individually interviewed many of the key players in badger/bTB, across government, scientific and campaigning roles. While I have used some quotations in the book, these interviews have primarily informed my underlying understanding, making it possible for me to make sense of the mass of documentary evidence available. Where possible I have digitised these sources and uploaded them into the qualitative analysis software NVivo, making the data searchable. However, much has remained stubbornly analogue.

The core aim of my research—and of this book—is to map out the contested terrain of debates over badgers and bTB since the late 1960s, so that we can better understand how the current situation has come about—to try and answer the question, 'How did we get into this mess?'[67] How did bTB transform from a well-controlled public health problem into a resurgent, poorly understood disease epidemic, understood either as an economic problem or a potential environmental risk? My work has been guided by two further research questions: What makes a scientific controversy happen 'in public'? Why have scientific debates over the connections between *M. bovis*, cattle and badgers become a public knowledge controversy, and why has this process accelerated? Finally, this has been an extraordinarily British controversy. BTB is a global disease problem, while the European badger (*Meles meles*) lives from the Iberian Peninsula to Iran in the east and north up to the Arctic Circle.[68] However, it is only in the UK and the RoI that causal links have been drawn between infection in badgers and domestic cattle, and only in Britain that proposals to cull wildlife to manage bTB have attracted such intense controversy. Why has this happened in this particular place (Britain) and time (the late twentieth and early twenty-first centuries)? While part of the answer lies in the specific geographical, ecological and agricultural factors contributing to the epidemiology of bTB in the UK, this cannot tell us the whole story.[69] To learn more, we need to first locate the disease (bovine tuberculosis) and then the animal (the badger) into their respective historical contexts before the two were brought together in the early 1970s. We will therefore take a detour into two backstories—first, the broader history of tuberculosis, including the story of how it came to be recognised, researched and partially brought under control. We will then explore the particular (and frankly peculiar) social and cultural history of badgers in Britain, before returning to the main account of the book.

1.3 Histories of Tuberculosis in Humans and Other Animals

People have written about and tried to treat the symptoms of what doctors today would characterise as 'tuberculosis' for a very long time before we called it that name. As documented by historians of medicine, how these symptoms were perceived, described, categorised and made sense of has changed over time. A disease—understood as a collection of physical symptoms, organised and explained according to underlying models of anatomy, pathology and epidemiology—comes into existence when doctors and patients collectively agree that these belong together, to 'frame' it in that way and give it a name.[70] While the ancient Greeks wrote about a disease called 'phthisis', which included symptoms such as coughing, fever, cysts in the body, spitting blood, tiredness and wasting away, some descriptions sound much closer to what we would today call 'cancer'. Treatments (including sea travel, changes in diet and blood-letting) were very different, based as they were on humoral theories of disease. In the medieval world, phthisis gave way to 'consumption' and 'scrofula' (swellings or infections in the neck), but underlying disease models and treatments remained broadly similar. It was from the eighteenth century onwards—as doctors started systematically what happens inside the body, via anatomy, pathology and the invention of new instruments such as the stethoscope—that closer connections were drawn between consumption, respiratory symptoms and lesions in the lungs (tubercles). However, these associations did not fully solidify into the new disease of 'tuberculosis' until later, in the nineteenth century.[71]

The story of how TB came to be recognised as a disease in its own right is closely bound up with the stories of the birth of bacteriology and germ theory, as charismatic scientists such as Louis Pasteur and Robert Koch vied to establish their reputations through the investigation of microorganisms and their connections with infectious disease.[72] In 1882, Koch was the first to establish causal connections between microbes and disease, using an elegant series of experiments with guinea pigs and what he had identified down the microscope as 'tubercle bacilli'. Although the causes of human TB continued to be intensively debated, eventually germ theory became more established as it provided convincing explanations for the spread of disease and generated effective clinical approaches such as vaccination and aseptic surgery.[73] However, confusion persisted over the relationship between TB in humans and in animals. While veterinarians had demonstrated as early as 1860 that TB in cattle could be passed to humans, medical doctors were less convinced. The controversy was compounded in 1901 when Koch himself changed his position on the issue. Counter to his earlier view that TB was a unified disease, caused by a single type of bacillus, at a major international congress Koch argued that TB in humans and cattle were distinct diseases, caused by different bacteria (later classified as *M. tuberculosis* and *M. bovis*). Putting a 'bombshell' under the growing consensus that meat and milk needed to be regulated to prevent zoonotic transmission, he also cast doubt on the risks of humans contracting bTB, arguing that this regulatory effort was a waste of time.[74] Given his status at the time as one of the world's most famous scientists, Koch's intervention generated immense confusion and controversy, reopening the uncertainties around bTB and how it should be controlled. The longer-term impacts were varied: in European countries, where veterinarians had more professional power, measures to remove infected meat and milk from the food chain continued unabated.[75]

By contrast, in Britain Koch's intervention opened a new public controversy, mobilised by industry actors to contest the need for regulation. The government appointed a Royal Commission of experts to investigate the situation (the third since 1890): the investigation took eleven years to conclude that bTB was zoonotic after all. Afterwards, public uncertainties over bTB persisted, making it harder to regulate the disease.[76] During the interwar period, bTB control was implemented using 'accreditation'—milk thought to be 'clean' could be sold under a government-approved quality mark. By the end of the 1930s this idea had been extended to the 'attestation' of cattle herds—a quality mark for those cleared of the disease through the newly developed tuberculin test and slaughtering of infected animals.[77] Further measures such as meat inspection, milk pasteurisation and improving cattle health were also gradually implemented by local authorities and industry. However, these measures were implemented on a voluntary, self-regulatory basis, leading to a piecemeal approach. It was not until after the war, when international health bodies such as the World Health Organization (WHO) and Food and Agriculture Organization of the United Nations (FAO) launched international public health campaigns focusing on TB, including bTB as an exemplary zoonosis, that state-led and enforced control schemes started to come into effect.[78] In the UK, veterinarians had consolidated their roles as experts within government during wartime, and in line with broader state-led agendas for boosting agricultural productivity, a new Area Eradication Scheme was implemented in 1950. This scheme boosted financial rewards and compensation for participating farmers, but also made it compulsory for cattle herds to be tested for bTB and for positive 'reactors' to be slaughtered. It was systematically rolled out across the country, targeting one area at a time, until by 1960 the entire country had been declared 'attested'.[79]

During the 1960s the final eradication of bTB was confidently predicted (following dramatic drops in disease rates), while MAFF's attention turned towards the eradication of other animal diseases such as swine fever and brucellosis.[80] While the local persistence of the disease in some areas was of concern within MAFF, bTB was generally considered to be a success story, dropping off scientific, policy and public agendas. *M. bovis* had embedded itself deeply into systems of food production via these regulatory systems, meaning that by the late 1960s consumers could increasingly rely upon their milk and meat being free of infections, unadulterated, easy to obtain and cheaper than ever before. The implementation of these regulatory structures contributed to changes in practices for producing, distributing, standardising, processing and selling meat and milk, setting us up for today's large-scale, fast-moving intensive livestock production systems. The nuts and bolts of applying, measuring and administering bTB testing in cattle herds created a reliable income stream for rural veterinary practices and consolidated extensive structures for regulating, investigating and researching animal health within MAFF, which we will explore further in Chap. 4. By the end of the 1950s, veterinarians were firmly embedded as core trusted experts in MAFF, while bTB testing had created routine reinforcements of the connections between farmers and clinical veterinarians.[81] By 1971 human and animal health agendas had largely moved on from bTB—widely regarding it as a solved problem—but tuberculous badgers were found in Gloucestershire. These animals had also been the focus of protracted uncertainty and public debate in Britain. However, the participants and key issues of Britain's badger debate had been, until then, entirely disconnected from the agricultural and public health concerns of bTB.

1.4 The Great British Badger Debate

Viewed from the outside, the extent to which British people have become exercised over the fate of an animal that many have never seen, much less interacted with, appears deeply strange. This was made clear to me early in this project, when giving talks to continental European audiences, to be met by blank stares and polite requests to explain exactly what kind of animal this 'badger' was. The extent to which the badger/bTB controversy is deeply embedded in British (and particularly English) history and culture is highlighted in media coverage of the topic, where journalists often reference Kenneth Grahame's classic children's novel *The Wind in the Willows* (1911) to help them talk about animal health. While agriculture today only creates a relatively small proportion of the UK's GDP and national employment, ideas about agriculture, landscape and rurality continue to have political and cultural significance. Many industrialised countries have their own version of the 'rural idyll', but the British version holds animals at its heart: the livestock which have shaped and reshaped our landscape; and the wildlife which are admired, cherished, reviled and excluded from this space.[82] Several scholars have pointed towards the historical legacies of the Industrial Revolution as the origins of this paradox. As human populations grew and migrated to the cities to take up new jobs, people's immediate environments and social conditions changed very rapidly, while agricultural landscapes also changed as food production increased and human tolerance for wild animals plummeted.[83] This period of rapid change created a range of social, political and cultural counter-responses, including campaigns against cruelty, for improving health and for political representation for all. While most of these movements were directed towards people, some (e.g. the abolition of slavery; women's suffrage) sought to extend the circle of full 'humanity', while others were concerned with protecting non-humans, including animals, landscapes and cultural heritage. These social movements initiated ongoing traditions of political campaigning on behalf of animals and the environment, including anti-vivisection, vegetarianism, campaigns to protect the countryside and against blood sports.[84] In art, philosophy and literature, Romanticism turned away from the wonders and horrors of the Industrial Revolution to instead create idealised images of Britain's unspoilt agrarian past, including imaginaries of the 'natural sublime', the 'rural idyll' and greater sympathy for animal suffering.[85] These ideas have left their mark ever since, as government agendas over rising populations and agricultural productivity have contested with those of conservationists, environmentalists, and animal welfare and animal rights campaigners.

The badger came to have such an unusual significance in British culture today via its multiple links into this history of loss and change.[86] As noted above, the European badger (*Meles meles*) has a very broad species range. However, there are some unusual aspects to their ecology and behaviour in the British Isles. To start with, in these countries most large predators (such as wolves and bears) have died out, leaving the badger as one of the largest wild mammals left in these ecosystems. Badgers are omnivorous, nocturnal foragers that in Britain live in large groups, building complex underground 'setts'; they defend well-defined, stable territories. Population densities are significantly higher than in mainland Europe, particularly in the south and western regions of the UK; and it is likely that these specificities contribute to the unusual disease ecology of bTB in Britain and the RoI.[87] Even though the badger is not unique to the UK, it is often seen by this country's inhabitants as 'that most ancient Briton of English beasts'—iconic and symbolic of the nation.[88] Biologists recognise it as one of only thirty surviving 'native' mammal species in the British Isles, and badgers have widespread associations with ideas of Britishness and the land, perhaps due to the long-standing nature of sett occupation. This can be seen in the usage of 'badger' or older versions of the word such as 'brock' in family and place names, while images of the animals continue to feature in heraldry and advertising.

The usage of badger as a verb—'to badger' (pester or harass) points us towards another, darker set of associations. Badgers have been the target of human practices of hunting, digging (using dogs and spades to extract the animals from underground) and baiting (forcing them to fight with dogs) for many centuries. The animals were eaten, their fat was used as a liniment, and other body parts were used in sporrans and shaving brushes. While these practices are now illegal in Britain and Ireland, badgers are still hunted in continental Europe, a factor which probably contributes to lower population densities.[89] The oldest British cultural reference I have found is in the c. tenth-century Exeter Book. This manuscript includes many Old English riddle-poems: number 15 tells the story of a heroic animal that lives underground in a hill, fighting and defending its family against digging invaders.[90] In the sixteenth century, the Tudors legally designated badgers as 'vermin'—nuisance animals—placing a generous bounty of twelve old pence per head.[91] Understandings of vermin at this time were significantly different to our own: while such animals were associated with disease, prior to germ theory this was via theories of 'miasma' and beliefs about witchcraft. Vermin animals were more directly seen as nuisances because they were creatures likely to destroy crops or steal human food supplies: it is probably for this reason that they were not only killed, but were treated as criminals, sometimes undergoing trials.[92] The badger at this time was admired—as many hunted animals were—but also reviled and killed if it got in people's way. Even though the beginnings of modern 'science' were forming, many people's ideas about animals were shaped as much by stories, fables and metaphor as by direct experience or observation. Figure 1.3 depicts a woodcut from Topsell's *The History of Four-footed Beasts and Serpents* (1658). It's recognisably a badger, yet the image is also highly stylised and appears in the book alongside 'real' (bears, cats, beavers) and 'imaginary' (unicorns, dragons, manticores) animals.[93]

Ideas about badgers started to change in the early nineteenth century as questions of animal cruelty—and what to do about it—were debated in earnest. While most early welfare legislation was focused on domestic animals, the 1835 Cruelty to Animals Act made it illegal to 'keep or use any

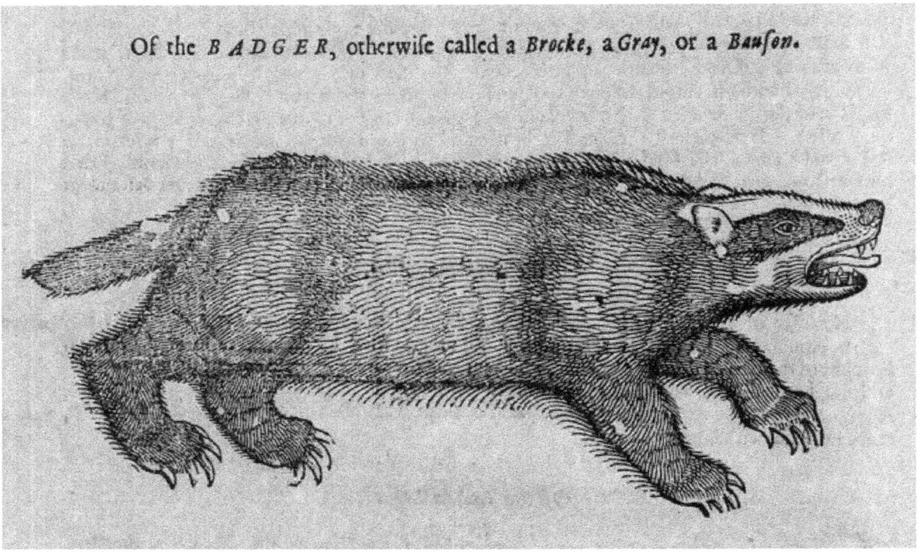

Fig. 1.3 'Of the BADGER, otherwise called a Brocke, a Gray or a Bauson' (Topsell et al., *The History of Four-footed Beasts and Serpents*, 1658)

House, Room, Pit, Ground, or other Place for the Purpose of running, baiting, or fighting any Bull, Bear, Badger, Dog, or other Animal (whether of domestic or wild Nature or Kind)'.[94] The Act was broadly aimed at outlawing popular sports in which animals were made to fight for entertainment, but specifically mentioned badgers as a target of these practices. While the impact was not immediate, the Act had the effect of drawing a line between legitimate hunting and illegitimate baiting, not eliminating but certainly driving the latter underground.[95] Early natural history accounts contain a disorienting mix of condemnations of baiting, descriptions of badger behaviour and detailed instructions on how to dig them out during a hunt.[96] It was during the final decades of the nineteenth and early decades of the twentieth centuries that badgers started to be more actively debated, certainly if the archives of British national newspapers are anything to go by. While they were far from a major preoccupation, intermittent exchanges started to appear alongside routine reporting of badger-hunts. The rise of natural history as scientific practice as well as a popular leisure activity was starting to transform people's understandings of wildlife.[97] These exchanges—often between naturalists and zoologists on the one hand and landowners or people involved with hunting on the other—sketched out two very different animals. People who were observing badgers wrote of an entirely new creature: one which was clean and tidy, played and cared for its fellows, kept to itself unless provoked, and performed 'useful' jobs for humans such as eating wasps' nests. However, other correspondents were not convinced, countering this idea of the Good Badger with their own Bad Badger—a figure familiar from the past. They argued that badgers should not be tolerated, much less cared for or protected, because the animals continued to be a nuisance. The Bad Badger was guilty of a series of misdemeanours, including crushing and damaging crops, 'taking' young rabbits, poultry, ground-nesting birds, and by some accounts even lambs, as well as evicting foxes and interfering with fox-hunts.[98]

The rehabilitation of the badger continued through the twentieth century, as the continuing popularity of natural history combined with the rise of new sciences such as ecology to inspire new artistic and literary representations of wildlife. The most iconic examples involving badgers were published within a few years of one another: Kenneth Grahame's *The Wind in the Willows* (1908) and Beatrix Potter's *The Tale of Mr. Tod* (1912). Like many of Potter's *Tales* (written to teach children the basics of natural history) *Mr. Tod* is a grim tale of predation, in which Tommy Brock the badger is of a decidedly villainous and criminal disposition, fitting into the older Bad Badger tradition.[99] While *The Wind in The Willows* has undergone a continual process of adaptation ever since, the character of Mr Badger is still recognisable (for Brits, at least): wise, old, grumpy and a bit anti-social, but also caring and fierce in the defence of his friends. Over time, Mr Badger appears to have melded with the naturalists' Good Badger, subsequently giving rise to many descendants who populate children's fictions (and toy boxes) to this day. A further phase in the rehabilitation of the badger took place alongside the rise of popular natural history as mass media content and new professional roles in the second half of the twentieth century.[100] Badgers were a particular source of fascination for several of the early photographers and filmmakers involved in the creation of the BBC Natural History Unit during the 1940s and 1950s. While they are notoriously shy, these animals have limited eyesight and a strong sense of routine, making them surprisingly easy to observe. They also provided a technical challenge—pushing on the development of night-time photography and live television broadcasts.[101] The Good Badger therefore became a modern media star not only as a fictional character, but also through the deeply compelling form of the nature documentary.[102]

As we will explore in Chap. 7, 2013 was an extraordinary year for the public controversy over badger culling and bTB. Press coverage reached unprecedented levels, as pilot culls implemented by the then Coalition government were met by widespread protests and controversy over whether they were 'safe, effective and humane'.[103] The Secretary of State for Defra was widely ridiculed for stating that 'the badgers are moving the goalposts' in response to journalistic questioning about the government's response to scientific criticism. A host of public figures ventured their opinions on whether badgers should be culled, in a debate that had by then clearly divided along partisan lines (Labour against, Conservatives for). In the middle of all this, founder of the Glastonbury Festival, national hero to many, and Somerset dairy farmer Michael Eavis decided to intervene, on behalf of his agricultural colleagues:

> The Somerset farmer, who keeps 400 dairy cows and has a badger sett at Worthy Farm, said he was 'not inviting' gunmen to kill his badgers but he was in favour of the cull 'in certain circumstances' when there is 'a heavy loss of dairy cattle'. 'As a dairy farmer I am not on the side of the badger', he told the Guardian, in his first public comments on the controversy over badgers' role in causing bovine TB in cattle. 'They've also uprooted all the orchids, and killed or eaten all the hedgehogs. They're still treated like a protected species, but they're actually quite a damaging animal.'[104]

Eavis is not generally known for inviting controversy for its own sake, despite deeply held political beliefs. What is striking about his comments is how other problems caused by badgers become foregrounded, with concerns about bTB and the impacts of the disease on cattle and farmers coming afterwards. As I have documented elsewhere and will return to at the other end of this book, Eavis is far from alone in his opinion that the Bad Badger is still alive and kicking. In today's controversy over badgers and bTB, participants for and against culling continue to mobilise the Good Badger and the Bad Badger in very similar ways to debates over a century ago. At that time, naturalists were only beginning to observe these animals in the wild, while debates over bTB were still mired in controversy over connecting diseases in humans to those in cows—wildlife was not even on the table. The Good Badger today continues to be lauded, now as a loved charismatic 'native' species and victim of human persecution. While accusations of stealing lambs have mostly receded, the Bad Badger continues to be accused of damaging crops, undermining buildings and eating other loved animals (principally hedgehogs). The rhetoric on both sides continues to focus on badgers' roles in human society and whether we love or hate them, rather than addressing the deep complexities of managing an infectious disease which moves between humans, domestic animals or wildlife in unpredictable ways.

While many aspects of the controversy are unique to the UK, this contested social dynamic (between the 'good' and 'bad' versions of an animal) is not. Instead it fits into a broader pattern of what anthropologist John Knight has described as 'pestilence discourses', seen across many cultures.[105] Pest animals are represented as dirty, violent, reproducing out of control and intruding on human spaces. While some creatures are kept solidly in this role (e.g. flies, rats), sometimes this varies across cultures (primates), while others occupy an in-between space where they are regarded differently by different groups of people within the same culture. When this is the case, the proper role of the animal can be fiercely contested and is often subject to change over time. Striking examples include the multiple roles played by pigeons (loved companions/charismatic wildlife/ dangerous vermin), or the dingo in Australia, which in different parts of the country is a reviled invasive species or a protected and valued participant in indigenous ecosystems and cultures.[106] The curiously plastic and deeply felt nature of the pest category is part of a larger complex of changing social roles assigned to and played by animals; contributing to our earlier exploration of the 'roles and traces' of animals in the history of medicine discussed above.[107] Pestilence discourses have both cause and consequence beyond the realm of language: such animals often have forms of life that bring them into conflict with humans, with often lethal consequences for the animals. At times this involves direct threats to people (e.g. creatures that are predatory, poisonous or disease vectors), but more often foraging on human food supplies, or just getting in the way. Researchers characterise these situations as 'wildlife conflict', recognising that they are as much or even more about conflict between humans about animals, as between humans and animals.[108] As I have argued elsewhere, changes in badgers' legal status and social roles, alongside long-standing continuities in debates over the Good/Bad Badger are strongly suggestive of a long-standing wildlife conflict, which precedes and drives today's knowledge controversy over bTB.[109] Through the rest of this book, I will trace the continuing development of Britain's 'badger debate' since the middle of the last century and explore how it has come to be thoroughly entangled with the politics of livestock health in Britain.

1.5 Vermin, Victims and Disease: An Overview

This book falls into a disciplinary gap—between historical research focusing on the past proper, with most 'modern' history going up to the 1950s at best—and social science, which tends to explore recent events, and rarely pays attention to change over time.[110] With some honourable exceptions,[111] the literature on bTB, conservation and the politics of animal welfare follows a similar pattern, meaning that this project navigates relatively unexplored terrain. Therefore, some tough decisions have been made about the scope of the project and this book barely scratches the surface of what remains to be learned. Principally, this is a history of the badger/bTB knowledge controversy, rather than a broader history of bTB or of wildlife politics. This focus on the controversy and on how knowledge about the problem was built has led to more attention being paid to those people regarded as 'experts' by the state—veterinarians and scientists—and the individual campaigners who challenged those expert views.

One group who have ended up dropping out of view (despite also being 'experts', of a different kind) are the farmers who raise, care, slaughter and grieve for cows infected with *M. bovis*, and whose ambivalent relationship with badgers is also at the heart of the problem.[112] This might sound strange, but it is partly *because* farmers are so important that I have set them aside in this research. My interest in the knowledge controversy, which has largely taken place in Whitehall, various government research facilities and in mass media, means that it would not be possible to do justice to the complexities of this history as it has played out on farms and in rural communities across the country. Such a project would require a different combination of research methods than the ones I have used, most likely employing a local, oral and community history approach. It would also need to be more fully grounded in the maturing literature on the social science of animal health, which is now exploring at depth the experiences, understandings and suffering of farmers involved in animal disease crises.[113] This decision has also been motivated by more pragmatic considerations: the files I consulted in the UK National Archives and the Zuckerman papers mention farmers less often than you might imagine, a telling absence speaking of their lack of direct engagement with policy. I was also unable to gain access to the post 1945 archives of the National Farmers Union (NFU). Given these constraints, I have sought to draw out farming perspectives whenever I can, as well as noting when, where and how other actors do (or do not) engage with farmers.

Structure of This Volume. Part One: Contexts. Chapter 1 introduces the specific combination of historical and cultural contexts which act as a backdrop to the debate. Chapter 2 starts by recounting the twists and turnabouts of how the UK went from a single badger, found dead of bTB in 1971, to a major government research programme and national-scale culling policy by 1975.

Part Two: Reframing Bovine TB (1965–1995). This section takes a thematic approach to the middle years of the controversy, with chapters on three interacting but identifiably different epistemic communities—*animal health*, *disease ecology* and *badger protection*. Chapter 3 explores the worlds, work and caring practices of farmers and veterinarians, drawing out the history and development of veterinary approaches to disease control policy in Britain. It then traces how government veterinarians worked with others to understand the badger/bTB situation (interspersed with episodes of public controversy) in the context of organisational tensions over the place of applied research in government. Chapter 4 conducts a similar exploration of the worlds of scientists responsible for pest control research within government, drawing out how they had already developed considerable experience of wildlife disease and of negotiating the British 'badger debate' by the early 1970s. This obscure niche within government—carved out by applied ecologists—turns out to have been surprisingly influential, not only on the badger/bTB debate, but on British wildlife conservation and animal welfare science, policy and practice. Chapter 5 moves on to the complex and overlapping groups concerned with badger protection, who had succeeded in making the animal into 'a mammal of interest'[114] to a widening circle of campaigners, media audiences and members of Parliament by the end of the 1960s. This chapter draws out the rapidly shifting negotiations between multiple 'cultures of care' through this period, whereby an early consensus that gassing the animals was the most 'humane' solution rapidly disintegrated, creating deeply entrenched oppositions to government policy that persist to this day.

Part Three: Contesting Animal Health (1996–Present). This brings these perspectives back together to explore an entirely new round of contestation over badgers and bTB. I will use the metaphor of the 'backstage' and 'frontstage' of policymaking to analyse the interactions between policy and public spheres since the mid-1990s.[115] This account will start in Chap. 6 with the winding down of MAFF's twenty-year research programme and policy regime, and the commissioning of senior ecologist Professor (now Lord) John Krebs to review 'the scientific evidence' and 'to make recommendations' on this basis.[116] This chapter will address relationships between science and policy since the 1990s, exploring repeating cycles of raised and broken expectations around science, technology and bTB. It will also provide an analysis of legitimacy rivalries within policy between the multiple epistemic communities. Chapter 7 will pick up the public face of these disputes, returning to the campaigners and lobby groups involved in badger/bTB. While this knowledge controversy has always had a public face, from 2010 onwards the issue started to attract much more mainstream media and political attention, culminating in a peaking of the issue in 2013. This chapter will chart the public expansion and increasing polarisation of the controversy, placing it into wider political contexts leading up to the Brexit referendum of 2016. Chapter 8 will summarise my arguments about TB in humans and other animals; wildlife conflicts; care as a driver of controversy; and expectations, science and policy. It will close by looking to the future of badger/bTB, making some suggestions about possibilities for moving forwards with this long-standing and notorious policy failure.

Notes

1. Francisco Olea-Popelka et al., 'Zoonotic Tuberculosis in Human Beings Caused by Mycobacterium Bovis—A Call for Action', *The Lancet. Infectious Diseases* (September 2016). For the global history of (human) TB see Christian W. McMillen, *Discovering Tuberculosis: A Global History, 1900 to the Present* (New Haven and London: Yale University Press, 2015).
2. Farm Crisis Network, 'Stress and Loss: A Report on the Impact of Bovine TB on Farming Families' (2009); Defra, 'A Strategy for Achieving Officially Bovine Tuberculosis Free Status for England' (London: HMSO, 3 April 2014).
3. For BSE see David Miller, 'Risk, Science and Policy: Definitional Struggles, Information Management, the Media and BSE', *Social Science & Medicine* 49(9) (November 1999): 1239–55; Patrick Van Zwanenberg and Erik Millstone, *BSE: Risk, Science and Governance* (Oxford: Oxford University Press, 2005). For the twentieth-century history of FMD see Abigail Woods, *A Manufactured Plague: The History of Foot-and-Mouth Disease in Britain* (Sterling, VA: Earthscan, 2004). For the 2001 FMD outbreak and its consequences, see K. Bickerstaff and P. Simmons, 'The Right Tool for the Job? Modeling, Spatial Relationships, and Styles of Scientific Practice in the UK Foot and Mouth Crisis', *Environment and Planning D: Society and Space* 22 (2004): 393–412; J. Law, 'Disaster in

Agriculture: Or Foot and Mouth Mobilities', *Environment and Planning A* 38(2) (2006): 227–39; Maggie Mort et al., 'Animal Disease and Human Trauma: The Psychosocial Implications of the 2001 UK Foot and Mouth Disease Disaster', *Journal of Applied Animal Welfare Science* 11(2) (28 May 2008): 133–48.

4. Jennifer A. Davidson et al., 'Epidemiology of Mycobacterium Bovis Disease in Humans in England, Wales, and Northern Ireland, 2002–2014', *Emerging Infectious Diseases* 23(3) (March 2017): 377–86.
5. Lam Yee Man, 'Is Risk a Drive for Change? Pollution and Risk Displacement in 1970s to 1980s Hong Kong', *Nature and Culture* 11(2) (1 June 2016): 165–95.
6. For the classification and phylogeny of the MTBC, see Sabrina Rodriguez-Campos et al., 'Overview and Phylogeny of Mycobacterium Tuberculosis Complex Organisms: Implications for Diagnostics and Legislation of Bovine Tuberculosis', *Research in Veterinary Science* 97(S) (2014): S5–19. For 'zoonotic TB': WHO, 'WHO | Roadmap for Zoonotic Tuberculosis' (2017).
7. For biomedical overviews of bTB, see Charles O. Thoen, James H. Steele and John B. Kaneene, *Zoonotic Tuberculosis: Mycobacterium Bovis and Other Pathogenic Mycobacteria* (Hoboken, NJ: John Wiley & Sons, 2014); M. Chambers et al., *Bovine Tuberculosis* (Wallingford, Oxfordshire: CABI, 2018).
8. Peter J. Atkins, *A History of Uncertainty: Bovine Tuberculosis in Britain, 1850 to the Present* (Winchester: Winchester University Press, 2016), 318. For a fuller exploration from the perspective of *M. bovis*, see also Philip A. Robinson, 'Performativity and a Microbe: Exploring Mycobacterium Bovis and the Political Ecologies of Bovine Tuberculosis', *BioSocieties* (6 June 2018).
9. In date order, the reviews are: S. L. Zuckerman, 'Badgers, Cattle and Tuberculosis' (London: HMSO, 1980); George M. Dunnet, David M. Jones and John P. McInerney, 'Badgers and Bovine Tuberculosis: Review of Policy' (London: HMSO, 1986); J. R. Krebs et al., 'Bovine Tuberculosis in Cattle and Badgers: Report by the Independent Scientific Review Group' (London: Ministry of Agriculture, Fisheries and Food, 1997); H. Charles J. Godfray et al., 'Independent Scientific Review of the Randomised Badger Culling Trial and Associated Epidemiological Research' (CSL, 4 March 2004); John Bourne et al., 'Bovine TB: The Scientific Evidence, Final Report of the Independent Scientific Group on Cattle TB', Independent Scientific Group on Cattle TB (London: Defra, 2007); David King et al., 'Bovine Tuberculosis in Cattle and Badgers' (London: Defra, 30 July 2007); H. Charles J. Godfray et al., 'A Restatement of the Natural Science Evidence Base Relevant to the

Control of Bovine Tuberculosis in Great Britain', *Proceedings of the Royal Society B: Biological Sciences* 280(1768) (2013): 1–18; Ranald Munro et al., 'Pilot Badger Culls in Somerset and Gloucestershire Report by the Independent Expert Panel' (London: Defra, 5 March 2014); H. Charles J. Godfray et al., 'Bovine TB Strategy Review: Report to Rt Hon Michael Gove MP, Secretary of State, Defra' (London: Defra, 2018).

10. Source: Web of Knowledge and PubMed databases, search for 'badger AND bovine tuberculosis'.
11. See, e.g. Atkins, *A History of Uncertainty*; Philip A. Robinson, 'A History of Bovine Tuberculosis Eradication Policy in Northern Ireland', *Epidemiology and Infection* 143(15) (2015): 3182–95; Keir Waddington, *The Bovine Scourge: Meat, Tuberculosis and Public Health, 1850–1914* (Woodbridge: Boydell & Brewer, 2006); Patrick Barkham, *Badgerlands: The Twilight World of Britain's Most Enigmatic Animal* (London: Granta Books, 2014); Stephan Price, *Thinking through Badgers: Researching the Controversy over Bovine Tuberculosis and the Culling of Badgers* (Wilmington, DE: Vernon Press, 2017); Dominic Dyer, *Badgered to Death: The People and Politics of the Badger Cull* (Kingston Upon Thames: Canbury Press, 2016).
12. Krebs et al., 'Bovine Tuberculosis in Cattle and Badgers', 7–8.
13. Bourne et al., 'Bovine TB', 14. For overall costs of the RBCT, see Defra, 'Total Cost of the Randomised Badger Culling Trial—A Freedom of Information Request to Department for Environment, Food and Rural Affairs', WhatDoTheyKnow, 5 September 2011.
14. Angela Cassidy, '"Big Science" in the Field: Experimenting with Badgers and Bovine TB, 1995–2015', *History and Philosophy of the Life Sciences* 37(3) (2015): 305–205.
15. Defra, 'Bovine Tuberculosis : The Government's Approach to Tackling the Disease and Consultation on a Badger Control Policy' (London: Department of Environment and Rural Affairs, 2010).
16. George Eustace, 'Bovine TB: Written Statement—HCWS720' (House of Commons, 24 May 2018).
17. Rebecca Giesler and Elena Ares, 'Badger Culling in England', *House of Commons Library Briefing Paper*, House of Commons Library Briefing Paper, 6837 (12 April 2018).
18. Atkins's data was collated from several sources: directly from AHVLA/AHPA; the UK Chief Veterinary Officer's Annual Report series; and the Parliamentary Select Committee on Agriculture's 5th Report Agriculture Committee, 'Badgers and Bovine TB, Vol. II: Fifth Report of Session 1998–1999 (HC 233-II)', Agriculture Committee Reports (London: House of Commons: HMSO, 20 April 1999).
19. As Atkins (*A History of Uncertainty*, 301) discusses, MAFF/Defra have frequently changed how they record bTB statistics, making long-term

comparisons problematic, to say the least. To gain a fuller picture, I recommend comparing this graph with those of Krebs et al., 'Bovine Tuberculosis in Cattle and Badgers', 13; Godfray et al., 'A Strategy for Achieving Bovine Tuberculosis Free Status for England', 16; Simon J. More et al., 'Further Description of Bovine Tuberculosis Trends in the United Kingdom and the Republic of Ireland, 2003–2015', *Veterinary Record* 183(23) (15 December 2018): 717.

20. Matt Lobley, Michael Winter and Rebecca Wheeler, *The Changing World of Farming in Brexit UK* (New York: Routledge, 2018).
21. Karen Sayer, 'Animal Machines: The Public Response to Intensification in Great Britain, c. 1960–c. 1973', *Agricultural History* 87(4) (2013): 473–501; Jon Agar, 'Transition: Sea Change in the Long 1960s', in *Science in the 20th Century and Beyond* (Cambridge: Polity, 2012), 403–32; Michael Tichelar, *The History of Opposition to Blood Sports in Twentieth Century England: Hunting at Bay* (New York: Taylor & Francis, 2016); Steven Griggs and David Howarth, 'Protest Movements, Environmental Activism and Environmentalism in the United Kingdom', in *The SAGE Handbook of Environment and Society* (London: SAGE, 2007), 314–24.
22. For accessible primers on the natural science of bTB (from several angles), I refer readers to (1) the TB Knowledge Exchange, run by my Exeter colleague Dr Andrew Robertson, 'TB Knowledge Exchange', TB Knowledge Exchange, 2018; (2) the multi-agency funded TB Hub: http://www.tbhub.co.uk/ and TB Advisory Service: http://www.tbas.org.uk/; (3) the badger/bTB briefing pages of the British Veterinary Association: https://www.bva.co.uk/News-campaigns-and-policy/Policy/Farm-animals/Bovine-tuberculosis/; and (4) a recent briefing published by the Zoological Society of London ZSL, 'Eradicating TB from Cattle and Badgers—A Review of Evidence' (London: Zoological Society of London, September 2018). For more detailed reviews see Godfray et al., 'A Strategy for Achieving Bovine Tuberculosis Free Status for England'; A. R. Allen, R. A. Skuce and A. W. Byrne, 'Bovine Tuberculosis in Britain and Ireland—A Perfect Storm? The Confluence of Potential Ecological and Epidemiological Impediments to Controlling a Chronic Infectious Disease', *Frontiers in Veterinary Science* 5 (2018): 109; C. Gortázar, J. F. Ruiz-Fons and U. Höfle, 'Infections Shared with Wildlife: An Updated Perspective', *European Journal of Wildlife Research* 62(5) (1 October 2016): 511–25; Robbie A. McDonald, 'Animal Health: How to Control Bovine Tuberculosis', *Nature* 511(7508) (July 2014): 158–59; Olea-Popelka et al., 'Zoonotic Tuberculosis in Human Beings Caused by Mycobacterium Bovis'; Thoen, Steele and Kaneene, *Zoonotic Tuberculosis*; Chambers et al., *Bovine Tuberculosis*.
23. WHO and FAO, 'JOINT WHO/FAO Expert Group on Zoonoses: Report on the First Session', *World Health Organization Technical Report*

Series 40 (May 1951): 1–47; J. W. R. Pearce, L. P. Pugh and Sir John Ritchie, *Animal Health: A Centenary, 1865–1965: A Century of Endeavour to Control Diseases of Animals* (London: Ministry of Agriculture, Fisheries & Food, HMSO, 1965).

24. Ernest G. Neal, *The Badger*, New Naturalists Monographs 1 (London: Collins, 1948); Ernest G. Neal, 'The National Badger Survey', *Mammal Review* 2(2) (1972): 55–64.
25. Warwick Anderson, 'Nowhere to Run, Rabbit: The Cold-War Calculus of Disease Ecology', *History and Philosophy of the Life Sciences* 39(2) (2017): 13–13; Susan D. Jones, 'Population Cycles, Disease, and Networks of Ecological Knowledge', *Journal of the History of Biology* 70(2) (2017): 357–91.
26. Godfray et al., 'A Strategy for Achieving Bovine Tuberculosis Free Status for England', 1.
27. Godfray et al., 'A Strategy for Achieving Bovine Tuberculosis Free Status for England', 67–69.
28. Jon Bielby et al., 'Localised Badger Culling Increases Risk of Herd Breakdown on Nearby, Not Focal, Land', ed. Emmanuel Serrano Ferron, *PLoS ONE* 11(10) (October 2016): e0164618–e0164618; ZSL, 'Eradicating TB from Cattle and Badgers—A Review of Evidence'; More et al., 'Further Description of Bovine Tuberculosis Trends in the United Kingdom and the Republic of Ireland, 2003–2015'; Carly Rozins et al., 'Social Structure Contains Epidemics and Regulates Individual Roles in Disease Transmission in a Group-Living Mammal', *Ecology and Evolution* 8(23) (2018): 12044–55; Lucy A. Brunton et al., 'Assessing the Effects of the First 2 Years of Industry-Led Badger Culling in England on the Incidence of Bovine Tuberculosis in Cattle in 2013–2015', *Ecology and Evolution* 7(18) (1 September 2017): 7213–30.
29. McDonald, 'Animal Health: How to Control Bovine Tuberculosis'; J. M. Broughan et al., 'A Review of Risk Factors for Bovine Tuberculosis Infection in Cattle in the UK and Ireland', *Epidemiology & Infection* 144(14) (October 2016): 2899–2926.
30. More et al., 'Further Description of Bovine Tuberculosis Trends in the United Kingdom and the Republic of Ireland, 2003–2015'; Andrew James Kerr Conlan et al., 'The Intractable Challenge of Evaluating Cattle Vaccination as a Control for Bovine Tuberculosis', ed. Neil M Ferguson, *ELife* 7 (5 June 2018): e27694; Eamonn Gormley et al., 'Oral Vaccination of Free-Living Badgers (Meles Meles) with Bacille Calmette Guerin (BCG) Vaccine Confers Protection against Tuberculosis', ed. Ann Rawkins, *PLoS ONE* 12(1) (January 2017): e0168851–e0168851.
31. Christian Gortazar et al., 'The Wild Side of Disease Control at the Wildlife–Livestock–Human Interface: A Review', *Frontiers in Veterinary*

Science 1 (January 2015): 1–12; More et al., 'Further Description of Bovine Tuberculosis Trends in the United Kingdom and the Republic of Ireland, 2003–2015'.

32. Annie Potts, 'Kiwis against Possums: A Critical Analysis of Anti-Possum Rhetoric in Aotearoa New Zealand', *Society & Animals* 17(1) (February 2009): 1–20; G. Enticott, 'Navigating Veterinary Borderlands: "Heiferlumps", Epidemiological Boundaries and the Control of Animal Disease in New Zealand', *Transactions of the Institute of British Geographers* 42(2) (November 2016): 153–65.
33. Allen, Skuce, and Byrne, 'Bovine Tuberculosis in Britain and Ireland—A Perfect Storm?'
34. For overviews, see Wyn Grant, 'Intractable Policy Failure: The Case of Bovine TB and Badgers', *The British Journal of Politics & International Relations* 11(4) (2009): 557–73; Atkins, *A History of Uncertainty*; Robinson, 'A History of Bovine Tuberculosis Eradication Policy in Northern Ireland'; Peter J. Atkins and Philip A. Robinson, 'Bovine Tuberculosis and Badgers in Britain: Relevance of the Past', *Epidemiology and Infection* 141(7) (January 2013): 1437–44; R. M. Bennett, 'The Political Economy of Bovine Tuberculosis in Great Britain', *Revue Scientifique et Technique de l'OIE* 36(1) (1 January 2017): 105–14.
35. Grant, 'Intractable Policy Failure: The Case of Bovine TB and Badgers'.
36. For 'knowledge controversies' see David Bloor, *Knowledge and Social Imagery* (2nd edition) (1976; repr., Chicago: University of Chicago Press, 1991); S. J. Whatmore, 'Mapping Knowledge Controversies: Science, Democracy and the Redistribution of Expertise', *Progress in Human Geography* 33(5) (July 2009): 587–98; Andrew Barry, 'Political Situations: Knowledge Controversies in Transnational Governance', *Critical Policy Studies* 6(3) (October 2012): 324–36.
37. For normal science, see Thomas S. Kuhn, *The Structure of Scientific Revolutions: 50th Anniversary Edition* (Chicago and London: University of Chicago Press, 2012). For science in the making, Bruno Latour, *Science in Action: How to Follow Scientists and Engineers through Society* (Cambridge, MA: Harvard University Press, 1987).
38. For an accessible introduction to STS ideas, see Sergio Sismondo, *An Introduction to Science and Technology Studies* (Chichester, UK: Wiley-Blackwell, 2010).
39. B. V. Lewenstein, 'From Fax to Facts—Communication in the Cold-Fusion Saga', *Social Studies of Science* 25(3) (1995): 403–36; Massimiano Bucchi, *Science and the Media: Alternative Routes to Scientific Communications* (New York: Routledge, 1998).
40. Brian Wynne, 'Misunderstood Misunderstanding: Social Identities and Public Uptake of Science', *Public Understanding of Science* 1 (1992):

281–304; S. Epstein, 'The Construction of Lay Expertise: AIDS Activism and the Forging of Credibility in the Reform of Clinical Trials', *Science, Technology & Human Values* 20(4) (October 1995): 408–37; H. M. Collins and R. Evans, 'The Third Wave of Science Studies: Studies of Expertise and Experience', *Social Studies of Science* 32(2) (2002): 235–96; Whatmore, 'Mapping Knowledge Controversies: Science, Democracy and the Redistribution of Expertise'; Morgan Meyer, 'Caring for Weak Ties—The Natural History Museum as a Place of Encounter between Amateur and Professional Science', *Sociological Research Online* 15(2) (2010): 9.

41. Angela Cassidy, 'Evolutionary Psychology as Public Science and Boundary Work', *Public Understanding of Science* 15(2) (April 2006): 175–205; Angela Cassidy, 'The (Sexual) Politics of Evolution: Popular Controversy in the Late 20th-Century United Kingdom', *History of Psychology* 10(2) (May 2007): 199–226.
42. Adam Spencer, 'One Body of Evidence, Three Different Policies: Bovine Tuberculosis Policy in Britain', *Politics* 31(2) (2011): 91–99; Warren Pearce, Anna Wesselink and Hal Colebatch, 'Evidence and Meaning in Policy Making', *Evidence & Policy: A Journal of Research, Debate and Practice* 10(2) (May 2014): 161–65; Mark B. Brown, 'Politicizing Science: Conceptions of Politics in Science and Technology Studies', *Social Studies of Science* 45(1) (December 2015): 3–30; Paul Cairney, 'The UK Government's Imaginative Use of Evidence to Make Policy', *British Politics* (5 January 2018).
43. 'Epistemic' means systems for building knowledge—for overviews, see Morgan Meyer and Susan Molyneux-Hodgson, 'Introduction: The Dynamics of Epistemic Communities', *Sociological Research Online* 15(2) (2010): 1–7; Peter M. Haas, 'Introduction: Epistemic Communities and International Policy Coordination', *International Organization* 46(1) (1992): 1–35.
44. Haas 'Introduction', 3.
45. See Claire A. Dunlop, 'Pathologies of Policy Learning: What Are They and How Do They Contribute to Policy Failure?' *Text* (January 2017). For the bTB case as pathological, also see Claire A. Dunlop, 'Epistemic Communities', in *Routledge Handbook of Public Policy*, ed. Eduardo Araral et al. (New York: Routledge, 2012), 229–44; Claire A. Dunlop, 'Contestation and Contingency in Advisory Governance', in *Rethinking Governance*, ed. Mark Bevir and R. A. W. Rhodes (New York: Routledge, 2016), 15.
46. For communities of practice, see Susan Leigh Star, 'Power, Technology and the Phenomenology of Conventions: On Being Allergic to Onions', *The Sociological Review* 38(S1) (1 May 1990): 41. For amateur/professional epistemic communities, see Meyer, 'Caring for Weak Ties'; Meyer

and Molyneux-Hodgson, 'Introduction: The Dynamics of Epistemic Communities'.

47. Bloor, *Knowledge and Social Imagery*, 7; Sismondo, *An Introduction to Science and Technology Studies*.
48. E.g. Nik Taylor and Richard Twine, *The Rise of Critical Animal Studies: From the Margins to the Centre* (New York: Routledge, 2014).
49. Garry Marvin, *Bullfight* (Champaign, IL: University of Illinois Press, 1994); Garry Marvin, 'English Foxhunting: A Prohibited Practice', *International Journal of Cultural Property* 14(3) (2007): 339–60; Garry Marvin and Susan McHugh, 'In It Together: An Introduction to Human–Animal Studies', in *Routledge Handbook of Human–Animal Studies*, ed. Garry Marvin and Susan McHugh (New York: Routledge, 2014), 1–9 (see p. 9); Garry Marvin and Susan McHugh, 'Interviewee: Garry Marvin; Interviewer: Susan Mchugh', *Antennae: The Journal of Nature in Visual Culture* 39 (Spring 2017): 7–20.
50. On symmetry, see Trevor J. Pinch and Wiebe E. Bijker, 'The Social Construction of Facts and Artefacts: Or How the Sociology of Science and the Sociology of Technology Might Benefit Each Other', *Social Studies of Science* 14(3) (1 August 1984): 399–441; H. M. Collins, 'In Praise of Futile Gestures: How Scientific Is the Sociology of Scientific Knowledge?' *Social Studies of Science* 26(2) (1996): 224–29; Bloor, *Knowledge and Social Imagery*, 158–85.
51. On neutrality in STS and 'futile gestures', see Collins, 'In Praise of Futile Gestures'.
52. My thanks to Sara Bea for her thoughts on the importance of such refusals: Sara Bea, 'The Good, the Bad and the Difficult: Sharpening STS Tools to Navigate Conflicting Normativities in the Medical Practice of Deceased Organ Donation', in *EASST2018: Meetings—Making Science, Technology and Society Together* (European Association for the Study of Science and Technology Conference, University of Lancaster, 2018).
53. See also Donna J. Haraway, 'The Promises of Monsters: A Regenerative Politics for Inappropriate/d Others', in *Cultural Studies*, ed. Lawrence Grossberg, Cary Nelson and Paula A. Treichler (London: Routledge, 1992), 295–337; Donna J. Haraway, *When Species Meet* (Minneapolis: University of Minnesota Press, 2007); Gail Davies et al., 'Science, Culture, and Care in Laboratory Animal Research: Interdisciplinary Perspectives on the History and Future of the 3Rs', *Science, Technology, & Human Values* 43(4) (2018): 603–21; Kristin Asdal, '"Interested Methods" and "Versions of Pragmatism"', *Science, Technology, & Human Values* 43(4) (7 May 2018): 748–55, for similar approaches.
54. Annemarie Mol, *The Logic of Care: Health and the Problem of Patient Choice* (New York: Routledge, 2008).
55. Mol, *The Logic of Care*, 25.

56. J. Law and A. Mol, 'The Actor Enacted: Cumbrian Sheep in 2001', in *Material Agency: Towards a Non-Anthropocentric Approach* (Dordrecht: Springer International, 2008), 57–77; Annemarie Mol, Ingunn Moser and Jeannette Pols, eds, *Care in Practice: On Tinkering in Clinics, Homes and Farms* (Bielefeld: Transcript Verlag, 2010); Thom van Dooren, 'Care: Living Lexicon for the Environmental Humanities', *Environmental Humanities* 5(2) (2014): 291–94; Amanda Rees, 'Animal Agents? Historiography, Theory and the History of Science in the Anthropocene', *BJHS Themes* 2 (January 2017): 1–10; Haraway, *When Species Meet.*
57. For 'good' farmers and veterinarians see Rhiannon Naylor et al., 'The "Good Farmer": Farmer Identities and the Control of Exotic Livestock Disease in England', *Sociologia Ruralis* 58(1) (2016): 3–19; Orla Shortall et al., 'Broken Biosecurity? Veterinarians' Framing of Biosecurity on Dairy Farms in England', *Preventive Veterinary Medicine* 132 (2016): 20–31; Tone Druglitrø, '"Skilled Care" and the Making of Good Science', *Science, Technology, & Human Values* 43(4) (2018): 649–70; Orla Shortall et al., 'True Cowmen and Commercial Farmers: Exploring Vets' and Dairy Farmers' Contrasting Views of "Good Farming" in Relation to Biosecurity', *Sociologia Ruralis* 58(3) (2018): 583–603.
58. For care and knowledge work in laboratories, see Anne Kerr and Lisa Garforth, 'Affective Practices, Care and Bioscience: A Study of Two Laboratories', *The Sociological Review* 64(1) (1 February 2016): 3–20. For museums and amateur–expert interactions Meyer, 'Caring for Weak Ties'. For good science and care, Druglitrø, '"Skilled Care" and the Making of Good Science'; Davies et al., 'Science, Culture, and Care in Laboratory Animal Research'.
59. Beth Greenhough and Emma Roe, 'Exploring the Role of Animal Technologists in Implementing the 3Rs: An Ethnographic Investigation of the UK University Sector', *Science, Technology, & Human Values* 43(4) (2018): 694–722; Davies et al., 'Science, Culture, and Care in Laboratory Animal Research'.
60. Angela Cassidy et al., 'Animal Roles and Traces in the History of Medicine, c.1880–1980', *BJHS Themes* 2 (January 2017): 11–33; Abigail Woods et al., *Animals and the Shaping of Modern Medicine: One Health and Its Histories* (Cham, Switzerland: Palgrave Macmillan, 2018).
61. Rees, 'Animal Agents?'
62. Etienne Benson, 'Animal Writes: Historiography, Disciplinarity, and the Animal Trace', in *Making Animal Meaning*, ed. Linda Kalof and Georgina M. Montgomery (East Lansing: Michigan State University Press, 2011), 3–16.
63. See, e.g., John Knight, 'Introduction', in *Natural Enemies: People–Wildlife Conflicts in Anthropological Perspective*, ed. John Knight (New York: Routledge, 2000), 1–36; Hal Herzog, *Some We Love, Some We*

Hate, Some We Eat: Why It's So Hard to Think Straight about Animals (San Francisco: Harper Collins, 2010).

64. Norman K. Denzin and Yvonna S. Lincoln, eds, *The SAGE Handbook of Qualitative Research*, fifth edition (Thousand Oaks, CA: SAGE, 2017), chap. introduction. See Preface, p. iii for further details.
65. A Strauss and J Corbin, 'Grounded Theory Methodology: An Overview', in *Handbook of Qualitative Research*, ed. N. K. Denzin and Y. S. Lincoln (Thousand Oaks, CA: Sage, 1994), 273–85.
66. Caroline Overy and E. M. Tansey, *A History of Bovine TB c.1965–c. 2000*, Wellcome Witnesses to Twentieth Century Medicine 55 (London: Queen Mary University of London, 2015).
67. David Reynolds, 'Case Study: TV History: Probing People's Comfortable Assumptions', *History and Policy* (18 August 2016); Richard E. Neustadt and Ernest R. May, *Thinking in Time: The Use of History for Decision Makers* (New York: Simon and Schuster, 1986).
68. Timothy J. Roper, *Badger* (London: Collins, 2010), 12.
69. See, e.g., Catherine M. O'Connor et al., 'An Ecological and Comparative Perspective on the Control of Bovine Tuberculosis in Great Britain and the Republic of Ireland', *Preventive Veterinary Medicine* 104(3–4) (May 2012): 185–97; S. D. Fitzgerald and J. B. Kaneene, 'Wildlife Reservoirs of Bovine Tuberculosis Worldwide: Hosts, Pathology, Surveillance, and Control', *Veterinary Pathology* 50(3) (May 2013): 488–99; Davidson et al., 'Epidemiology of Mycobacterium Bovis Disease in Humans in England, Wales, and Northern Ireland, 2002–2014'; Matthew J. Silk et al., 'Using Social Network Measures in Wildlife Disease Ecology, Epidemiology, and Management', *BioScience* 67(3) (1 March 2017): 245–57.
70. Charles E. Rosenberg, 'Disease in History: Frames and Framers', *The Milbank Quarterly* 67 (1989): 1–15; Charles E. Rosenberg and Janet Lynne Golden, *Framing Disease: Studies in Cultural History* (New Brunswick, NJ: Rutgers University Press, 1992).
71. For an introduction to the history of TB see Helen Bynum, *Spitting Blood: The History of Tuberculosis* (Oxford: Oxford University Press, 2012). For global perspectives, see McMillen, *Discovering Tuberculosis.*
72. For the history of bacteriology see e.g. M. Worboys, 'Germ Theories of Disease and British Veterinary Medicine, 1860–1890', *Medical History* 35(3) (July 1991): 308–27; Christoph Gradmann, *Laboratory Disease: Robert Koch's Medical Bacteriology* (Baltimore: Johns Hopkins University Press, 2009); Jacob Steere-Williams, 'Performing State Medicine During Its "Frustrating" Years: Epidemiology and Bacteriology at the Local Government Board, 1870–1900', *Social History of Medicine* 28(1) (September 2014): 82–107.

73. Waddington, *The Bovine Scourge.*
74. Waddington, *The Bovine Scourge*, 113–17, provides an excellent account of Koch's 'confusion'; see also Atkins, *A History of Uncertainty*, 1–75.
75. Alan L. Olmstead and Paul Rhodes, *Arresting Contagion: Science, Policy, and Conflicts over Animal Disease Control* (Cambridge, MA: Harvard University Press, 2015); Tatsuya Mitsuda, 'Entangled Histories: German Veterinary Medicine, c.1770–1900', *Medical History* 61(1) (January 2017): 25–47.
76. Worboys, 'Germ Theories of Disease and British Veterinary Medicine, 1860–1890'; Waddington, *The Bovine Scourge.*
77. Atkins, *A History of Uncertainty*, 203–36.
78. Susan D. Jones, 'Mapping a Zoonotic Disease: Anglo-American Efforts to Control Bovine Tuberculosis before World War I', *Osiris* 19 (January 2004): 133–48; Olmstead and Rhodes, *Arresting Contagion*; Robinson, 'A History of Bovine Tuberculosis Eradication Policy in Northern Ireland'; Atkins, *A History of Uncertainty.* For the twentieth-century restatement of zoonosis, placing TB at the top of the list, see WHO and FAO, 'JOINT WHO/FAO Expert Group on Zoonoses; Report on the First Session'.
79. The most complete historical account of this process can be found in Atkins, *A History of Uncertainty.* However, accounts from government vets indicate that national attestation was far from straightforward, suggesting there is much more to learn about the period between 1945 and 1965 when bTB was brought under control—see Andrew J. Proud, 'Some Lessons from the History of the Eradication of Bovine Tuberculosis in Great Britain', *Government Veterinary Journal* 16 (2006): 11–18.
80. Pearce, Pugh and Ritchie, *Animal Health*; Abigail Woods, 'A Historical Synopsis of Farm Animal Disease and Public Policy in Twentieth Century Britain', *Philosophical Transactions of the Royal Society of London. Series B, Biological Sciences* 366(1573) (July 2011): 1943–54.
81. G. Enticott, 'The Local Universality of Veterinary Expertise and the Geography of Animal Disease', *Transactions of the Institute of British Geographers* 37(1) (June 2011): 75–88; Rhiannon Fisher, '"A Gentleman's Handshake": The Role of Social Capital and Trust in Transforming Information into Usable Knowledge', *Journal of Rural Studies* 31 (July 2013): 13–22.
82. The 'rural idyll' is generally understood as an idealised version of the countryside or rural life; see Jeremy Burchardt, *Paradise Lost: Rural Idyll and Social Change in England since 1800* (London: I.B. Tauris, 2002); J. Wallwork and John A. Dixon, 'Foxes, Green Fields and Britishness: On the Rhetorical Construction of Place and National Identity', *British Journal of Social Psychology* 43(1) (2004): 21–39; John Horton,

'Producing Postman Pat: The Popular Cultural Construction of Idyllic Rurality', *Journal of Rural Studies* 24(4) (1 October 2008): 389–98. For landscape and animals in Britain, see David Matless, *Landscape and Englishness* (Islington: Reaktion Books, 1998); John Sheail, '"One and the Same Historic Landscape": A Physical/Cultural Perspective', *International Journal of Heritage Studies* 13(4–5) (2007): 321–34; Jessica Sellick and Richard Yarwood, 'Placing Livestock in Landscape Studies: Pastures New or Out to Graze?' *Landscape Research* 38(4) (August 2013): 404–20; Karen Victoria Lykke Syse, 'Stumbling over Animals in the Landscape: Methodological Accidents and Anecdotes', *Nordic Journal of Science and Technology Studies* 2(1) (December 2016): 20.

83. Roger Lovegrove, *Silent Fields: The Long Decline of a Nation's Wildlife* (Oxford: Oxford University Press, 2007); Sheail, 'One and the Same Historic Landscape'; André Magnan, 'Food Regimes', *The Oxford Handbook of Food History*, 16 October 2012.
84. See, e.g., Hilda Kean, *Animal Rights: Political and Social Change in Britain since 1800* (Islington: Reaktion Books, 1998); Emma Griffin, *Blood Sport: Hunting in Britain since 1066* (New Haven: Yale University Press, 2007).
85. David Perkins, *Romanticism and Animal Rights* (Cambridge: Cambridge University Press, 2003).
86. I have explored these themes at depth in earlier publications: see Angela Cassidy, 'Vermin, Victims and Disease: UK Framings of Badgers in and beyond the Bovine TB Controversy', *Sociologia Ruralis* 52(2) (April 2012): 192–204; Angela Cassidy, 'Badger–Human Conflict: An Overlooked Historical Context for Bovine TB Debates in the UK', in *Understanding Conflicts about Wildlife: A Biosocial Approach*, ed. Catherine M. Hill, Amanda D. Webber and Nancy E. C. Priston (Oxford: Berghahn Books, 2017).
87. Roper, *Badger*; Andrew W. Byrne et al., 'The Ecology of the European Badger (Meles Meles) in Ireland: A Review', *Biology & Environment: Proceedings of the Royal Irish Academy* 112(1) (January 2012): 105–32; O'Connor et al., 'An Ecological and Comparative Perspective on the Control of Bovine Tuberculosis in Great Britain and the Republic of Ireland'; Johanna Judge et al., 'Abundance of Badgers (Meles Meles) in England and Wales', *Scientific Reports* 7(1) (2017): 276.
88. E. Thomas, 'The Combe', in *Poems* (London: Selwyn & Blount, 1917).
89. H. I. Griffiths, David H. Thomas and Europe Council of 'The Conservation and Management of the European Badger (Meles Meles)' (Strasbourg: Council of Europe Publishing, 1997); Roper, *Badger*.
90. Kristopher Poole, 'Foxes and Badgers in Anglo-Saxon Life and Landscape', *Archaeological Journal* (April 2015): 1–34; Corinne Dale,

The Natural World in the Exeter Book Riddles (Woodbridge: Boydell & Brewer, 2017), 40; Marie Nelson, 'Old English Riddle No. 15: The "Badger": An Early Example of Mock Heroic', *Neophilologus* 59(3) (1975): 447–50.

91. Lovegrove, *Silent Fields*, 230.
92. M. Fissell, 'Imagining Vermin in Early Modern England', *History Workshop Journal* 47(47) (March 1999): 1–29; Lucinda Cole, 'Of Mice and Moisture: Rats, Witches, Miasma and Early Modern Theories of Contagion', *Journal for Early Modern Cultural Studies* 10(2) (2014): 65–84.
93. Edward Topsell et al., *The History of Four-Footed Beasts and Serpents* (London: Printed by E. Cotes, for G. Sawbridge [etc.], 1658), 26–27. See Public Domain Review, 'The History of Four-Footed Beasts and Serpents (1658)', The Public Domain Review (2015), for an overview of this colourful source; for 'real' and 'imaginary' medieval and early modern animals, see Boria Sax, *Imaginary Animals: The Monstrous, the Wondrous and the Human* (Islington: Reaktion Books, 2013).
94. '1835: 5 & 6 William 4 c.59: Cruelty to Animals Act' (2017).
95. Griffin, *Blood Sport: Hunting in Britain since 1066*, 146–48.
96. See e.g. Alfred E. Pease, *The Badger—A Monograph* (London: Lawrence and Bullen Ltd, 1898).
97. Richard W. Burkhardt, *Patterns of Behavior: Konrad Lorenz, Niko Tinbergen, and the Founding of Ethology* (Chicago and London: University of Chicago Press, 2005); Lynn K. Nyhart, *Modern Nature: The Rise of the Biological Perspective in Germany* (Chicago: University of Chicago Press, 2009).
98. For a fuller account of the Good Badger and the Bad Badger, see Cassidy, 'Vermin, Victims and Disease'; Cassidy, 'Badger–Human Conflict'.
99. Tess Cosslett, *Talking Animals in British Children's Fiction, 1786–1914* (Aldershot: Ashgate, 2006); Beatrix Potter, *The Tale of Mr. Tod* (Frederick Warne & Co., 1908).
100. Jean-Baptiste Gouyon, 'The BBC Natural History Unit: Instituting Natural History Film-Making in Britain', *History of Science* 49(4) (2011): 27; Jean-Baptiste Gouyon, 'Science and Film-Making', *Public Understanding of Science* 25(1) (1 January 2016): 17–30.
101. See Cassidy, 'Vermin, Victims and Disease', and Cassidy, 'Badger–Human Conflict', also Chaps. 4 and 5 on popular natural history.
102. Brett Mills, 'Towards a Theory of Documentary Representation for Animals', *Screen* 56(1) (1 March 2015): 102–7; Brett Mills, *Animals on Television: The Cultural Making of the Non-Human* (London: Palgrave Macmillan, 2017).

103. For 'safe, effective and humane', see Munro et al., 'Pilot Badger Culls in Somerset and Gloucestershire Report by the Independent Expert Panel'. Chapter 7 will explore how badger/bTB knowledge became more 'public' and increasingly polarised since 2010.
104. Simon Hattenstone and Patrick Barkham, 'Michael Eavis Throws Support behind Badger Cull', *The Guardian*, 21 June 2013.
105. See Knight, 'Introduction', in *Natural Enemies*, and rest of volume.
106. For pigeons, see Colin Jerolmack, *The Global Pigeon* (Chicago: University of Chicago Press, 2013); for dingoes see S. Healy, 'Deadly Dingoes: "Wild" or Simply Requiring "Due Process"', *Social Studies of Science* 37(3) (2007): 443–71; Karen F. Hytten, 'Dingo Dualisms: Exploring the Ambiguous Identity of Australian Dingoes', *Australian Zoologist* 35(1) (January 2009): 18–27.
107. Cassidy et al., 'Animal Roles and Traces in the History of Medicine, c.1880–1980'; Woods et al., *Animals and the Shaping of Modern Medicine.*
108. Good overviews can be found in Catherine M. Hill, 'Perspectives of "Conflict" at the Wildlife–Agriculture Boundary: 10 Years On', *Human Dimensions of Wildlife* 20(4) (2015): 1–6; S. Pooley et al., 'An Interdisciplinary Review of Current and Future Approaches to Improving Human–Predator Relations', *Conservation Biology* 31(3) (2016): 513–23; Sarah L. Crowley, Steve Hinchliffe and Robbie A. McDonald, 'Conflict in Invasive Species Management', *Frontiers in Ecology and the Environment* 15(3) (2017): 133–41.
109. Cassidy, 'Badger–Human Conflict'.
110. D. Inglis, 'What Is Worth Defending in Sociology Today? Presentism, Historical Vision and the Uses of Sociology', *Cultural Sociology* 8(1) (March 2013): 99–118.
111. E.g. Atkins and Robinson, 'Bovine Tuberculosis and Badgers in Britain'; Robinson, 'A History of Bovine Tuberculosis Eradication Policy in Northern Ireland'; Atkins, *A History of Uncertainty.*
112. For the ambiguities of farmers' relationships with their livestock animals, see, e.g., Rhoda Wilkie, *Livestock/Deadstock: Working with Farm Animals from Birth to Slaughter* (Philadelphia: Temple University Press, 2010).
113. For farming and trauma during the 2001 FMD outbreak, see Ian Convery et al., 'Death in the Wrong Place? Emotional Geographies of the UK 2001 Foot and Mouth Disease Epidemic', *Journal of Rural Studies* 21(1) (January 2005): 99–109; Law, 'Disaster in Agriculture: Or Foot and Mouth Mobilities'; Mort et al., 'Animal Disease and Human Trauma'. For the social ramifications of bTB, see Farm Crisis Network, 'Stress and Loss: A Report on the Impact of Bovine TB on Farming Families'; G. Enticott et al., 'Farming on the Edge: Farmer Attitudes to Bovine Tuberculosis in Newly Endemic Areas', *Veterinary Record* 177(17)

(2015): 439; Damian Maye et al., 'Animal Disease and Narratives of Nature: Farmers' Reactions to the Neoliberal Governance of Bovine Tuberculosis', *Journal of Rural Studies* 32 (August 2014): 401–10; Lindsay Hamilton, Nick Evans and James Allcock, '"I Don't Go to Meetings": Understanding Farmer Perspectives on Bovine TB and Biosecurity Training', *Veterinary Record*, Online First (7 January 2019).

114. Robert A. Lambert, 'The Grey Seal in Britain: A Twentieth Century History of a Nature Conservation Success', *Environment and History* 8(4) (2002): 450.

115. Sarah Ayres, Mark Sandford and Tessa Coombes, 'Policy-Making "Front" and "Back" Stage: Assessing the Implications for Effectiveness and Democracy', *The British Journal of Politics and International Relations* 19(4) (1 November 2017): 861–76.

116. Krebs et al., 'Bovine Tuberculosis in Cattle and Badgers: Report by the Independent Scientific Review Group', 10.

2

History of bTB

During the early 1970s, the British Ministry of Agriculture, Fisheries and Food (MAFF) moved from the discovery of a single dead badger to a full-scale wildlife culling policy; as well as from optimism to panic about bTB in only four years. In this chapter, we will investigate this rapid transition, introducing many of the dramatis personae who were to shape debates over badgers and bTB for many years to come. These included MAFF field officers, veterinarians and scientists who first became aware of and were charged with investigating the problem; naturalists and zoologists knowledgeable about wildlife; senior policymakers and politicians who acted upon this knowledge; animal protection activists and campaigners; and the organisms themselves—mycobacteria, cows and badgers. The chapter will demonstrate how attending to the multiple and changing roles assigned to badgers, as well as following the 'traces' they have left behind in historical documents, can help us understand how the history of bTB has been shaped by animals and humans alike.[1] It will follow this fast-moving situation as people started unravelling the complex connections between wild badgers, cattle and *M. bovis.* To do this, we must explore the immediate social, political and policy contexts into which the idea of tuberculous badgers was received, investigated, understood and contested. At this time, Britain was entering an extended period of political, economic and social instability: a wider backdrop which helps explain the decisions made about a then-obscure animal and a no-longer prominent cattle disease. One facet of the changes overtaking British society involved a shift in relationships between science and society, including new environmental and animal advocacy movements. In the years leading up to the reshaping of the badger's social role into that of disease victim, there had been a series of incidents involving environmental damage, wildlife and infectious diseases. This chapter will show how they formed part of a developing atmosphere of anxiety and dissent over human–animal relations, in which the previously unconnected concerns of animal health and the long-standing British 'badger debate' came together.

2.1 Animal Anxieties in the Early 1970s

The 1970s is widely remembered as a period of political and economic instability, as well as social change, in Britain and across the world: an era increasingly used as a historical touchstone for understanding our own unstable and uncertain times. The decade saw the entry of the UK into the newly formed European Economic Community, explosions of political violence in Northern Ireland; serial crises in labour relations; and the 1973 oil crisis, eventually leading to the 'three-day week' and widespread recession. The 1970s is also notorious for rapid changes in government, whereby the UK saw five different administrations, swinging back and forth between left- and right-wing party control. In 1970, the Labour ministry of Harold Wilson—which had held power since 1964—was voted out, to be replaced by a Conservative government led by Edward Heath. The Heath government came in with a reforming agenda, taking the UK into the EEC and attempting to curb trade union power while deregulating the economy. Heath's government rapidly came unstuck and by 1974 he was forced to call a general election: this resulted in a hung parliament and Labour forming a minority government, once more under Harold Wilson. Wilson served as prime minister for a further two years before resigning and passing the leadership to James Callaghan in 1976. Over the following few years the economy worsened, culminating in the 1978–1979 'Winter of Discontent', during which widespread strikes led to shutdowns in public services. Callaghan's government eventually ended in a vote of no confidence from members of Parliament, resulting in the 1979 general election, where the Conservative party, now led by Margaret Thatcher, was elected to power in a landslide victory.[2]

The 1970s is also known for the acceleration of social changes starting in the previous decade, including the emergence of women's liberation and gay rights movements; widespread tensions over immigration and race; and intense conflicts over labour rights. Alongside these debates, the anti-war and anti-nuclear movements of the 1960s turned towards broader concerns about environmental damage, joining forces with older, more established conservation movements. Environmental politics became more radical, with the formation of new international NGOs such as Greenpeace and Friends of the Earth alongside countless local groups, many of whom put into practice direct forms of protest learned from other campaigns.[3] Similarly, while the UK had long-standing traditions of political action against animal cruelty, including anti-vivisectionism and anti-blood-sports campaigning, animal politics also took a more radical turn at this time. New forms of activism emerged, including the disruption of fox and other hunts in the field (sabbing) and releasing animals from laboratories: it was also around this time that distinctions between long-standing 'animal welfare' and more radical 'animal rights' agendas started to emerge.[4] These changing attitudes were not only expressed via radical politics, but in more everyday practices, such as an increasing popularity of vegetarianism and veganism,[5] and more significantly for this story, an upswing in involvement with natural history, conservation and environmental groups.[6] Threaded through all of this was a debate about the roles that science should play in society, involving practicing scientists and other intellectuals involved in radical politics in the USA and UK. While sociobiology, nuclear weapons/energy and industrial pollution formed the core topics of concern (none of which are directly relevant here) radical science movements drew upon and contributed to the other social movements of the time, creating newly critical attitudes towards technocracy and ideas of scientific progress across these movements.[7] It is also worth noting that public and media reactions to key 'galvanising events' for the new environmental politics in the UK, including Rachel Carson's *Silent Spring* (1962), the Smarden toxic chemical spill (1963) and the Torrey Canyon oil spill (1967), all turned upon literary and visual imagery of suffering animals affected by pollution.[8] As historian Jon Agar has argued, these intertwined debates about environmental impacts, science and society took place during a 'long 1960s' in the history of science and technology, starting in the late 1950s and ending in the mid-1970s, over which science–society relations fundamentally changed.[9]

As we will see here, alongside Smarden and the Torrey Canyon, this period also saw a series of incidents involving animals, suffering, infectious diseases, science and British agricultures and environments. An international outbreak of myxomatosis (a painful, lethal and highly infectious viral disease affecting rabbits) had reached the UK in 1953. While the worst had passed within a few years, 'rabbit clearance societies' charged with culling infected animals remained active until well into the 1970s.[10] While myxomatosis will be explored more fully in Chap. 4, it is worth noting here that the disease lingered in the popular imagination, particularly via Richard Adams's deeply influential children's novel *Watership Down*. Between October 1967 and June 1968 there was also a major outbreak of foot and mouth disease (FMD), a virus affecting livestock. While FMD does not kill outright, it is painful, debilitating, affects productivity and is highly infectious—this is why we try and control it.[11] Attempts at preventing the 1967–1968 outbreak were particularly unsuccessful, with MAFF having to call in the army after only twelve days, and, as in 2001, very large numbers of infected animals were killed in a very short time, with devastating impacts on agriculture.[12] Finally, since the 1940s Europe had experienced a slowly spreading epizootic of rabies, which seemed to particularly affect wild foxes. By 1969, it had reached Germany and eastern France, creating concerns about disease spread from the continent to the UK. When a terrier imported from Germany (named Fritz) escaped in Surrey, biting several people and subsequently dying of rabies, MAFF reacted strongly, imposing movement restrictions on dogs in the area, and conducting a 'mass extermination' of local wildlife.[13] Following this there were several rabies panics during the early 1970s, and like myxomatosis, the disease cast a shadow on popular culture, spawning a whole subgenre of speculative fiction playing on fears of infection.[14] Between them, myxomatosis, FMD and rabies contributed to a wider sense of unease about animals, the environment, government and science, where events involving infectious disease appeared to act as a particular touchstone for articulating people's fears and political concerns. This formed the immediate context in which veterinarians, naturalists and scientists tried to understand the connection between badgers and bTB, and policymakers and politicians decided what to do about it.

2.2 Becoming Tuberculous: Understanding and Acting on Bovine TB in Wildlife

In April 1971, a Gloucestershire dairy farmer brought the dead body of a wild badger found on his land into the local government Animal Health office in Gloucester. Roger Muirhead, a local MAFF veterinary officer, conducted a post-mortem examination of the animal. He reported pathological lesions caused by tuberculosis, and identified its causal bacterium, *Mycobacterium bovis*, in fluids taken from the badger's lymph glands. The diagnosis was subsequently confirmed by scientists at the government's Central Veterinary Laboratory, and was immediately communicated to other officials and experts within MAFF.[15] Within four years this individual had stimulated a major research programme into 'TB in cattle and badgers', involving parallel laboratory, clinical, experimental and field investigations, all conducted by Ministry scientists and field officers, which would continue right the way through to 1997. This animal also precipitated a series of laws regulating the protection and management of wild badgers, which in adapted form remain in force today. Finally, this event led to the rapid formulation of new policy for managing bTB, whereby badgers on farms suffering bTB breakdowns were gassed in their setts with sodium cyanide, a technique already in use for rabbit control. Given that at the time relatively little was known about the pathology, microbiology and epidemiology of bTB in wildlife, or about the ecology and behaviour of badgers, why did MAFF move from the traces of one sick animal to a national-scale wildlife culling policy in such a short space of time?[16]

I will now unpack this narrative, often repeated in today's debate, to fully investigate how MAFF moved so rapidly from a single incident in an obscure corner of the countryside, to viewing badger/bTB as a national problem which must be rapidly dealt with. Using internal civil service correspondence, now held in the National Archives, alongside public media coverage from the time, I will relate how MAFF's veterinarians, scientists and field officers started piecing together the puzzling relationships between *M. bovis*, cattle and badgers. I will also explore the perspectives and actions of external actors, including other parts of government, naturalists, farmers and badger protection campaigners as they helped, harassed, pressured, confirmed and contested the Ministry's developing knowledge of the problem. Along the way, I will introduce many of the dramatis personae who will feature through the rest of this book. These include MAFF field officers, veterinarians and scientists who first became aware of and were charged with investigating the problem; naturalists and zoologists with much-needed expertise about wildlife and ecosystems; senior policymakers and politicians who acted upon this knowledge; animal protection activists and campaigners; and the organisms themselves—mycobacteria, cows and badgers.

As discussed in Chap. 1, the research underpinning this book has set out to take a more animal-centred approach to the history of bTB. I will follow government scientists, veterinarians and field officers as they followed the traces left by this unfortunate animal and its compatriots, struggled to understand their significance, and to decide what action should be taken. I will also introduce the other actors who were involved with badgers, cows and *M. bovis* at the time, exploring the other traces and roles that these organisms had already left while interacting with people. These traces—and the varying interpretations of them made by different people—provided contexts which people outside of MAFF used to make sense of the news. I will explore their varying responses to this news, and their relationships with government ministers, civil servants, veterinarians and scientists over the following few years. While some of these responses were similar to the oppositional dynamics seen in today's controversy, others took a collaborative approach to what they saw as a shared problem, creating a less contested and more collective approach to the situation. By following the activities of those immediately involved in these early investigations, alongside their public and private responses to these rapidly unfolding events, I will demonstrate how these first few years profoundly shaped the dynamics of the badger/bTB controversy, which have continued to play out since that time.

A Dead Badger on a Farm

By the end of the 1960s MAFF had been trying to control bTB in cattle for several decades, initially for the purposes of public health—because the meat and milk of affected cattle were a major source of tuberculosis in humans—and latterly to boost cattle health and productivity. National programmes for managing transmission risks had significantly reduced TB rates in animals and humans in the UK. Politicians and veterinarians were united in confidently anticipating the eradication of bTB from the UK, and MAFF had declared several regions in the UK to be 'attested', with cattle herds testing free of the disease.[17] These successes were publicly celebrated, with the Minister of Agriculture announcing it would come to pass 'within five years or less' in 1957.[18] While the eradication of bTB was announced by MAFF 'for all practical purposes' in October 1960, the situation behind the scenes was much murkier. Pockets of localised infection were persisting, particularly in Gloucestershire and Cornwall, with some farms experiencing repeated outbreaks.[19] Ministry veterinarians were deeply concerned by this, and found they were unable to explain the source of these infections. Therefore, MAFF's Veterinary Investigation

Service dispatched a team to the remote West Penwith peninsula in Cornwall to conduct a full epidemiological investigation of bTB in the area. Despite their detailed investigation, in which they mapped bTB outbreaks and examined all possible sources of disease, including fencing, animal housing, slurry, delays in TB testing following the 1967–1968 FMD outbreak, cattle movement, other livestock and wildlife (including badgers), they came to no firm conclusions.[20]

Independently of this investigation, Roger Muirhead, an MAFF Veterinary Officer stationed in the Gloucestershire countryside near Wooton under Edge (another area of persistent infection), had found an animal trace which would send shockwaves through the Ministry, veterinarians, scientists, wildlife advocates, as well as farmers still struggling with bTB.

> In April 1971 the owner of a large farm lying in the Cotswolds a few miles to the east of the head of the Wortley valley, brought into the Divisional Office a badger which he had found dead on his farm. Examination revealed generalised tuberculosis. A slide revealed numerous acid fast organisms taken from a mesenteric lymph gland which were subsequently typed by the Central Veterinary Laboratory as *Mycobacterium bovis*.[21]

Shortly afterwards, a second badger was found and shot on a nearby farm also suffering persistent outbreaks, this time in calves: this animal was also found to be infected with bTB. In June 1971, Muirhead and his superiors in the local Animal Health office for Gloucestershire met with their local counterparts in the Infestation Control Division (ICD)—responsible for dealing with animal threats to agricultural production—to inform them of the situation. The news was passed on to MAFF's South West regional office in Bristol, as well as to ICD's scientific teams at the Pest Infestation Control Laboratories (PICL). Their initial response was sceptical: 'has the cowman been tested?' wrote one, suggesting that the source of these outbreaks was most likely human.[22] On the whole, ICD scientists and field officers regarded the evidence at this stage as 'circumstantial', indicating bTB infections in badgers and cattle in the same area, but saying nothing about the direction of transmission, nor whether the disease was being carried by other wildlife.[23] PICL officers had reason to be sceptical: for many years they had received regular correspondence from members of the public implicating the animals in disruptive 'pest' activities such as spoiling and raiding crops, destabilising riverbanks and stealing poultry. Whenever these complaints were investigated, ICD field officers concluded that the culprits were either wildlife species such as foxes, or occasionally aberrant old or sick individuals described as 'old rogue badger[s]'.[24] ICD also had primary responsibility within MAFF for managing infectious diseases in wildlife: it is for these reasons that Muirhead and his veterinary colleagues turned immediately to them for help.

An initial summary of the situation from Muirhead was circulated to relevant government experts in and outside of MAFF by the end of the year. Dr Archibald McDiarmid of the Agricultural Research Council was less circumspect than ICD: while he thought it likely that badgers had caught bTB from cattle and that this was a localised problem, he recommended that badgers in the area be 'eliminated' as soon as possible.[25] Following further meetings between Animal Health and ICD, the two divisions agreed to collaborate on a joint field survey of the immediate area, mapping bTB incidence on a farm-by-farm basis alongside sett locations. The survey also sought to obtain more bodies and samples from local wildlife—not just badgers but also foxes, rabbits, rats and so on—to look for the presence of *M. bovis* in other species.[26] The news about these unpredictably infected animals also moved rapidly up the hierarchies of government, and by February 1972 ministers had been briefed. Their responses were brisk, with the Parliamentary Secretary (junior minister) commenting, 'Fond as I am of badgers, I am quite clear that we could not permit a situation to continue in which they were proved carriers of TB.'[27]

But what had prompted Muirhead to conduct a post-mortem on that badger carcass in the first place? In Cornwall, local veterinary officers had suggested that the animals might have been a source of TB as early as 1962, while Muirhead himself wrote that farmers in Gloucestershire had long held similar opinions.[28] Following the initial case, Muirhead had collected further badger carcasses with the help of local farmers: as such his investigations had been public knowledge in the area throughout 1971, and by March 1972 the news had reached the local press.[29] Ministry officers were therefore under pressure from this quarter from the very beginning, and while they emphasised the uncertainties involved, farmers in both Gloucestershire and Cornwall had no such doubts and campaigned publicly and privately for action to be taken against badgers.[30] MAFF were well aware of the 'explosive'[31] situation, stressing in their briefing to ministers that 'pressure is likely to grow for something to be done about the problem.' At the same time, they also drew attention to the strong feelings that badgers provoked, negative in some cases, but positive in many others: 'The status of the badger in children's books and in the nature-lover's heart ensures that he is not an animal to be trifled with.'[32] While we have already explored some of the contexts which contributed to the badger being granted this simultaneously vilified and elevated status, the late 1960s had seen an intensification of the badger debate. Vigorous campaigns to grant badgers special legal protections were in full swing. It was highly likely that civil servants had badger protection campaigns in mind when they recommended that 'in order to avoid major political repercussions', alongside the field survey work, the Ministry should meet with 'wildlife interests' in order to consult their views and enrol their help with research investigating the problem.[33] These actions, alongside the volume of press clippings held in MAFF archives, attest that civil servants were fully aware (and wary of) the public ramifications of the news.

While ICD had some knowledge of badgers relating to their contested role as pests, as well as considerable experience of wildlife disease relating to myxomatosis, at the time MAFF's veterinarians had minimal knowledge about these or many other wild animals. More widely, relatively little was understood about badger physiology, behaviour and ecology: the person with most expertise on badgers at the time was widely acknowledged to be Dr Ernest Neal, a retired schoolmaster living in Taunton. Neal gained his PhD in 1960 and had been a nationally renowned expert on the animals since publishing his classic work of popular natural history *The Badger* in 1948, while also conducting groundbreaking nature photography for the BBC. Neal was therefore top of the invitation list for MAFF's meeting with 'wildlife interests', held on 16 March, alongside representatives of the Council for Nature (the umbrella body for conservation organisations), naturalists in Gloucestershire and the Nature Conservancy (the government body responsible for scientific advice on conservation, part of the Department of the Environment). While Neal was unable to make this initial meeting, he conferred extensively with MAFF officers and scientists (including Roger Muirhead and Harry Thompson of ICD), later travelling to Gloucestershire to meet with them and observe badgers at one of the affected setts.[34] This strategy of including and enrolling wildlife groups initially paid off. Neal had been working for some years with the UK Mammal Society on a nationwide Badger Survey, and the local Recorder for the Society volunteered to help with MAFF's work.[35] The conservationists consulted 'responded in a friendly and sympathetic way to the problem'[36] and, following the initial meeting, it was agreed that 'badgers in one, and if necessary up to 3, of the known infected sets should be slaughtered and the carcases examined'.[37]

However, not all 'wildlife interests' were as sympathetic as Neal, nor as convinced that the evidence was clear enough to warrant culling. When members of the Nature Conservancy (shortly to be renamed Nature Conservancy Council, or NCC)[38] heard about the situation in August 1971, they were immediately concerned 'that a widespread purge of Badgers will occur' when the news became public.[39] Unlike MAFF, the scientists of NCC were primarily concerned with the protection and conservation of environments, animals and plants. At the time, NCC members were debating internally whether badgers should be their concern: while some argued that populations were relatively abundant and were therefore not interested, others argued that the animals were under 'threat' from badger digging and hunting.[40] Following the news about TB in badgers, NCC members recast the role of the badger into that of vulnerable victim to be protected, rather than pest or disease transmitter to be controlled. After consulting with Muirhead and Thompson, zoologist J. F. D. Frazer of the NCC summarised their scepticism:

> The evidence for the badger as a source of infection is therefore somewhat flyblown. If anything, badgers are more likely to have been infected from the cattle in the first place. There is no evidence of badgers breathing in the calves' faces or spitting on the grass. Nor, as far as we know, has there been any check on the farmer, his family and his cowman—man being a major host of bovine tuberculosis.[41]

Unlike government veterinarians, who employed epidemiological methods of tracing disease outbreaks through geographical associations (Fig. 2.1), the zoologists and ecologists of the NCC saw only the coincidental colocation of sick badgers and sick cows, which proved nothing about the ultimate source of infection. Despite, or perhaps because of, these concerns, following the meeting in March 1972, the NCC offered the help of a regional officer to 'present the Conservancy's views in the planning of the extended Badger survey'.[42] NCC scientists believed they should have a hand in 'steering' the research,[43] and that it should be conducted jointly by MAFF and themselves.[44] They were also in favour of a 'control' or comparison sampling of badgers from a non-tuberculous area, which their own internal minutes recorded: however, the outcomes circulated more widely by MAFF omitted this point.[45]

While the situation was effectively public knowledge in the Wooton area from the start, MAFF officers shared the NCC's concerns about the

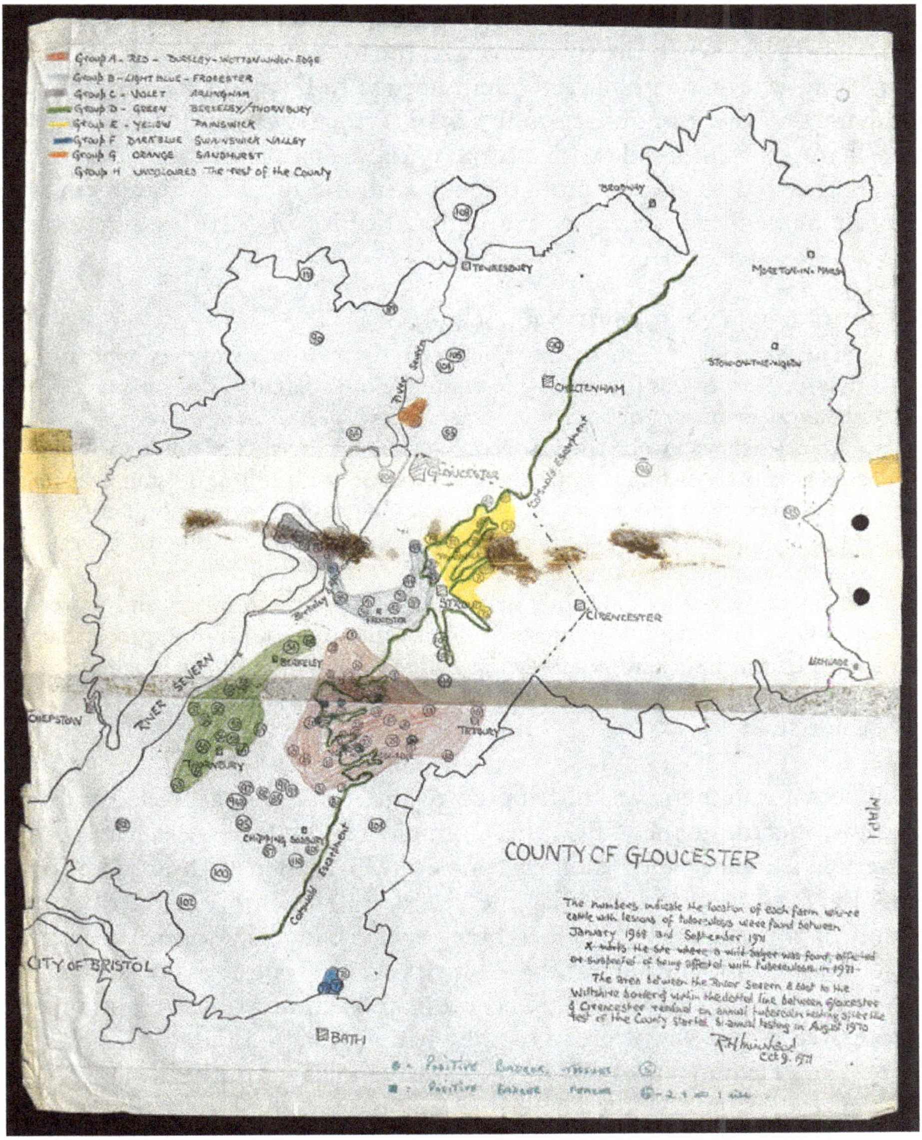

Fig. 2.1 Map initially prepared by Roger Muirhead in September 1971, held in MAFF FT 41/88. Note strikethrough of original 'X marks the spot' notation and replacement with multiple outbreaks

consequences for badgers and had worked to keep it out of the news through 1971. When the story broke in the local press in March 1972, all parties agreed that a public statement needed to be made.[46] An attempt at preparing a note for publication in *Habitat* (the newsletter of the Council for Nature) foundered in extensive editing, and it became clear that MAFF needed to engage more directly with the media. A statement was rapidly agreed and issued by the regional office of MAFF's agricultural advisory service, ADAS:

> TUBERCULOSIS IN WILD BADGERS
>
> The Veterinary Arm of the Ministry's Agricultural Development and Advisory Service has identified the existence of tuberculosis of bovine type in badgers in an area of South Gloucestershire.
>
> This is believed to be the first record of the occurrence of tuberculosis in badgers and accordingly while there is at present no full understanding of the significance of the disease in this species, a possible connection between badger infection and a continuing tuberculosis problem in some of the cattle in the area is being investigated.
>
> A meeting was held recently between officers of the Ministry and representatives of the Wildlife interests to discuss the situation. It was agreed that measures will be taken to survey the badger population of the area and to study the epidemiology of the disease in badger sets which are believed to be infected.

The above statement was distributed to the local press as well as interest groups, including the NFU, the Country Landowners Association, the Veterinary Society and wildlife groups on 23 March, with an additional caveat: 'It is to be hoped that the release of this information does not result in the indiscriminate slaughter of wild badgers. Control measures are under consideration by the Ministry in the one area known to be involved and any private and un co-ordinated action would be quite inappropriate.'[47] The news spread rapidly, with coverage in national newspapers, the farming press and broadcast media. Muirhead and Neal participated in interviews where they emphasised the local nature of the problem and again requested that badgers be left unmolested.[48] Unlike the local and farming press, national newspapers were more concerned about the potential 'death sentence' for badgers than the implications for farmers.[49] Further problems developed when the findings of the West Cornwall investigation were published, reaching no firm conclusions regarding the role of badgers. The news was received badly by Cornish farmers, who campaigned for immediate action, claiming to have 'studied' the animals for many years and be certain that they were the source of infection.[50]

2.3 Following Badgers, Tracing Bacteria

It was initially envisaged that MAFF's survey of badgers and bTB in Gloucestershire would take three months,[51] enabling them to learn more, clarify the situation and take swift action. Three ICD officers were assigned the job of recording the locations of badger setts, alongside positive TB reactors in cattle and farms. The officers also took samples of badger faeces and collected the bodies of badgers and samples from other wildlife they found in the area. They were assisted by representatives of the NCC and the Mammal Society, with veterinary officers including Muirhead conducting post-mortems, and experts at the Central Veterinary Laboratories in Weybridge conducting microbiological testing. However, these field investigations were far from straightforward. Badgers were a poorly understood, nocturnal species that lived underground in inaccessible rural areas. As the survey proceeded, the time, space, personnel and costs involved rapidly escalated, as MAFF field officers got to grips with the logistics of finding and following these unfamiliar creatures: 'They have had the arduous and painstaking task of finding as many setts as possible in a part of Gloucestershire which is well populated by badgers and where steep wooded hillsides make searching quite tiring.'[52] The field officers persisted, continuing to follow traces of badger bodies, bodily fluids, tracks and behaviour, and to document these traces using maps, photographs, post-mortem and microbiological reports, and numerical data.

As these badger traces were found and recorded, they were mapped onto the geography of the area, alongside the locations of key bTB outbreaks on farms—as part of the official MAFF survey and by Roger Muirhead as part of his ongoing personal investigations (Fig. 2.1). As the name suggests, the Wooton Under Edge area sits on the Cotswold Escarpment, a geological formation running through the county. It creates spectacular scenery and steep wooded hillsides, today much beloved by tourists, but also makes ideal badger country—easy for the animals to both dig and hide in. As MAFF built up a picture of the local situation, their understanding of the scale of the problem changed: not only were almost all other wildlife samples coming back clear, but increasing numbers of TB-positive badgers were being found. These were brought to MAFF officers by members of the public: as word spread, farmers and naturalists started presenting badger carcasses for inspection on a regular basis. By 1974 MAFF were calling on members of the public to do this whenever they encountered a dead badger, as the animals were (and still are) frequent victims of road traffic accidents.[53] Muirhead's hand-drawn map (reproduced in Fig. 2.1) reflects this rapidly changing situation. An initial statement, 'X marks the spot where a wild badger, affected or suspected of being affected with tuberculosis in 1971', has been crossed out, to be replaced with a more complex mapping of seven potential outbreak areas, outlined in different colours and labelled 'Groups A–G'. While the field officers in Gloucestershire were still conducting these initial investigations, the Cornwall veterinary investigation team had returned to the area—and reported finding *M. bovis* in badger faeces samples.[54]

As the survey proceeded and the situation became increasingly public, senior MAFF officials and ministers considered what action should be taken, and how. Once more they turned to ICD, the only people in MAFF with experience of 'badger control'. While the initial setts near Wooton had been destroyed by excavation during the summer of 1972, this procedure was both time-consuming and expensive.[55] Therefore, other options for killing tuberculous badgers were explored, to decide what to do as more infected animals were found across an increasingly wide area. Because badgers were not legally defined as pests, it was illegal to use cyanide to 'gas' the animals—the standard procedure for destroying rabbits and moles. While a marksman could be employed to target a 'rogue' individual, this required 'much patience' and was therefore too costly; available traps were bulky and unreliable; leaving snaring as the only other 'legal but cruel' option.[56] ICD officers therefore adapted the design of snare traps, developing a procedure which was quicker and in their view more humane. However, animal welfare campaigners disputed this claim.[57] These pressures drove policy needs for a new regulatory framework to manage people's behaviour towards badgers in the event of bTB infection: in turn this created another new animal role, as subjects of government legislation. In 1973, the government passed the Badgers Act. On the one hand the Act responded to the lobbying of badger advocates, granting the animals specific protections against killing or cruelty. At the same time, it created a framework by which government could licence individuals to 'to kill or take' the animals for research or conservation purposes, as well as 'for purposes of preventing the spread of disease'.[58]

Once the Act had passed in December 1973, at the NFU's request, Ministry officials planned a series of 'Open Days', where techniques for badger control would be demonstrated for farmers and landowners, to ensure that licensees would be able to kill the animals in the proper way.[59] Therefore when such an event was announced, to be held at Brock Hill on Scrubbett's Farm, Gloucestershire, over 50 farmers attended, alongside representatives of the NFU, conservation groups and the RSPCA; plus officers from PCD, Animal Health, Rowland Moyle (a junior MAFF minister) and Peter Hardy (the MP who had sponsored the Badgers Act). Shooting, snaring, live-trapping and digging techniques were demonstrated, killing ten animals in total.[60] While well attended, the event did not go according to plan. Badger protection campaigners Ruth and David Murray came along and objected to the use of snares, subsequently arguing that MAFF officers should be prosecuted under the Badgers Act, as the Act 'prohibited cruel ill treatment of badgers and that snaring was inherently cruel'. While officers reported that there was a consensus from attendees that badger control was necessary, they also felt that it 'was a specialist job and ought to be left to the Ministry. This was hardly the object of the exercise.'[61] As well as complaining at the event itself, the Murrays took photographs and instigated investigations by RSPCA and the local police, who shortly afterwards cautioned the Regional Pests Officer in charge of the event.[62] When legal advice ruled that snaring was not in fact illegal (provided it was carried out properly) and the police dropped all charges, Ruth Murray then pursued a private prosecution of the incoming Labour Minister for Agriculture, Frederick Peart.[63] Even though neither attempt was successful, the demonstration and its consequences provided an ongoing source of media coverage, bringing badger/bTB to the attention of wider audiences.[64] More prominent badger protection campaigners such as Lord Arran picked up on the bTB issue and included it in their ongoing animal advocacy, leading to questions asked in both Houses of Parliament.

2.4 A Change of Direction?

Following the Scrubbett's Farm disaster, MAFF cancelled a planned second 'Open Day' demonstration, and all parties urgently re-examined how best to cull badgers.[65] Wildlife experts such as Ernest Neal and Harry Thompson believed that barring the legal obstacles, using cyanide gas would be the most effective and humane option.[66] The technology had been developed during the 1930s, with the influential 1951 Scott Henderson Committee concluding it was 'an extremely effective and humane method of control and should be used in preference to any other method for destroying animals which live underground'.[67] Policymakers were already exploring whether the law could be changed, and following the argument at the demonstration 'it was agreed both by Mrs. Murray and by farmers present that the Ministry ought to take the lead in dealing with the badger situation and that it should use cyanide gas for the purpose of slaughtering badgers'.[68] In response to a question in Parliament about the incident, the Agriculture Minister stated that MAFF was to 'reappraise' policy in relation to badger control and bTB. Peter Hardy wrote to ministers expressing his concerns about snaring, alongside a willingness to support any proposed legal changes.[69]

By this time, the original field survey had been completed and the work extended as many more infected badgers had been found in Gloucestershire, while investigations continued in Cornwall and *M. bovis* had also been found in badger samples from Wiltshire and Dorset. Two 'comparison' surveys had been carried out in areas with lots of badgers but low rates of bTB in cattle, neither of which had found the disease in badgers. While other wildlife had initially been investigated for signs of infection, with the exception of two rats and two moles, these samples had tested negative for bTB.[70] Despite the challenges involved, MAFF's field officers, veterinarians and scientists had worked together to follow, document and interpret the traces left by *M. bovis* in badgers and other animals. In the process, their understanding of the problem had changed: from a relatively isolated and anomalous incident amenable to sett-by-sett solutions, to a rapidly escalating region-wide disease outbreak. By the end of 1974, bTB had been found in approximately 17% of the badger carcasses that had been examined (in Gloucestershire) and 6% of faeces samples (gathered more widely).[71]

MAFF started formulating a more systematic plan for investigating the still highly uncertain relationships between badgers, cattle and bTB. The SVS successfully lobbied for an expansion of staff and resources to handle bTB in investigation centres in Gloucester, Truro and Wiltshire. This included the relocation and promotion of specialist veterinary staff—in pathology and epidemiology—to support Roger Muirhead's work in Gloucestershire; to conduct cross-species transmission experiments at the Central Veterinary Laboratories in Weybridge; and to develop veterinary epidemiological research on the problem.[72] PICL and NCC initially proposed an expansion of the field surveys into a jointly conducted research programme on badger ecology and behaviour. While the project was approved, it instead continued the existing MAFF-only partnership of ICD officers, PICL scientists and SVS research and field staff.[73] The idea of conducting some kind of experiment in the field was raised: what would happen if badgers were systematically removed from a larger area and prevented from returning for a long period of time?[74] Prompted in part by NCC's scepticism, the experiment was intended 'to prove or disprove the significance of the badger in the perpetuation of bovine tuberculosis in cattle'.[75] The proposed experiment would also investigate 'sett reoccupation'—the tendency of other badgers to move into a sett when the residents had been killed.[76] This idea converged with veterinary arguments for removing badgers from severely affected areas (including Steaple Leaze in Dorset and Thornbury in South Gloucestershire) to create the idea of 'clearance trials' which could fulfil both agendas.[77]

MAFF's reappraisal included a coherent rethink of policies which had up until then been developed on an ad hoc basis in the face of a rapidly changing situation. There was a distinct policy shift: from a relatively 'hands-off' stance whereby MAFF officers investigated bTB outbreaks and then advised farmers and landowners on what to do if tuberculous badgers were found, to one where the state took ownership of investigations and of badger control. The first step was to change the law to enable badger gassing without making it legal for anyone with a grudge against the animals to do likewise, and to scope out the costs of government conducting the culls.[78] A consensus formed that this was the best way forward, supported by badger specialists such as Thompson, Neal and Murray, alongside key actors in Gloucestershire including the local Trust for Nature Conservation and the local branch of the NFU. The latter even wrote to MAFF's Regional Office to underline this mutual support.[79] Following a meeting involving the heads of Animal Health, PICL, SVS, RSPCA, BVA, NCC, NFU and the Council for Nature, it was agreed to insert a relevant clause into an existing wildlife protection bill Peter Hardy was putting through Parliament.[80]

MAFF held a press conference to announce their new approach, which included new procedures in the event of an 'unexplained' breakdown of bTB (i.e. where no other source of infection could be found, implicating badgers). MAFF veterinarians would investigate the farm and test badger bodies and faeces for *M. bovis*. If these were positive, then ICD officers would come in and destroy the animals: this was known as a 'fire-brigade operation'. The clearance trials were announced at the same time, but without mentioning experiments—instead they were framed in terms of bTB control.[81] Detailed plans were drawn up and MAFF started to recruit new staff and plan their training and working procedures to implement the new culling policy.[82] Once Hardy's bill had passed into law, ICD immediately started testing gassing equipment, and publicly invited a range of actors to join a new Consultative Panel. The Panel comprised key individuals such as Ernest Neal and leading conservationists; MAFF personnel including Thompson and the Chief Veterinary Officer (CVO); and representatives of a range of organisations including NFU, BVA, NCC and the RSPCA.[83] The Panel was charged with keeping under review:

a. the evidence relating to bovine tuberculosis in badgers, including its incidence and its relationship to bovine tuberculosis in cattle; and
b. the operations to be undertaken by the Ministry in order to eradicate bovine tuberculosis from badgers and to monitor its existence in the badger population.[84]

This inclusive approach, bringing all parties into ongoing dialogue about the problem, was essentially a formalisation of what MAFF officers had been doing from the very beginning, when Muirhead, Thompson and Neal worked closely together to help each other understand an unprecedented situation and advise MAFF on what to do about it. Early acknowledgements of the uncertainties involved faded into the background, to be replaced by the language of action, as seen here from the CVO: 'Further research and investigation confirmed that badgers infected with bovine tuberculosis were playing an important role in perpetuating the disease in these areas. With much regret therefore we had to obtain powers to take effective action to eliminate this reservoir of infection.'[85]

2.5 Looking, Seeing, Knowing and Acting

By following the scientists, veterinarians, policymakers, naturalists and politicians who struggled to make sense of the traces left by *M. bovis*, we can now see how and why MAFF moved from one dead animal to a full-scale culling policy so quickly. What had initially appeared to be an isolated and anomalous incident (to be dealt with locally and without too much fuss) transformed with alarming rapidity into a situation with a great deal more biological, geographical and political significance. The relationships between badgers, cows and *M. bovis* had not changed. However, once MAFF officers started looking for traces of bTB in badgers they found more and more, creating a conceptual connection that became more widely visible. What this meant varied according to the roles that people had already assigned to badgers: for those who already saw them as pests, it was easy to also see them as diseased. For those committed to convincing others that badgers were victims of human persecution, the appearance of bTB provided another reason to defend them. These differing interpretations meant that the new role created for badgers—of disease vector—was immediately contested. For veterinarians looking to diagnose the source of unexplained outbreaks, geographical proximity confirmed this role, but for zoologists and ecologists used to working with experimental methodologies, the evidence was less clear-cut. The discovery of tuberculous badgers meant that animal protection and conservation agendas started working together directly in ways that had rarely happened before in Britain. This realignment will be discussed at greater length in Chap. 5. Aside from the Murray prosecutions, this disagreement stayed out of the public sphere and was rarely voiced-even in MAFF's internal meetings. Instead, most of the experts involved—including naturalists, conservationists, PICL scientists and government veterinarians—worked hard to convey coordinated messages about the situation.

Local political pressures would also have been a factor driving such a rapid policy shift. Most immediately these came from farmers and local veterinary officers dealing with positive bTB tests, many of whom were already convinced that badgers were to blame: this was backed up by pressure from the NFU at local and national level. At the same time, policymakers were keen to work closely with badger advocates and naturalists trying to protect the animals, attempting to head off public controversy. These pressures were in turn shaped by a shared policy context in which actors both internal and external to MAFF were used to participating in an inclusive approach to policymaking.[86] Prior to 1971, MAFF's main experience of dealing with infectious disease in wildlife had been myxomatosis, and so it was to their colleagues in ICD and PICL that veterinarians immediately turned for help. As we saw earlier, the previous few years had seen a series of other incidents involving animals, infectious disease and environmental problems, including early attempts at eradicating invasive species, myxomatosis, a rabies scare, the 1967–1968 outbreak of FMD and the Torrey Canyon oil spill. These incidents drew upon and contributed to the emergence of newer, more radical forms of environmental and animal advocacy, as well as to a wider atmosphere of unease around human–animal relations, within which MAFF officers felt a pressure to take action as rapidly as possible.

The broader political contexts of the early 1970s must also be considered, as they shaped both the immediate politics around badgers that MAFF officers were negotiating, and the policy decisions which they were charged with implementing. When Muirhead first reported to his superiors about bTB in badgers, MAFF was busy negotiating changes to agricultural policy relating to the UK's impending entry into the EEC. Beyond the Ministry, by 1972 the Heath administration was already in trouble, and by the spring of 1974 had fallen from power. Given these pressures, the brisk ministerial response to the news is not that surprising. Neither bTB nor badgers were high on political priorities, and ministers would be unlikely to have had the time or inclination to request a closer examination of the evidence linking the two. The aftermath of the Scrubbett's Farm demonstration combined with wider political turmoil to bring badger/bTB to the attention of a much wider circle of people than before. In March 1974 the Labour party had just managed to form a minority government under Harold Wilson, reinstalling Fred Peart as the third Minister of Agriculture to hold the position since 1970. Media coverage of Ruth Murray's attempts to prosecute Peart provided a strong incentive for Labour to draw a line under the previous few years and present a new policy approach. The decision to move from providing advice while relying on farmers to carry out badger control, to MAFF taking charge of research and culling operations was a bottom-up one borne of a consensus amongst scientists, naturalists and farmers. However, this policy shift, from one where government assumed an advisory role, to one in which it took control of and responsibility for all aspects of bTB control, was also highly congruent with the broader political differences between the Conservative Heath administration and the Labour Wilson government.

Between 1971 and 1975, bTB in badgers rapidly changed from a completely unknown and unanticipated problem, to one visible to a relatively restricted group of people, to an embarrassingly public problem which politicians were keen to be seen as taking decisive but consultative action on. Although legislative changes and the commencement of culling operations in 1975 reinforced the badger's role as a threatening vector of disease, MAFF's expanded research effort tacitly acknowledged that its role in propagating bTB was not yet settled. In the years that followed, the circumstantial nature of the evidence was one important source of scientific and policy controversy, but the multiple and contradictory roles assigned to badgers in the early 1970s and publicised via policy documents and in national and local media also drove ethical, political and emotional responses, which fuelled debates over tuberculous badgers that are still ongoing today. The events of these few short years brought together a diverse range of actors, some of whom had pre-existing patterns of interaction and others who established new cooperative and adversarial relationships which were to profoundly shape the badger/bTB debate for years to come.

Notes

1. Benson, 'Animal Writes: Historiography, Disciplinarity, and the Animal Trace'; Cassidy et al., 'Animal Roles and Traces in the History of Medicine, c.1880–1980'; Woods et al., *Animals and the Shaping of Modern Medicine*.
2. For overviews of the twists and turns of British society and politics through the 1970s, see Dominic Sandbrook, *State of Emergency: The Way We Were. Britain, 1970–1974* (London: Penguin, 2011); Lawrence Black, Hugh Pemberton and Pat Thane, eds, *Reassessing 1970s Britain* (Manchester: Manchester University Press, 2013). For a contrasting view of the 1970s 'crisis', see also Emily Robinson, Camilla Schofield, Florence Sutcliffe-Braithwaite, Natalie Thomlinson, 'Telling Stories about Post-war Britain: Popular Individualism and the 'Crisis' of the 1970s', *Twentieth Century British History* 28(2) (June 2017): 268–304.
3. Jon Agar, 'What Happened in the Sixties?' *The British Journal for the History of Science* 41(4) (July 2008): 567; Sandbrook, *State of Emergency*, 176–221; Mark Wilson, 'The British Environmental Movement: The Development of an Environmental Consciousness and Environmental Activism, 1945–1975' (PhD, Northumbria University Newcastle, 2014), 232–307.
4. Kean, *Animal Rights*, 201–5; Robert Garner, *Animals, Politics and Morality* (Manchester: Manchester University Press, 2005); Griffin, *Blood Sport*, 182–201.
5. Kean, *Animal Rights*, 203–4.
6. David Evans, *A History of Nature Conservation in Britain* (New York: Routledge, 1997), 136–42; Tim Sands, *Wildlife in Trust: A Hundred Years of Nature Conservation* (London: Elliott & Thompson, 2013), 69–92.
7. Agar, 'What Happened in the Sixties?' 577.
8. For 'galvanising events', *Silent Spring*, the Smarden spill and Torrey Canyon disaster, see G. Kroll, 'The "Silent Springs" of Rachel Carson: Mass Media and the Origins of Modern Environmentalism', *Public*

Understanding of Science 10 (2001): 403–20; J. F. M. Clark, 'Pesticides, Pollution and the UK's Silent Spring, 1963–64: Poison in the Garden of England', *Notes and Records: The Royal Society Journal of the History of Science* 3 (15 February 2017): 297–327; Timothy Cooper and Anna Green, 'The "Torrey Canyon" Disaster, Everyday Life, and the "Greening" of Britain', *Environmental History* 22(1) (January 2017): 101–26.

9. Agar, 'What Happened in the Sixties?' 568–69; Agar, 'Transition: Sea Change in the Long 1960s'.
10. Peter W. J. Bartrip, *Myxomatosis: A History of Pest Control and the Rabbit* (London: I.B.Tauris, 2008).
11. Woods, *A Manufactured Plague*.
12. Woods, *A Manufactured Plague*, 108–26.
13. Neil Pemberton and Michael Worboys, *Mad Dogs and Englishmen: Rabies in Britain, 1830–2000* (Basingstoke: Palgrave Macmillan, 2007).
14. Pemberton and Worboys, *Mad Dogs and Englishmen*, 182–86.
15. R. H. Muirhead, 'Bovine Tuberculosis in Wild Badgers in South Gloucestershire', *State Veterinary Journal* 27(1) (1972): 197–205.
16. A briefer account of this sequence of events can be found in Cassidy et al., 'Animal Roles and Traces in the History of Medicine, c.1880–1980', 27–32.
17. W. D. Macrae, 'The Eradication of Bovine Tuberculosis in Great Britain', *J Roy Agric Soc Engl* 122 (1961): 64–71.
18. Anon 'Cattle Tuberculosis "Over in Five Years"', *Times*, 6 June 1957, 7.
19. Sir John Ritchie, 'Bovine TB at Bay', *Times*, 3 April 1963; Atkins, *A History of Uncertainty*, 237–52.
20. R. A. Richards et al., 'Inquiry into Bovine TB in West Cornwall' (London: Ministry of Agriculture, Fisheries and Food, 1972).
21. Muirhead, 'Bovine Tuberculosis in Wild Badgers in South Gloucestershire', 198.
22. C. J. Armour, 13 September 1971, NA MAF 109/381, item 14.
23. R. J. Clark, 3 March 1972, NA MAF 109/381, item 17.
24. See Sect. 4.3 for more on the 'old rogue badger'; also Grant, 'Intractable Policy Failure: The Case of Bovine TB and Badgers'.
25. A. McDiarmid, 'Comments on Report concerning tuberculosis in Badgers', 11 January 1972, NA MAF 287/752, item 10.
26. 'Bovine tuberculosis—badgers in Gloucestershire. Note of a meeting at Tolworth', 16 February 1972, NA MAF 287/752, item 31a.
27. M. H. Sullivan, 21 February 1972, NA MAF 287/572, item 40.
28. R. F. Symes, 6 September 1971, NA MAF 109/381, item 13, also Muirhead, 'Bovine Tuberculosis in Wild Badgers in South Gloucestershire'.
29. Anon., 'Badgers May Spread TB in Cows', *Gloucester Citizen*, 17 March 1972, NA MAF 145/21, item 95.

30. Anon., 'Exterminate Badgers Plea', *Gloucester Citizen*, 6 November 1973; in NA MAF 109/294, item 34; F. Butcher, 'TB time-bomb under a county's dairy farmers', *Farmer's Weekly*, 22 June 1973, 51.
31. 'Telegram from Knowles Bristol', NA MAF 109/294, item 14.
32. 'Note for the Minister', 17 February 1972 NA MAF 287/752, item 38.
33. Ibid.
34. H. V. Thompson, 9 May 1972, NA MAF 109/381, item 44.
35. A. Killingley, 9 June 1972, NA MAF 287/752, item 110. See Neal, 'The National Badger Survey', for the National Badger Survey.
36. H. V. Thompson, 30 May 1972, NA MAF 287/752, item 97.
37. 'Bovine TB—badgers in Gloucestershire—notes from a meeting held on 16 March 1972 at Tolworth', NA MAF 287/752, item 62.
38. The Nature Conservancy was a government body founded in 1949, responsible for administering National Parks, and conducting research on conservation issues. In 1973 it was split into the Nature Conservancy Council (NCC) responsible for parks and scientific advice, and the Institute for Terrestrial Ecology (ITE); John Sheail, *Nature in Trust: The History of Nature Conservation in Britain* (Glasgow: Blackie, 1976), 224. National Archives records transition smoothly from NC to NCC, and so I will refer to NCC throughout.
39. J. W. Blackwood, 27 August 1971, NA FT 41/88 (item numbers absent in FT (NCC) files).
40. J. F. D. Frazer, 'NOTE FOR THE RECORD', 6 February 1973, NA FT 1/60.
41. J. F. D. Frazer, 'In Confidence: Badgers and Bovine TB Investigation', 8 September 1971, NA FT 41/88.
42. D. A. Cadwalladr, 24 March 1972, NA MAF 109/381, item 28b.
43. P. A. Gay, 'BADGERS AND BOVINE TB IN GLOUCESTERSHIRE', 23 March 1972, NA FT 41/88.
44. 'TB in Badgers: note of a meeting held Monday 11th June', 4, NA FT 41/88.
45. J. F. D. Frazer, 'Tuberculosis and Badgers', 17 March 1972, NA FT 41/88; cf. 'Notes For the Minister', NA MAF 287/752, item 54.
46. Anon., 'Badgers May Spread TB in Cows', *Gloucester Citizen*, 17 March 1972, NA MAF 145/21, item 95.
47. D. Barber, 'TUBERCULOSIS IN WILD BADGERS', 23 March 1972, NA MAF 109/381, item 23.
48. H. V. Thompson, 'Letter to RJ Clarke', 18 April 1972, NA MAF 109/381, 37; R. Muirhead, 'Letter to Dr. Gay of NCC', NA MAF 109/381, 81a.
49. B. Silcock, 'Infected Badgers Face Extermination', *Sunday Times*, 23 April 1972; in NA MAF 287/752, 104.
50. Anon., 'National Pet or Pest?' *Peninsular West*, 4 April 1973, 4–5; in NA FT 41/88.

51. A. P. Stevens, 'Memo to RJ Clark', 20 March 1972, NA MAF 109/381, 20.
52. R. J. Clark, 18 July 1972, NA MAF 145/21, item 109.
53. 'Itinerary for the Parliamentary Secretary's visit to the South West Region. Appendix 2', NA MAF 109/383, item 90. This was formalised into a nationwide project which we might today describe as 'citizen science', and ran until 1997; MAFF, 'Bovine Tuberculosis in Badgers. Report by the Ministry of Agriculture, Fisheries and Food' (London: Ministry of Agriculture, Fisheries & Food: HMSO, November 1976); J. Gallagher and J. Nelson, 'Cause of Ill Health and Natural Death in Badgers in Gloucestershire', *The Veterinary Record* 105(24) (15 December 1979): 546–51.
54. Richards et al., 'Inquiry into Bovine TB in West Cornwall', sec. 4.3.
55. E. J. Coombe, 'Memo to R. Clarke', 11 August 1972, NA MAF 109/381, 89.
56. 'Minutes of the Divisional Pest Officers Conference', 25–26 May 1960, NA MAF109/381, item 10/2; A. P. Stevens, 'Letter to D.W.M. Herbert', 12 February 1974 NA MAF 109/381, item 67.
57. A. Warne, 'Memo: Instructions to Pest Staff and Field Officers', 4 December 1973, NA MAF 109/383, 23.
58. 'Badgers Act' (1973), 4.
59. P. Riddick, 'Letter: Badgers and Bovine TB', 28 March 1974, NA MAF 109/383, item 63.
60. R. J. Clark, 'Memo: BADGERS IN AREAS WITH BOVINE TUBERCULOSIS: A DEMONSTRATION OF CONTROL METHODS', 26 April 1974, NA MAF 109/383, item 75; R. J. Clark, 'Report on Badger Control Demonstration—Glos', 9 May 1974, NA MAF 109/383, item 85.
61. R. J. Clark, NA MAF 109/383, item 85.
62. R. G. Symes, 'Badger Aftermath', 10 May 1974, NA MAF 109/383, item 91; R. J. Clark, 'BADGER CONTROL DEMONSTRATION: POLICE INVESTIGATION OF COMPLAINT OF CRUELTY TO BADGERS', 23 May 1974, NA MAF 109/383, item 109.
63. R. J. Clark, 'Mr. Harrison Jones—telephone memo', 2 July 1974, NA MAF 109/295, item 50; Foot and Bowden Solicitors, 'Letter to George Adam Turrell', 11 November 1974, MAF 109/295, item 74.
64. Anon., 'Protest on Badger Cruelty', *Daily Telegraph*, 13 May 1974, in NA MAF 109/384, item 4; D. Slight, 'Peart Named in Badger Rumpus', *Daily Mirror*, 14 May 1974, in NA MAF 109/384, item 6; anon., 'Butchered! They have no right to do this to God's creatures', *Cotswold Star*, no. 32, June 1974, 1.
65. Anon., 'Reprieve for the Badgers', *The Citizen*, 11 June 1974, in NA MAF 109/295, item 40.
66. For further details on the origins and usage of sodium cyanide in mammalian pest control, see Sect. 4.1.

67. J. Scott Henderson, 'Report of the Committee on Cruelty to Wild Animals. Cmd 8266, June 1951' (London: Home Office/Scottish Home Department, June 1951). See also Sects. 4.3 and 5.1.
68. D. W. M. Herbert, 'Minute: Bovine Tuberculosis and Badgers', 28 February 1974, NA MAF 109/294, item 77/1; Harrison Jones, 'Telex to WT Barker Tolworth', 14 May 1974, NA MAF 109/295, item 6.
69. Hansard, *HC* Deb 20 May 1974 vol. 874 cc20–1; P. Hardy, 'Letter to Parliamentary Secretary, MAFF', 14 May 1974, NA MAF 109/295, item 8a.
70. A. C. L. Brown, 'Animal Health 1974: Report of the Chief Veterinary Officer' (London: Ministry of Agriculture, Fisheries and Food, 1975), 46–47.; also W. T. Barker, 'Badgers and BTB: briefing papers to Ernest Neal', 14 May 1974, NA MAF 109/295, item 7.
71. Brown, 'Animal Health 1974', 46.
72. 'Memo: TB in Badgers, Research at CVL, Weybridge', 22 January 1975, FT 41/90. For early MAFF bTB pathology research see e.g. J. Gallagher et al., 'Pulmonary Tuberculosis in Free-Living Lechwe Antelope in Zambia', *Tropical Animal Health and Production* 4(4) (December 1972): 204–13; R. H. Muirhead, J. Gallagher and K. J. Burn, 'Tuberculosis in Wild Badgers in Gloucestershire: Epidemiology', *Vet Rec.* 95(24) (1974): 552–55; J. Gallagher, R. H. Muirhead and K. J. Burn, 'Tuberculosis in Wild Badger (Meles Meles) in Gloucestershire—Pathology', *Veterinary Record* 98(1) (1976): 9–14; Gallagher and Nelson, 'Cause of Ill Health and Natural Death in Badgers in Gloucestershire'. For the CVL transmission experiments see T. W. Little, P. F. Naylor and J. W. Wilesmith, 'Laboratory Study of Mycobacterium Bovis Infection in Badgers and Calves', *The Veterinary Record* 111(24) (1982): 550–57. For epidemiology see F. A. Stuart and J. W. Wilesmith, 'Tuberculosis in Badgers: A Review', *Rev. Sci. Tech. Off. Int. Epiz.* 7(4) (1988): 929–35.
73. J. H. Seymour, 'Memo: TB-Badgers', 30 August 1974, NA MAF 109/295, item 80; Brown, 'Animal Health 1974', 15; MAFF, 'Bovine Tuberculosis in Badgers. Report by the Ministry of Agriculture, Fisheries and Food', sec. Appendix 7.
74. K. Williams, 'Memo: Eradication of Bovine TB—Badgers', 26 September 1974, NA MAF 109/295, item 95.
75. H. V. Thompson, 'Letter to RJ Clark', 25 July 1974, NA MAF 109/383, item 154; Prest, I. 'Note: The badger and bovine tuberculosis', 3 May 1974, FT 41/89.
76. L. Goldthorpe, 'Letter to CEH Sparrow, Glos. Trust for Nature Conservation', August 1974, NA MAF 109/383, item 156.
77. L. Goldthorpe, 'Badgers. Ref LP/N4214A', 26 June 1974, NA MAF 109/295, item 49a; K. Williams, 'Eradication of Bovine Tuberculosis—Badgers', 26 September 1974, NA MAF 109/295, item 95. For a published summary of MAFF clearance trials see R. S. Clifton-Hadley et al.,

'The Occurrence of Mycobacterium Bovis Infection in Cattle in and around an Area Subject to Extensive Badger (Meles Meles) Control', *Epidemiology and Infection* 114 (1995): 179–93.

78. A. P. Hardiment, 'Memo: TB Badgers', 22 July 1974 NA MAF 109/383, item 156.
79. P. Riddick (NFU), 'Letter re Badgers and Bovine TB', 12 August 1974, NA MAF 109/295, item 79.
80. D. Barwick, 'Meeting to Discuss Legislation to Permit the Gassing of Badgers', 29 January, 1975, NA FT 41/90.
81. MAFF, 'MAFF Press Notice: New Powers to Gas Badgers', 5 February 1975.
82. H. A. Carn, 'Memo: Badgers—Safety of Staff', 5 August 1975, NA MAF 109/384, item 73.
83. MAFF, 'MAFF Press Release: Consultative Panel on Badgers and Tuberculosis', 24 September 1974.
84. Brown, 'Animal Health 1974', 15.
85. Brown, 'Animal Health 1974', 2.
86. Grant, 'Intractable Policy Failure: The Case of Bovine TB and Badgers'.

PART II

Rethinking bTB

3

World and Work of Animal Health Epistemic Community

By 1975, the existence of tuberculous badgers—and the idea that they could be responsible for the persistence of TB in British cattle herds—had solidified from a relatively obscure idea of some farmers and veterinarians into a still uncertain but rapidly cohering fact. This knowledge—and the risks it posed for human, domestic and wild animals—spurred the previously unrelated communities involved with badgers and with bTB to work together. In turn, this created new collaborative networks committed to understanding the new problem of badger/bTB. The Ministry for Agriculture, Fisheries and Food (MAFF) had moved from a local veterinary officer finding a single dead badger during the spring of 1971 to major investment in research and a national-scale culling policy. While policymakers' attempts at inclusive working, enlisting the help of farmers, landowners, naturalists and badger advocates had been strikingly successful, fractures were appearing. This middle section of the book will investigate what happened next, with the aim of understanding how and why participants in today's knowledge controversy over badgers and bTB have come to have such dramatically different perspectives. To that end, the next three chapters will investigate in depth the knowledge, expertise, working practices and practical goals of three key 'epistemic communities' that developed around badger/bTB over the following twenty years: ***animal health***, ***disease ecology*** and ***badger protection***.[1] In turn, each will be placed into the broader historical and institutional contexts of their formation in mid-twentieth-century Britain prior to the connection of badgers and bTB.

This chapter will explore the worlds and work of the *animal health* epistemic community, comprising field and research veterinarians, policy-makers and politicians in MAFF; veterinarians in clinical practice; farmers; and their representatives. It will pick up from the longer history of tuberculosis outlined in Chap. 1, to overview the development of frameworks for regulating bTB in the UK. It will place these frameworks into the broader contexts of veterinary disease control, caring and ethical practices, mid-twentieth-century animal health policy, and the internal organisation of the Ministry. We will then return to the story of badger/bTB with MAFF's 'Bovine TB in Badgers' research and policy programme, launched in 1975, and follow the veterinary investigations carried out under this remit. As MAFF's researchers started investigating the traces left by *M. bovis* in wild and domestic animal bodies, its policy of culling badgers by 'gassing' was becoming controversial. The incoming Conservative government of 1979 hoped to settle criticisms by inviting an 'authoritative expert'—Lord Solly Zuckerman—to review the situation. Instead, Zuckerman's report drew further media attention to the issue, creating wider public controversy than before. In the final part of this chapter, we will explore the less famous 'son of Zuckerman' Dunnet review, published in 1986 and conducted by a multidisciplinary team of scientists.[2] Even though the criticisms made by the Dunnet group were downplayed by MAFF, their recommendations were implemented, contributing to policy change and the fading of bTB away from public scrutiny during the late 1980s.

3.1 Animal Health and Cultures of Caring for Livestock

The practices of epistemic communities—as they work together to build reliable knowledge aimed at achieving shared policy goals—can also be understood as a product and producer of shared 'cultures of care', as discussed in Chap. 1.[3] Shared understandings of what constitutes 'good care' co-produce shared understandings of 'good work', in human health, laboratory science, farming and veterinary practice.[4] I will use these frameworks to analyse the intersecting cultures of care that have mutually shaped the working practices of the British state as it has sought to understand and regulate animal health over the past two centuries. Just as Dutch healthcare workers in the twenty-first century must balance their embodied, everyday, flexible and adaptive but ultimately disempowering 'logics of care' for patients with formalised, market-based but empowering 'logics of choice', which engage with the economic constraints of healthcare, the epistemic communities of badger/bTB have had to perform similar balancing acts.[5] These interactions profoundly shape who makes policy and practical decisions about care and what decisions get made under any given set of circumstances.

This chapter will explore the particular cultures of care[6] developed by the epistemic community involved with British animal health policy, and how they in turn have shaped MAFF's policies for controlling bTB over the past century. Originating in the interactions of farming and veterinary practices of care for individual animals, herds, owners and wider economic interests, *animal health* care involves long-established procedures and policies for preventing the spread of infectious disease in animals. Often described as 'stamping out', these involve the slaughter of infected individuals and their immediate contacts, while also controlling the movement of other animals in affected areas.[7] Variations on this practice are still deployed worldwide to manage infectious diseases in livestock, from bTB to foot and mouth disease (FMD) to influenza. For those accustomed to the elaborate, patient-focused, life-preserving techniques of modern human medicine, this way of working can be a shock. While veterinary care of companion animals in rich countries increasingly converges with human medical practice, using complex surgical and technological interventions, the underlying ethical basis of most animal health practice is quite different. Unlike human medicine, which tends to prioritise the preservation of *life*, farmers and veterinarians place a greater emphasis on preventing animal *suffering*. In practice this means that sick animals in pain or distress are more likely to be killed (euthanised, put down, put to sleep), rather than undergoing stressful, painful or expensive treatments.[8] Veterinary care is also influenced by the wishes of the patient's owner (rather than patients themselves, who are legally property), particularly because animal healthcare tends to be a commercial enterprise, creating different dynamics around the 'logics of choice' and patient agency.[9] This can make ethical decision-making for veterinarians morally and emotionally fraught, guided as it must be by owners' relationships with their animals (from deep emotional connections through to bald assessments of financial value).[10] These decisions often bring to the fore clear tensions between the 'theory' of veterinary scientific evidence and the 'practice' of veterinary clinical and farming animal care, which must be negotiated on an ongoing basis.[11]

Such trade-offs have also been shaped by the type of animal involved and the societal roles that it has been assigned by the human society it lives in. While pets are cared and mourned for, other animals are not so fortunate. The balancing of life/death and care/suffering changes for livestock and working animals; is deeply contested for wild animals; and those designated as pests receive hostility rather than any form of care.[12] The history of the profession also reflects our changing relationships with animals: while in Britain today the majority work with companion 'small animals' and there are such things as wildlife veterinarians, these are relatively recent trends.[13] The origins of the veterinary profession instead lie in providing medical care for animals doing important work. It was the importance of horses (as military, transport and agricultural muscle) which led to the founding of the first veterinary schools in France and Britain in the late eighteenth century.[14] Veterinarians did not become routinely involved in the treatment of farm animals until later, following a series of battles to establish their professional status (distinct from doctors and from those involved with animal husbandry).[15]

The arrival of rinderpest in the UK in 1865 devastated British horses and livestock, creating a major driver for the establishment of the veterinary profession, embedding and intertwining their work into the affairs of the state via concerns about agricultural productivity and (human) public health.[16] The government formed a Veterinary Department to deal with the problem, setting the course towards developing structures for state interventions to control animal disease. Even though British veterinarians struggled with disciplinary rivalries with human public health experts, following a series of reforms, they established themselves as a legally recognised profession in 1881.[17] In 1893 the position of Chief Veterinary Officer (CVO) was created and has been filled ever since—given that the Chief Scientific Adviser was a mid-twentieth-century invention, this probably makes the CVO the most long-standing expert advisory role in British government.[18] Over the following decades, veterinarians extended their purview beyond rinderpest and establishing a network of veterinary inspectors qualified to identify diseased meat and animals. They developed dual roles: initially field-based, problem-solving 'practical men', and latterly laboratory and research-oriented 'scientific experts'. Following the end of the First World War, veterinary services were consolidated under the newly formed Ministry of Agriculture and Fisheries, bringing together the previously separated roles of policy enforcement and disease diagnosis.[19] Key government institutes for animal health research were established at this time, including the Central Veterinary Laboratory (1917) and Pirbright Experimental Station (1924).[20] While vets have maintained their professional role within government, they have experienced an ongoing process of internal reorganisation, repeatedly bringing together and separating their policy-implementing and scientific-researching functions.[21]

As well as the obvious risks of zoonosis (in diseases like bTB), infectious diseases affecting livestock alone (such as FMD) are managed partly for welfare reasons, but also because they bring with them economic risks. These manifest in the death of infected animals as well as suppressed productivity (of, for example, meat and milk). Therefore, policy decisions about infectious diseases in livestock were, and still are, motivated by a further logic—of cost, operating in the financial interests of animal owners and the wider economy. Therefore, veterinarians and policymakers concerned with *animal health* look beyond the individual patient to think about welfare and the spread of disease across herds, flocks and wider populations, further modifying practices of care.[22] As 'stamping out' was elaborated, it required the detection of disease carriers as well as sick animals, driving the development of technologies for diagnosis and surveillance of microorganisms. This eventually led to what is described today as 'test and slaughter' regimes for animal disease control (which do as the name suggests: positive animals and their herd-mates are culled), an elaboration of the stamping-out approach. By the mid-twentieth century, stamping-out regimes were considered within animal health to be reliable, tried and tested. However, they were not always successful and continued to be controversial, particularly in relation to proposed alternative solutions such as vaccination. During FMD outbreaks in Britain in the 1950s, proponents of vaccination objected to what they saw as 'barbaric and medieval' and 'unscientific' disease control policies.[23] While MAFF prevailed at the time, continuing with stamping out in their struggles with the much larger FMD outbreak of 1967–1968, the vaccination controversy returned during 2001, when around 6 million animals were slaughtered, creating a spectacle that made the consequences for animals dramatically visible to wider publics.[24]

The animal health epistemic community is not only comprised of veterinarians, policymakers and politicians, but also farmers: bound by these regulatory systems and (partly) in whose interests they had been developed in the first place. As I discussed at the beginning of this book, the voices of farmers themselves are often conspicuously absent from archival MAFF correspondence about bTB. When they do feature it is usually as correspondence with the National Farmers Union (NFU), which paradoxically is regarded by policy scholars as an exemplary 'policy insider'—a non-governmental body with close working connections with policymakers.[25] Animal health cultures of care (balancing care, choice and cost) inside government in the UK have therefore formed in dialogue with the parallel cultures of care of farmers—albeit mediated through the NFU. We already know that 'good care' is co-produced by ideas and practices of 'good farming'—fundamentally farmers need their animals to thrive, but must also see livestock through to slaughter and ultimately make enough money to live.[26] Agricultural workers constantly negotiate animal agency, expressed as a willingness or otherwise to cooperate with being herded, milked, confined, mated and medically treated.[27] This constant negotiation—with the agency of their charges, as well the uncertainties of wider environments—has created cultures of care which help manage these uncertainties. Good farming is often bound up with ideas of *stewardship*: long-term care of a specific place, including the plants and animals living there. Farming care is—like traditional medical care—embedded, relational and fundamentally parental, in that the carer holds most of the power and agency in the relationship. It often involves understandings of human–environment relations which see people as holding responsibility for maintaining and controlling the 'balance of nature'.[28] Social research into the difficult, distressing and dirty work of killing animals shows how farmers must try to manage these contradictions, negotiating paths between emotional connection and disconnection.[29] While such negotiations are far from easy, it does seem that for most farmers at least, the death of their animals at slaughter for meat production is understood as a 'good death'—one which happens at the right time, without excessive cruelty and to serve an ultimate purpose—to provide people with food and income for the farm.[30]

The premature illness and/or death of livestock can therefore disrupt the delicate balance of human–animal relations on a farm. This is where farming, veterinary and animal health policy cultures of care come into conflict, particularly when the last is practised to protect populations.[31] When livestock animals are slaughtered to prevent the spread of infectious disease, the deaths happen in an untimely and disorderly fashion, while control over the situation (a key aspect of farming care) is removed to the state. The following quote is from an anonymous account published in *Farmers Weekly* in 1973, but barring minor details it could easily be from the present day:

> Within 14 days, we had Ministry orders that the whole milking herd had to be slaughtered. One calf was slaughtered and found to have had nothing wrong, so the other 46 were given a second chance. A further test has been ordered for them and we are waiting for that. If they go down I don't know what I shall do. These are all I have left from a 10 year policy using nominated bulls on my best cows. As a result of what has happened, I have my fixed costs relentlessly going on, and until I restock I have no income apart from interest on the compensation payment.[32]

Despite financial compensation, the abrupt ending of their animals' lives, cessation of these relationships and disruption of day-to-day life was, and continues to be, a source of intense distress to many farmers. The loss of an entire herd entails a further disruption of farming 'stewardship' care, as herds also represent past and future care of lineages and land.[33] State disruption to these routines of care engenders a sense of helplessness and resignation, making it harder to persuade farmers to take action to control the spread of infection in farm spaces. Paradoxically this can also be used to justify taking action against badgers, while others express distress and scepticism in the face of state culling policies.[34] Stamping out has tended to be adopted by richer countries with the resources to implement it, easily controlled borders (enabling them to exclude reinfection from elsewhere in the world), and the political or economic clout to only trade with others adopting similar regimes.[35] In the colonial era it was implemented to the benefit of settler farmers and undermined traditional, locally developed husbandry practices; these inequities persist in today's regimes of global and veterinary public health.[36] This pattern is also present domestically, whereby the costs and benefits of such policies have tended to work in favour of landowners, larger farms and elite breeders, and against smaller-scale producers.[37] While in recent years there has been a greater emphasis on government working in 'partnership' with farmers to reshape disease control policies, it is questionable to what extent this has made any difference to these feelings of helplessness in the face of infectious disease.[38] Even though bTB is a manifest disease problem for humans and animals elsewhere in the world, in the UK it rarely poses direct health risks. As we will explore later in the book, while these risks can be minimised, the regulatory policies that make this possible have brought with them new economic, social and emotional risks, in turn fuelling public contestation of those policies.

3.2 MAFF's 'Bovine Tuberculosis in Badgers' Research Programme

To pick up our story from the end of Chap. 2, by 1975 MAFF had announced a new approach to the transformed problem of bTB in badgers, comprising a state-led culling policy; an inclusive Consultative Panel advising policymakers; and major investment in new research. While public statements emphasised MAFF's decisive policy action, the scale of the proposed research effort tacitly acknowledged how little was understood about the situation. The 'Bovine Tuberculosis in Badgers' research programme involved work across several sites by multiple disciplinary specialists. It expanded and formalised the preliminary work on field epidemiology, pathology, bacteriology, immunology, transmission, the effectiveness of culling, and the behaviour and ecology of badgers. The latter work was mostly conducted by field biologists located in MAFF's Infestation Control Division and will be discussed in the next chapter. Here we will concentrate on the veterinary side of MAFF's research effort. To understand fully how these multiple policy and research actors were working together at the time, we need to take a brief detour into the wonderful world of UK government research and organisational structures within and beyond MAFF. Mirroring wider political turmoil, the early 1970s was a period of extensive change within civil service research. Financial tensions combined with wider debates about research–policy relations within government led to the commissioning and publication of the Rothschild Report in 1971, which proposed that 'applied' research be relocated from the (independent) research councils into relevant ministries.[39] In parallel, these drivers had instituted major changes in government agricultural research, with MAFF forming a new umbrella organisation, the Agricultural Development and Advisory Service (ADAS) the same year. ADAS brought the State Veterinary Service (SVS) together with other agricultural experts, including the Infestation Control Division (ICD), crop research, and the pre-existing National Agricultural Advice Service, which provided expert advice to farmers. This move separated the SVS from the policy-facing Animal Health Division. ADAS combined advisory, research and policy implementation roles: this structure continued until another round of reorganisation (and privatisation) during the late 1980s.[40] The organisation of the SVS itself remained broadly unchanged, comprising three subsections: field services, veterinary investigations (field epidemiology) and the Central Veterinary Laboratory

(CVL). The SVS was overseen by the CVO and centralised management, but all three divisions maintained considerable autonomy: the CVL in its main location in Weybridge, and the field and investigation services through MAFF's network of regional offices.[41]

Roger Muirhead, the SVS Veterinary Officer who had found tuberculous badgers, worked out of MAFF's divisional office in Gloucester. After 1975 regional investigations were further supported and supplemented by the SVS, with new veterinary investigation (VI) centres opening in Gloucester and Truro and new work initiated at the CVL. John Gallagher was relocated to Gloucester and started worked closely with Muirhead and other colleagues to formalise the existing data and publish their findings. Once they started looking for tuberculous badgers, they found more and more of them, spread across an increasingly wide area. Many of these animals had extensive lesions, some in the lungs but mostly in the lymph nodes and kidneys, containing huge numbers of bacilli.[42] The VI team at Gloucester also researched the viability of *M. bovis* bacilli in badger bodily fluids, carcasses, 'infected setts' and soil samples. After several months, they were unable to detect the bacteria, leading them to the conclusion that infected materials were likely to 'self-sterilise' in the field.[43] Instead they argued that the major transmission route from badgers to cattle was likely to be via pasture contaminated with infected urine and spit.[44] Further pathology investigations concluded that bTB was the major cause of sickness and death in badgers in Gloucestershire at the time, and highlighted the role of bite wounds for badger–badger transmission. The paper also drew attention to externally visible symptoms of bTB in badgers, such as emaciation and overgrown claws.[45]

At the CVL, a small 'colony' of wild badgers were brought in to study them under laboratory conditions. They were inoculated with *M. bovis* from infected cattle and groups of calves were inoculated vice versa, demonstrating that cross-infection was possible.[46] When the infected badgers were housed with calves, the cows became sick, surviving between six months and a year after exposure.[47] By 1976, MAFF had already concluded that 'badgers are susceptible to the disease and can play a significant role in transmitting infection to cattle'.[48] Badger immune responses to *M. bovis* were investigated, and CVL scientists quickly found that standard tuberculin testing did not work.[49] Towards the end of the decade, VI officers (field epidemiologists) and CVL researchers started working on techniques to identify different strains of *M. bovis* in cattle and badgers in different areas, suggested by variations in disease virulence.[50] Both groups contributed to ongoing efforts to identify and map bTB incidence, continuing to follow the traces of badgers and *M. bovis* in the environment. Samples of bodily fluids were tested for the bacterium, alongside the bodies of badgers killed during culling and research, plus those of animals that had been found dead either from disease or road traffic accidents (RTAs). From early in Muirhead's investigations in Gloucestershire, farmers and other members of the public had been bringing dead badgers to MAFF officers. In 1976, MAFF decided to capitalise on this enthusiasm, instituting a formal 'Badger Survey', requesting that any carcasses found by members of the public be brought to the nearest Ministry office, and recording the resulting data. This project—which would now be described as 'citizen science'—continued until 1990.[51]

Finally, veterinary researchers and field staff worked in collaboration with ICD on a series of 'clearance trials'—interventions designed to test the effect of clearing all badgers from a given area.[52] The first of these took place at Steeple Leaze Farm in Dorset, which had experienced unusually high rates of cattle disease. Under pressure from the farmer and local NFU, MAFF prioritised the case, with the trial starting as soon as gassing was legalised.[53] The second intervention took place around Thornbury, near Bristol and was described as 'an experimental badger clearance programme'.[54] The idea was to remove all badgers from an area clearly bounded by rivers and motorways, in order to prevent the animals 'recolonising', and observe the effects on bTB in cattle.[55] In both interventions all badger setts had to be gassed repeatedly as field officers discovered new animals moving into the area: the clearances lasted for about five years. Despite these difficulties, MAFF persisted with removing badgers from both intervention areas and by 1979 reported that badgers had been successfully cleared: crucially they also reported that there had not been any new outbreaks of bTB in cattle herds.[56] The new research programme reported to MAFF every year or so, summarising key findings and new lines of enquiry: a condensed version was included in the CVO's Annual Report. Aside from some early publications in the *Veterinary Record*, much of this work was not published in peer-reviewed journals until well into the 1980s, and not until 1995 in the case of the Thornbury clearance trial.[57] While these projects were long term by design, given MAFF's awareness of the sensitivity of the topic, perhaps there were qualms about making the finer details of this research public. It seems that during the 1970s the SVS considered this internal reporting and the advice of their own experts to be an adequate standard of evidence on which to build policy.

The *Bovine Tuberculosis in Badgers* reports were used to communicate the situation upward to senior civil servants and ministers in MAFF and outwards to the experts and external policy interests represented in the Consultative Panel. Initially MAFF stressed the Panel's role in reviewing and approving policy, and the group convened three times a year.[58] By 1975 MAFF had forged a consensus that the best route forward was to cull badgers using 'gassing': pumping a product called Cymag (sodium cyanide in powder form) into setts, where it reacts with moisture in the air to release hydrogen cyanide gas. The technique was already in use (by MAFF and private citizens) for 'pest control' of rabbits and moles and would have been widely familiar (Fig. 3.1 depicts a MAFF gassing crew and their gear *in situ* in Gloucestershire).[59] Once the law had been changed to make this possible, the policy was rapidly rolled

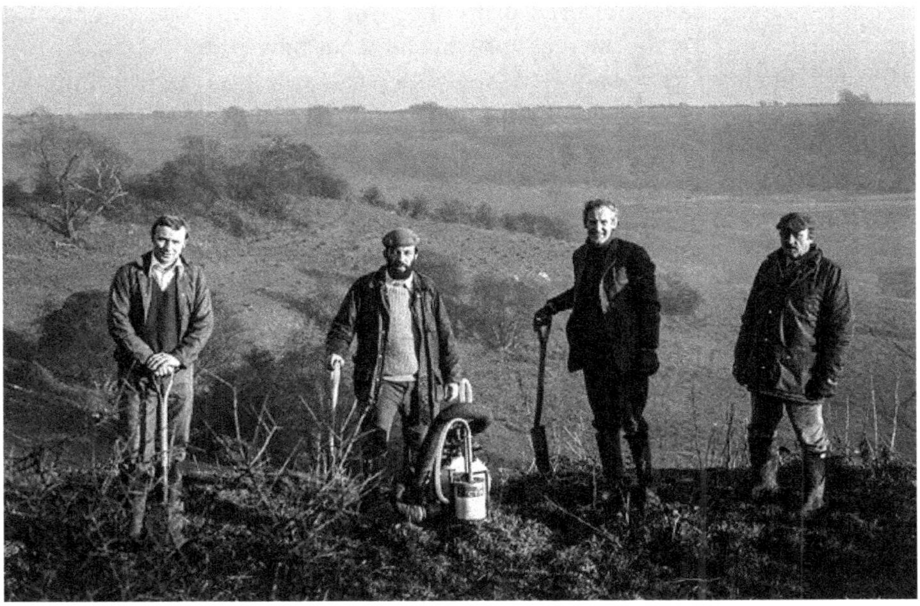

Fig. 3.1 'The badger brigade and their gassing machine near Dursley'—photograph by Jane Bown https://en.wikipedia.org/wiki/Jane_Bown. Source: 'New battle over the "bad" badgers—George Brock', *Observer*, 12 Dec. 1976, 3. Reproduced by permission of Guardian News and Media Ltd

out from 1976 onwards. The formal procedure, known as a 'fire brigade' operation, involved gassing all setts in the area of a bTB outbreak where 'no other source of infection has been revealed' and where local badger traces tested positive for *M. bovis*.[60] Thirty-three culling operations were conducted in 1976, rising to approximately fifty per year through 1977–1978.[61] By the end of the decade MAFF was upbeat about their progress and confident that their research had confirmed that badgers should be targeted.[62] They consolidated the culling policy, introducing further legislation granting officers powers of entry to private land in four Control Areas spread across the South West of England. This led to a drop-off of the locally focused 'fire brigade' operations and a shift to wider-scale culling towards the end of the decade.[63]

Outside of MAFF, others were not so confident. Privately, the scientists and officers of the Nature Conservation Committee (NCC)—a Department for the Environment body responsible for conservation research and policy—continued to be highly critical of MAFF's scientific standards.[64] Critically, the specialist consensus on gassing was not shared by wider publics or the media, and several local newspapers started campaigning against the policy.[65] Meanwhile, the UK was weathering the ongoing instabilities of the 1970s. Following the 1975 referendum on membership of the European Economic Community (EEC), MAFF had been heavily occupied with negotiating and implementing the Common Agricultural Policy system of agricultural subsidies and trade agreements. Following the collapse of the Conservative Heath government in 1974, Labour took power but continued to weather political instabilities, with the resignation of Harold Wilson in 1976, and a further three years of minority Labour government under the leadership of James Callaghan. Following a period of prolonged recession and industrial unrest known as the 'Winter of Discontent', a Parliamentary vote of no confidence in Callaghan's government was passed on 28 March 1979, triggering a General Election on 3 May. While bTB was still a relatively obscure issue in and of itself, badger advocates had skilfully reframed the disease in terms of gathering wider concerns over agricultural intensification, environmental damage and livestock welfare.[66] The incoming Conservative government, led by Margaret Thatcher, was elected on the strength of a modernising, reforming agenda. Badger/bTB had by that time been a thorn in the side of ministers and policymakers for nearly a decade. Was it time to think again?

3.3 'An Objective Look'

The incoming Conservative government awarded the position of Minister of Agriculture to Peter Walker (a core member of the Heath administration) who had overseen the creation of an entirely new dedicated Department of the Environment in 1970s. Following the election in the spring of 1979 and a summer of anti-gassing protests, including a particularly difficult confrontation on Dartmoor,[67] Walker announced that he had asked a fellow pioneer in environmental policy—Lord Solly Zuckerman—to review the situation:

> I have been concerned about the recent criticism of this Ministry's policy for dealing with badgers infected with bovine tuberculosis. The criticism has centred on the extent to which infected badgers are likely to pass on the disease to cattle and on the methods used to eradicate the disease. I have therefore asked Lord Zuckerman, President of the Zoological Society of London, to take an objective look at the problem and to give me his advice on the way it should be tackled in the future. I propose to make his findings public.[68]

Walker's press release invited anyone who wished to provide 'scientific evidence' to contact MAFF, and announced a moratorium on gassing 'beyond what is necessary to maintain freedom from the disease in areas that have already been cleared of it'.[69] Zuckerman was eminently well qualified: as well as his specialisms (zoology and physiology) and presidency of the Zoological Society of London, he had been involved with government enquiries on environmental pollution, FMD and rabies.[70] His position as the first Chief Scientific Adviser to the UK government (retired), member of the House of Lords and an integral part of 'the Establishment' made him the quintessential authoritative expert of the time. From Walker's perspective, Zuckerman could be trusted to provide a clear analysis of the situation (which had become more complex as research on the topic had progressed), advise ministers on the best course of action and help to calm burgeoning controversy over badger culling.

Zuckerman's archives show that five years earlier, HRH Prince Philip, Duke of Edinburgh (also President of the World Wildlife Fund), had enquired about badgers and bTB as part of his regular correspondence with Zuckerman.

> My Dear Solly,
>
> I hear that badgers are being blamed for the spread of various diseases among cattle and other domestic farm animals—particularly tuberculosis. Is this really possible? I'm afraid I don't really know by what means TB gets around.
>
> Yours ever, Phillip.[71]

Zuckerman made enquiries with MAFF, who passed on the information available internally at the time. He wrote back to Prince Phillip, forwarding the material with the statement 'It does look as though some guilt must attach to them [badgers].'[72] This exchange highlights Zuckerman's unusual position working across the worlds of science, policy, agriculture, conservation and elite society.[73] It also provides further evidence for the choice of Zuckerman to conduct the review, as a core and authoritative science-policy actor, who had recently stepped down from his formal role in government.

Zuckerman started to get correspondence almost immediately after the announcement, but he started work in earnest in the New Year, meeting with the CVO, senior MAFF officials and the Consultative Panel in London. He then visited the South West, where he consulted MAFF officers and policy teams in the area, alongside local farmers, naturalists and badger protection campaigners. While compiling the report, he consulted at least twenty individuals, collated submissions from nineteen external organisations, reviewed the scientific literature and received ninety-eight written submissions from individuals, including farmers, MPs, scientists external to MAFF, naturalists, animal welfare campaigners and members of the public.[74] The report was delivered to the Minister in August 1980 and was characteristically precise, comprising a review of the key scientific issues, followed by a section rebuffing various critiques of MAFF's policy and ending in a series of recommendations. Zuckerman maintained his earlier position: that MAFF's research had confirmed a connection between bTB in badgers and cattle, and that the current policy was the correct course of action and should continue. He drew upon medical analogies to support the various lines of veterinary enquiry which had been conducted; and cited the existing consensus that gassing was the most effective and humane technique available. Ever the scientist, Zuckerman acknowledged that there was still much to learn, recommending an expansion of MAFF's existing research. He also outlined key areas for further investigation, including specific research 'to devise improvements in the gassing procedures that have been used hitherto'.[75] MAFF regarded the report as a vindication and a return to business as usual, announcing the resumption of gassing with immediate effect.[76] To further support their case, MAFF released figures suggesting there had been a recent increase in bTB rates in cattle in the South West, alongside findings of a 'significant' number of infected badgers, which they attributed to the suspension of gassing.[77]

The publication of the report (in October 1980) prompted more press and other media than ever before (see Fig. 7.1). However, the media and public responses were very different to MAFF's. Zuckerman's role was usually reported quite neutrally, describing him as a scientist whose 'findings' supported the government's position. Others were more sceptical of his neutrality, using headlines such as 'RUN, BADGER, RUN: The scientists are after you!'[78] Following the initial report the story persisted as a series of organisations and public figures took the opportunity to get a wider airing for their criticisms of MAFF. While key groups such as the RSPCA and NCC (who had both privately raised concerns about gassing) publicly supported Zuckerman, other scientists and badger protection campaigners were highly critical.[79] The Mammal Society wrote to *Nature* to dispute Zuckerman/MAFF's claim that gassing had reduced bTB in cattle,[80] while ecologist Hans Kruuk commented that 'the evidence presented does not warrant the conclusions'.[81] Zuckerman was incensed and immediately defended himself, responding with commentaries in the *Sunday Times* and in *Nature*, in which he restated his main arguments and disputed the 'spurious criticisms' that had been made.[82] The argument continued on the pages of both *Nature* and *New Scientist* via letters and articles throughout 1981 and into 1982, drawing in a wide range of correspondents, including the CVO and Martin Kaplan—an eminent TB expert in the WHO.[83] The controversy was not limited to the scientific press and also took place in mainstream media coverage. This included further expert criticisms, badger persecution, more protests, a lengthy piece in the glossy *Observer Magazine* from BBC presenter Phil Drabble (including pictures of snared badgers and gassing operations) and scathing commentary from columnist Auberon Waugh.[84]

Zuckerman was incensed by these responses, firing off a series of letters to senior MAFF officials, the Minister, John Maddox (the editor of *Nature*) and scientific colleagues, including the head of the Natural Environment Research Council (Hans Kruuk's boss). In these letters he demanded retractions and suggested that Drabble (among others) be sued for libel. Zuckerman's correspondents advised him against this:

> … there is little doubt that it is defamatory, and defamatory of you. … But, having said this, I would very much discourage you against bringing a libel action in these circumstances. It is obviously an issue on which people feel very strongly and are therefore moved to extravagant and reckless utterance. With the picture of assassinated badgers in front of their eyes there is no knowing what a jury would do and it would only require three members of the jury to provoke a disagreement. Also it is the easiest thing in the world to work up hostility to members of the Establishment and certainly to Established scientists. Moreover, the motivation of the author is, on the face of it, not hostility to you but affection for badgers.[85]

This is quoted at length not only for a sense of the likely weight of public opinion at the time in a legal context, but also for the reference to 'the Establishment', at a time when traditional British power structures (including science) had been under widespread criticism for years. Zuckerman—as a senior scientist, government policy adviser and friend of the Royal Family—would have been seen by both friends and enemies as such—note also his formal suit in the *Private Eye* cartoon (Fig. 3.2).

By the end of 1981 the media coverage had faded away. However, another storm was quietly brewing for Zuckerman and MAFF. As requested, MAFF had commissioned scientists at the Chemical Defence Establishment (CDE), Porton Down, to conduct further research on the effects of cyanide on badgers. For several years, wildlife groups had been reporting stories of distressed animals emerging from gassed setts: at the urging of RSPCA's Wild Animals Committee, ICD, CDE and the RSPCA started discussing further research early in 1979.[86] MAFF had continued with gassing, based on long experience of its speedy and lethal effect on other mammals and, following the snaring imbroglio (see Sect. 2.3), lack of other options. Following the publication of Zuckerman's report, a contract was placed with CDE to carry out this work, which was completed by March 1982. The scientists at Porton applied standard laboratory dose–response techniques to determine the correct concentrations of hydrogen cyanide required to kill badgers. They used ferrets as a 'model organism': a sensible choice, given the two species' shared membership of the Mustelid family, the well-established tradition of working with ferrets in biomedicine, and the likely political implications of conducting laboratory experiments

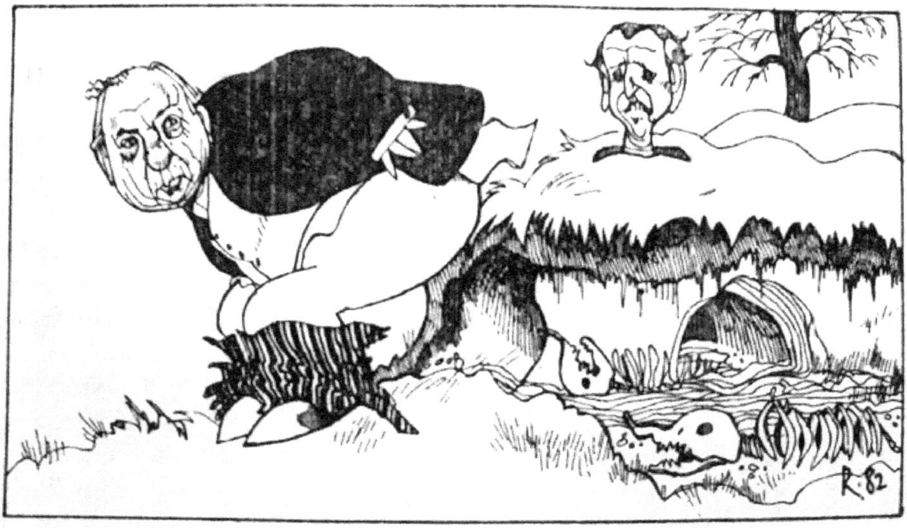

Fig. 3.2 Cartoon from *Private Eye*, January 1982. Zuckerman is depicted on the left, having 'gassed' a badger sett, while the Minister (Peter Walker) appears on the right, popping up for air (artist credit: Willie Rushton). Reproduced by kind permission of *Private Eye* magazine/The Estate of Willie Rushton[98]

on large numbers of badgers.[87] Three groups of about sixty ferrets were exposed to a cyanide spray in a sealed chamber, respectively for one, five and twenty-five minutes. The Porton scientists also exposed four wild badgers to cyanide, to directly observe the effects on *Meles meles.* The findings were dramatic: unbeknownst to anyone, it turned out that mustelids were unusually resistant to cyanide poisoning. The ferrets required extremely high doses to kill them and cyanide 'was not as effective at producing rapid unconsciousness as had previously been thought'.[88] The badger experiments were particularly alarming: only one animal died, slowly, and several showed obvious signs of distress before collapsing. Unlike other mammals, which tend to recover from a sublethal dose of cyanide with no ill effect, the ferrets and badgers that survived showed longer-term symptoms, including vomiting and paralysis.[89] Badgers were living up to their popular reputation as extraordinarily tough animals who are very difficult to kill.

Upon receipt of the CDE Porton research, MAFF convened an emergency meeting of senior officials. They agreed to continue with gassing but to warn the Minister 'of potential difficulties' while they sought a meeting with the CDE scientists to 'to ascertain their interpretation of the results and to explore, if necessary, alternative methods of control': a confidential summary of the situation was circulated to senior MAFF staff.[90] The meeting with CDE took place on 15 June, at which the generalisability of the experiments and the implications for policy were discussed. Some SVS staff were sceptical, suggesting that the effects of Cymag itself (sodium cyanide *powder*, not the hydrogen cyanide gas used in the CDE experiment) should be properly tested under field conditions. However, the CDE scientists defended their work, arguing that this would be impractical, expensive, unethical and likely to demonstrate even less effectiveness. They emphasised that they 'did not believe that hydrogen cyanide gassing was a humane way of killing badgers', conflating the two.[91] The implications of earlier work done by MAFF investigating Cymag distribution in real setts was also explored—it had been found that the poison ended up unevenly spread through the complex of tunnels. CDE believed it likely that in the field badgers were dying slowly from the lower doses, and that the problems of getting poisons into the furthest reaches of a sett meant that any other substance (e.g. carbon monoxide) would have similar problems.[92]

Following these deliberations, the civil servants rapidly reached agreement on what to do next and the Minister was briefed: 'There must be serious doubt as to whether hydrogen cyanide gassing of badgers is the most humane method of despatch. Nor can we be sure that badgers do not escape from gassed setts.'[93] In other words, MAFF policy team were concerned not only that gassing was cruel (and would be unacceptable for wider publics), but that it was not fully effective for disease control purposes. They recommended that gassing be suspended immediately. With snaring and gassing now ruled out, officials now turned towards an effective yet time-consuming procedure: combining cage-trapping and killing the animals with a direct shot. Peter Walker wrote to Lord Zuckerman on 28 June regarding the 'very disturbing' findings, requesting an urgent telephone call.[94] He then formally made the decision to stop gassing, and met with the Consultative Panel on 1 July to inform them of the situation, while MAFF announced the Minister's statement at the same time. This process had de facto excluded the Panel from decision-making. In their briefing notes to the Minister, animal health officers had considered the possibility of consulting the Panel and dismissed it on the grounds of urgency, assuming that they would agree with the decision to stop gassing immediately.[95] Over the course of the Zuckerman review process, the role of the Consultative Panel had shifted from needed policymaking partners to a legitimising rubber-stamp.

The immediate effect was to reopen the public controversy by prompting further media coverage and criticisms of government.[96] This policy reversal had the effect of undermining the authoritative report that MAFF and Zuckerman had thought would calm things down, even though it was a direct consequence of following scientific recommendations. Zuckerman's interventions in defence of MAFF had probably exacerbated this problem, by reinforcing the impression that his position was borne of a desire to defend government and the status quo. The *Mirror*'s editorial page was particularly damning: 'It has taken seven years of protests to stop this vile slaughter of one of God's loveliest creatures. All that time the cyanide killers were lying through their teeth when they said it didn't hurt. The arrogant know-alls at the Ministry of Agriculture and the RSPCA who wouldn't listen deserve to be put in badger sets themselves. And see how they like it.'[97] Instead of being treated as the senior scientist and respected government figure he had been through most of his career, Zuckerman found himself to be the target of invective and a figure of fun—as seen in the scatological response to the affair from *Private Eye* (Fig. 3.2).

From Zuckerman's correspondence, it seems that the hostile responses to the report took him entirely by surprise, and his zeal in rebutting critiques rapidly turned to dismay as he became more deeply entangled in the controversy. He wrote to a friend early in 1981, 'I have asked myself whether having now experienced this backlash I would have said yes so easily to Peter Walker's request when he put it over the telephone. I said yes, because I like Peter and because the way he explained the whole thing to me all that would be required would be a week's work: looking at documents and talking to people in his Department.'[99] Alongside formal submissions to the enquiry, Zuckerman received a large volume of private correspondence—which increased after the report was published. This included detailed scientific discussions, speculations, impassioned pleas both for and against culling, photographs of injured animals, jokes and a small but significant amount of personal abuse. Some of this material has been retained in the Zuckerman archive (in a folder marked 'Nut Letters'). It includes anti-Semitic abuse, accusations of Nazism, religious tracts and threats: for example, to put him on 'the other side of the bars' at London Zoo.[100] Robert Armstrong, Secretary of the Cabinet Office, wrote to Zuckerman,

> Dear Solly,
> I worry for you.
> When I was driving to Dorset yesterday, I found myself behind an exceedingly dirty truck; and in the dirt on the back of the truck someone had scrawled in bold capital letters the legend
> GAS LORD ZUCKERMAN.
> Mrs. Murray strikes again, I suppose.[101] But I really think that you should keep clear of the South West for the time being. I worry for you.
> A Happy New Year to you both.
> Yours ever, Robert.[102]

Around this time, Peter Walker wrote to Zuckerman apologising that, 'you are still in the thick of it'.[103] While Zuckerman initially replied with a relatively upbeat note, remarking, 'I sincerely hope that I shall be able to get shot of the badgers and the enthusiasts before too long', the controversy was taking its toll.[104] By this time he was well into his seventies and suffering increasing health problems, affecting his dealings with others: 'he began to be irritable and at times unreasonable, autocratic and impatient … He became less and less prepared to take into account other views than his own.'[105] A month later Zuckerman wrote to Walker again: 'I have really had enough. I have now given up the better part of a year to the matter, and this I can ill spare at my time of life when I have other things I wish to do', ending the letter, 'Please, please, take over …' Zuckerman urged Walker to encourage MAFF's 'veterinary and other scientists' to 'speak out' in the press.[106] Walker replied expressing sympathy: 'It is monstrous that you should continue to be pestered. Do, of course, pass all correspondence and complaints direct to us and we will deal with this.'[107] However, MAFF continued with their existing strategy of formal press releases, ministerial statements and technical reports, while scientists working within the Ministry confined their public communication to occasional letters to editors. Zuckerman continued to pursue badger/bTB throughout 1981, but following the suspension of gassing in 1982, he appears to have abandoned the argument.

So why did Zuckerman take the position that he did? Many of his opponents assumed or implied that he was politically motivated and certainly Zuckerman was at the heart of the political and scientific Establishment. However, Zuckerman's annotations of the submissions and correspondence with actors in badger/bTB do not support this idea, although they do offer considerable insight into his thinking. While he was widely known as the head of London Zoo and was deeply involved in the formation of British environmental science and policy,[108] he was an old-fashioned scientific polymath, with a primary training in medicine—although he never practised, moving immediately into research in anatomy, primatology and physiology.[109] However, as his secretary put it, Zuckerman 'did not suffer fools gladly'.[110] His post-report comment to Walker is key: 'I do hope that you agree that a channel has been given to me to stop the illiterate and unscientific campaign against MAFF's policies with regard to the badger.'[111] While he had considered all submissions and met with the full range of actors in badger/bTB, he regarded MAFF's veterinarians and scientists to have the most in-depth and legitimate expertise on the matter, reacting strongly against suggestions that the gassing policy was unacceptable to 'reputable scientists'.[112] As we will explore in the next two chapters, the main criticisms of the Zuckerman report came from scientists—mammologists and ecologists outside of government—and from naturalists and animal advocates who had remobilised existing campaigns for badger protection around bTB. As we know from other scholarship on Zuckerman's life and work, while one of his specialisms was in primatology, he had little respect for field biologists, ethologists and ecologists, regarding their work to be less rigorous than his own laboratory-based approach.[113]

As well as responding in the media and threatening to sue, Zuckerman wrote privately to ecologist Hans Kruuk's superiors at the Institute for Terrestrial Ecology (ITE) (a government research institute under the aegis of the NCC) questioning 'the propriety of him, as someone who is supported by public funds, criticising a ministerial decision based upon the advice of people who know far more about tuberculosis in cattle than he does'.[114] When this got nowhere Zuckerman then escalated to the director of the Natural Environment Research Council, complaining to them of 'the Institute of Celestial Ecology (Terrestrial Ecology is a fancy name for what an earlier generation of zoologists called "natural history")'.[115] He also wrote, 'As a zoologist and medical man I know of no one on its [the Mammal Society's] Council who, on the basis of experience, would be consulted on matters relating to the epidemiology of animal disease.'[116] Privately, he was also highly dismissive of the expertise represented by MAFF's Consultative Panel, which 'was obviously set up as a PR body, consisting as it does of farmers, badger enthusiasts, etc.'[117] This was also evident in his correspondence and comments about campaigners, who he also referred as 'enthusiasts'. Of naturalist Eunice Overend, he wrote, 'I have no doubts about Miss Overend's sincerity, but her "facts" happen to be wrong.'[118] Zuckerman was even ruder about Ruth Murray, using two full pages of his report to attack 'Mrs Murray's' position (Murray contested that badgers did not suffer from bTB), which he argued amounted to 'unsubstantiated assertions'.[119]

These comments reflect Zuckerman's own hierarchy of expertise, with 'medical men' like himself and MAFF's veterinarians at the top, field biologists way down the list and untrained 'enthusiasts' at the bottom.[120] As suggested by his self-description as a 'medical man', Zuckerman seemed to regard MAFF's veterinarians as equivalent to doctors and biomedical researchers, and as a senior policy adviser he would have been familiar with the 'stamping out' approach to disease control. An alignment with animal health cultures of care is also suggested by the prominence given to farmer testimony in the report, awarded an eight-page appendix.[121]

From his point of view, Zuckerman had done precisely what Walker had asked, in the same way he had always conducted such reviews in the past. While he had worked as the government's Chief Scientific Adviser from 1964 to 1971, upon his retirement he stood back from the day-to-day workings of government science and moved to Norfolk. This meant that by 1979 he would have been less directly exposed to the broader political changes of the time relating to science, the environment and policy. Even though (or perhaps because) Zuckerman had worked through the thick of the 1960s and 1970s 'sea change' in science-society, his reaction to 'enthusiast' criticisms of MAFF's research and policy was hostile and dismissive.[122] When his report was publicly and virulently contested, he was surprised, defensive, upset and eventually exhausted. Rather than resolving the matter, the report instead prompted further media attention and public disagreement between experts. Zuckerman was further drawn into the controversy, due to his position as a public scientist and his own combative nature, which combined explosively with the indirect nature of MAFF's public communications. This pattern—of developing controversy, leading to an expert review (anticipated to resolve the problem), which then creates further controversy—was to set a course for badger/bTB which persists into the present day.

3.4 Research Expansion, Policy Tinkering

Despite its association with the modernising Conservative Thatcher government, the Zuckerman report did not directly drive any change in bTB policy. Not only was Zuckerman a staunch supporter of the traditional animal health approach to disease control, the Minister Peter Walker (a moderate Conservative and member of the Heath administration) would also have been in favour of continuity. Instead it was Zuckerman's recommendation for further research, the CDE Porton scientists' entirely unexpected findings—and the unanimous conclusion that this made the gassing policy inhumane—which precipitated rapid policy change in 1982. Snaring had already been ruled out: with this finding taking gassing off the table, policymakers turned to the previously discarded option of cage-trapping. While the idea had been discarded due to the vulnerability of traps to 'interference', the tendency of the animals to get 'trap shy' and logistical complexities, trapping techniques had been refined in research contexts where catching live animals was necessary. Given the lack of alternatives, MAFF officials and the Consultative Panel rapidly agreed that trapping should be adopted to replace gassing as its main culling technique, developing standard procedures for field staff.[123] Beyond this technological change, MAFF's overall policy course continued, albeit modified into a 'clean ring' strategy—of removing badger social groups in an increasing circle around an outbreak until a layer of uninfected animals was found and removed.[124]

Zuckerman's other recommendations included that another review be published in three years' time; that MAFF's existing research programmes should continue; and that mechanisms be created for the 'freer exchange of information' between Ministry staff, private veterinarians, naturalists and academic scientists.[125] In 1982 MAFF set up a new Co-ordinating Group to pull together the various strands of bTB activity taking place across the department, as well as to 'act as a liaison point for outside research institutions and organisations involved in this work'.[126] The ongoing research investigations were now being published in academic journals, all of which seemed to confirm the association between bTB in badgers and cattle.[127] Collaborations between CVL and academic microbiologists had developed a method for identifying multiple strains of *M. bovis*, and tracing these suggested that the disease had jumped between the two species on more than one occasion.[128] By this time the 'clearance trials' were showing even more striking results. MAFF officers had had to go to considerable effort to clear badgers from these spaces, re-culling periodically until 1982. In the Thornbury study area, the area had been recolonised by 1989, but no infected badgers were found and there still were no herd 'breakdowns' (positive TB tests)—later SVS reported this effect persisting well into the 1990s.[129] Following the discovery of badgers' apparent lack of immune response to *M. bovis*, researchers at CVL focused on the key problem of diagnosis, developing new techniques for culturing the microbe in the lab, identifying multiple strains and attempting to apply BCG vaccinations to badgers.[130] While these diagnostic problems knocked on to veterinary scientists' abilities to understand the epidemiology of *M. bovis*, nonetheless knowledge about badger/bTB had become much more sophisticated since the early investigations in Gloucestershire a decade previously.

MAFF's overall capacity to monitor, follow and understand the spread of infectious disease in animals had improved greatly, with increasing numbers of VI field officers and the establishment of a specialist Epidemiology Unit. This enabled SVS to start collating its disease control data nationally, providing statistical expertise to support policy surveillance and epidemiological research alike.[131] As computers became cheaper and more widely used in government, the Unit adopted these technologies, creating a database to help them understand this increasing volume of data, including bTB surveillance data, the introduction of EEC standardised cattle testing and the new brucellosis eradication scheme.[132] As data from the various field studies came in, the epidemiologists were able to start building up a picture of the movements of *M. bovis* in wildlife and how it might relate to that in cattle populations. This data, analysed in-house and by externally funded researchers, had consistently found *M. bovis* in the badger population, but only sporadically in other wildlife or domestic species.[133] Veterinary epidemiologist John Wilesmith had been recruited by Veterinary Laboratories Agency (VLA) in 1976 and was central to the new epidemiological work on bTB, including statistical analyses associating badger sett density with outbreaks of 'unknown origin' in cattle herds.[134]

The application of computing to epidemiology continued and expanded following the Zuckerman report, the advent of mathematical modelling techniques and MAFF's creation of a fully staffed Computer Unit in the SVS.[135] With the advent of microcomputing, a Commodore 8096 PC was sent from CVL to Truro VI centre during 1982 so that staff could computerise badger data for later analysis.[136] Veterinary Officer Roger Sainsbury, stationed at MAFF's Divisional Office in Truro, was greatly pleased by its arrival. Sainsbury was an electronics and home computing enthusiast, who had initially trained himself via PC magazines and then with Open University courses.[137] He realised that the badger data could be helpful for MAFF field investigations and built a similar database for infected cattle. However, this data was not in a format that was useful for field staff:

> The vets were going out on field investigations with computer printouts of all the badgers and cattle infection that had been found locally. Sadly this was a complete waste of time, nobody looked at it. You couldn't visualise where the infected animals were on the ground. So it wasn't really very good ... So I thought a picture is worth 1000 words—why don't we try and display it graphically? I therefore wrote a TB mapping program which was much more useful. It was a very early example of a Geographical Information System (GIS). The locations of the cattle herds and badgers shown on the map acted as a key to find further information about these in the accompanying database.[138]

The program (TB Maps and Stats) projected MAFF's surveillance data for cattle and badgers onto the grid references of a map, creating a more sophisticated version of the hand-drawn mapping techniques used in Muirhead's early investigations (Fig. 2.1). The software was a great success and was rapidly integrated into the routine work of the SVS in areas where TB was a problem.[139] TB Maps and Stats remained in use by MAFF and its successor, the UK Department of the Environment and Rural Affairs (Defra) until 2006, when Animal Health's national VetNet database was phased out and replaced by a new system, SAM. The datasets, programmes and associated documentation for TB Maps and Stats are now held in the National Archives.[140]

MAFF's regional veterinary experts had adopted and adapted new computing technologies to help align this new data with their existing practices of disease mapping, deeply rooted in the history of epidemiology. Nineteenth-century pioneers of public health had established field practices of 'shoe-leather epidemiology',[141] in which investigators would travel to an area experiencing a disease outbreak to learn about local communities and the physical environment from 'physicians, chemists, veterinarians, farmers, politicians, and business owners'.[142] They would then map this information to help establish spatial relationships between disease victims and potential sources of infection, as in the famous case of John Snow and the Broad Street pump.[143] This spatial way of understanding and controlling the spread of infectious disease pointed the way towards establishing links between disease and contaminated milk—a key issue for controlling bTB.[144] Field knowledge and mapping were central to establishing the veterinary case for connections between cattle, badgers and

M. bovis. This is particularly apparent in Roger Muirhead's early case reports (Fig. 2.1), but similar techniques featured in the Cornwall investigation of 1972, and most of MAFF progress reporting on badger/bTB.[145] What geographers usefully describe as 'the spatiality of disease'[146] was not just important for epidemiological research: it also guided the underlying logic of implementing 'stamping out' across animal health policy.

In 1985 MAFF put into place the final recommendation of Zuckerman's report: that another expert review be conducted a few years later. Perhaps to avoid risking a repetition of Zuckerman's autocratic approach, MAFF invited a small committee to conduct the review. The new chair, Prof. George Dunnet, was an ecologist specialising in fisheries, well versed in MAFF and the complexities of science policy. He worked with David Jones, head veterinarian at the Zoological Society of London, and, signalling a key shift, an agricultural economist, Prof. John McInerney of the University of Exeter. This reflected the increasing importance of economics to MAFF, as it underwent further rounds of funding cuts through the 1980s. Over this decade, MAFF also instituted another round of restructuring and now privatisation, furthering government agendas of reducing the role of the state. The advisory role of ADAS was reduced and in 1987 it began charging for agricultural 'extension' advice services to farmers and industry. By the early 1990s MAFF's agricultural research and veterinary services were transformed into 'executive agencies', making it possible to sell their services to public and private users: ADAS, the Veterinary Medicines Directorate, the Central Veterinary Laboratories and the Central Science Laboratory. The Animal Health policy group was brought back together with the remaining parts of the SVS under the management of the CVO, to form a single Animal Health and Veterinary Group, which was promptly demerged once again in 1994, due to 'a lack of transparency in relations between its constituent parts and confused accountability in decision making'.[147]

It was in this context of renewed change within MAFF that the Dunnet review was published in the spring of 1986. While the report continued to support culling, it was with considerably less enthusiasm, and the Dunnet group instead challenged the existing scientific, veterinary and policy consensus within MAFF on several fronts. Core veterinary research on the pathology and immunology of the disease in badgers and cattle was accepted: that badgers caught bTB and were likely to act as a significant 'reservoir' for the disease in cattle, while other wildlife was not significantly involved. However, Dunnet et al. highlighted significant knowledge gaps in the distribution and broader epidemiology of the disease across the two species. Without 'extensive, long-term field studies, involving the killing of large numbers of badgers and cattle over an extensive area' (a prospect which they considered impractical), they argued it would be impossible to prove that the disease passed from badgers to cattle.[148] Furthermore, without an accurate diagnostic test for badgers, it was impossible to develop a better understanding of the incidence of bTB in their populations. Given these uncertainties, the Dunnet group argued that MAFF's 'clean-ring' strategy (based on the assumption that localised 'pockets' of infection in badgers could be cleared out) was not viable.[149] They also conducted their own analyses of MAFF's policy regime—first a time-series analysis of bTB incidence, which concluded that badger culling was not working well enough, and second an economic evaluation, which estimated that the costs of the culling policy outweighed the benefits to the tune of £7 million.[150] According to their analyses, badger culling would never be able to pay its own way.[151]

The report made recommendations based upon an assumption that a new, more suitable diagnostic test for bTB in badgers would be 'achievable' in three to five years.[152] Following their early immunological findings and the collaborative work on typing *M. bovis* strains, CVL researchers were exploring alternative tests which could detect antibodies to the bacterium.[153] Wider successes in the development of antibody-based diagnostic tests (known as ELISA) for a range of other animal infections may have contributed to this optimistic stance.[154] The Dunnet group recommended that an 'interim strategy' be implemented in the intervening period. Rather than the 'unattainable' goal of complete and permanent disease eradication in both species, they instead argued that policy should aim 'to limit the transmission of disease from badgers to cattle by dealing with identifiable and avoidable risks, quickly and effectively at a reasonable cost'.[155] The 'clean ring' strategy, based upon the long-standing MAFF tradition of stamping out, should be abandoned, and badgers should only be culled immediately on and around farms suffering a bTB outbreak where no other source of infection could be found. Finally, the Dunnett group recommended an expansion of research into the problem—while the most urgent priority was developing a diagnostic test for badgers, work on the population biology and epidemiology of the disease was also important.[156]

While MAFF accepted the Dunnett recommendations and the Minister immediate pledged to implement them, his statement downplayed the critical nature of the report.[157] Over the following years, culling was gradually scaled back, while research continued, with a marked increase in the number and range of collaborations with external partners and academic scientists.[158] However, this optimism was short-lived. While a functioning ELISA test was developed, its sensitivity was heavily affected by the progression of the disease. In other words, it worked best for older badgers with active symptoms of disease (e.g. tuberculous lesions), when what was really needed for policy was the opposite.[159] While the ELISA test was useful for research, it turned out not to be robust enough to change the policy assessments made by Dunnet et al. Therefore the 'interim strategy' remained in place, not for the envisaged five years, but instead for over ten. Meanwhile, a newly unfolding animal health crisis was occupying most of MAFF's attention. While the first case of Bovine spongiform encephalopathy (BSE) was identified in 1986, MAFF announced the existence of this entirely new disease in 1987, confirming that 132 new cases had already been found.[160] BSE was declared a notifiable disease in 1988 and a pandemic in 1989: given the completely unknown nature of the problem, the major part of MAFF veterinary research, investigation and surveillance teams were devoted to understanding and controlling this catastrophic new animal health problem. When BSE was found to be transmissible to humans, the public and political pressure on MAFF reached even greater heights, especially given their disastrous strategy of reassuring the public that British beef was 'safe'.[161] In the heat and light of an expanding and increasingly political animal health crisis, the chronic yet still unresolved problem of bTB faded into obscurity, where it was to stay for many years.

3.5 Managing M. bovis Through Animal Health Care

In this chapter, we have investigated how MAFF's veterinary scientists, field officers and policymakers got to grips with researching and acting upon the newly identified problem of bTB in badgers. Veterinarians have had a formal role as expert advisers within the British Government for over a century, making them central and long-standing members of the animal health epistemic community. As such, understanding how their working practices created reliable knowledge for policy—and were mutually shaped by caring practices—is critical to understanding their approach to badger/bTB. While animal health 'cultures of care' originated in partnerships between farmers, veterinarians and policymakers, 'stamping out' practices of disease control are still traumatic for farmers facing the loss of their animals. These tensions are caused by conflicts between practices of caring for specific farms and herds, and those needed for caring for entire populations and the wider economic interests of the country.

Having explored how care and caring practices operate in the epistemic community around animal health in Britain, we can see how they have guided processes of policymaking and veterinary research as MAFF struggled with the unexpectedly sticky problem of badger/bTB. The spatial logic of 'stamping out'—long established for managing infectious diseases including bTB—was applied to the new problem of tuberculous badgers. Research practices in the SVS were guided by an implicit multidisciplinarity, in which specialists in multiple fields—particularly laboratory and field investigators—worked in partnership on shared problems, while preserving disciplinary boundaries. The 'shoe-leather epidemiology' of regional veterinary officer Roger Muirhead was supplemented with further expertise from pathology and microbiological testing.[162] Once MAFF recognised the scale of the problem, this developed into a full-scale scale research programme, employing the above approaches, plus increasingly sophisticated work in fields such as immunology and epidemiology. As the programme moved into the 1980s, MAFF increasingly collected data on bTB and other infectious diseases, adopting new computing technologies to create centralised resources to collate the information. The lab–field loop was reinforced once more when regional veterinary investigators found ways of adapting PCs to converge this data with older field epidemiology practices of mapping, making it much more useful for day-to-day working practice.

We can also see how changes in government administrations—and their attendant political ideologies—have shaped changes in badger/bTB policy. Under the Conservative Heath government, MAFF took a laissez-faire, hands-off advisory approach to badger culling, which was rapidly brought under state control (and implementation) when Labour took power again in 1974. Despite its radical, modernising agenda, the inception of the Thatcher government did not bring change but an attempt to bolster support for existing MAFF policy, albeit in the guise of an expert review. It was scientific research, and the unexpected resistance of badgers to cyanide gassing, which forced policy change in 1982, and agendas such as privatisation affected MAFF more towards the end of the decade. The Zuckerman review had inadvertently started a cycle of broken expectations between science, policy and wider society which was to continue through the history of badger/bTB to the present day.

Notes

1. See Sect. 1.2; also e.g. Haas, 'Introduction'; Meyer and Molyneux-Hodgson, 'Introduction: The Dynamics of Epistemic Communities'; Dunlop, 'Epistemic Communities'.
2. Grant, 'Intractable Policy Failure: The Case of Bovine TB and Badgers', 561.
3. Davies et al., 'Science, Culture, and Care in Laboratory Animal Research'.
4. E.g. Mol, Moser and Pols, *Care in Practice.*
5. Mol, *The Logic of Care.*
6. See Sect. 1.2, also Davies et al., 'Science, Culture, and Care in Laboratory Animal Research'.
7. Worboys, 'Germ Theories of Disease and British Veterinary Medicine, 1860–1890'; Keir Waddington, 'To Stamp out "so Terrible a Malady": Bovine Tuberculosis and Tuberculin Testing in Britain, 1890–1939', *Medical History* 48(1) (January 2004): 29–48; Woods, *A Manufactured Plague*; Abigail Woods, 'Patterns of Animal Disease', in *Routledge History of Disease*, ed. Mark Jackson (New York: Routledge, 2016), 147–64; Paul Brassley, 'Murrains to Mad Cows: A Very Short History of Governments, People and Animal Diseases', in *Contested Countryside: Rural Politics and Land Controversy in Modern Britain*, ed. Jeremy Burchardt and Philip Conford (London: I.B.Tauris, 2008), 145–67.
8. J. Law, 'Care and Killing: Tensions in Veterinary Practice', in *Care in Practice: On Tinkering in Clinics, Homes and Farms*, ed. A. Mol, I. Moser and J. Pols (Bielefeld: Transcript, 2010), 57–69; Abigail Woods, 'From Cruelty to Welfare: The Emergence of Farm Animal Welfare in Britain, 1964–1971', *Endeavour* 36(1) (2012): 14–22; Henry Buller and Emma Roe, *Food and Animal Welfare* (London: Bloomsbury, 2016); Kerstin Weich and Herwig Grimm, 'Editorial', *Food Ethics* 1(3) (1 March 2018): 205–8.
9. Vanessa Ashall, Kate M. Millar and Pru Hobson-West, 'Informed Consent in Veterinary Medicine: Ethical Implications for the Profession and the Animal "Patient"', *Food Ethics* 1(3) (1 March 2018): 247–58.
10. Patricia Morris, 'Introduction: Euthanasia in Veterinary Medicine', in *Blue Juice: Euthanasia in Veterinary Medicine* (Philadelphia: Temple University Press, 2012), 1–18; Nora Schuurman, 'Performing Good

Death at the Veterinary Clinic: Experiences of Pet Euthanasia in Finland', *Area* 49(2) (2016): 208–14; Law, 'Care and Killing'.

11. Lindsay Hamilton, 'Bridging the Divide between Theory and Practice: Taking a Co-Productive Approach to Vet–Farmer Relationships', *Food Ethics* 1(3) (1 March 2018): 221–33.
12. Cassidy et al., 'Animal Roles and Traces in the History of Medicine, c.1880–1980'; Woods et al., *Animals and the Shaping of Modern Medicine*.
13. Andrew Gardiner, 'The Animal as Surgical Patient: A Historical Perspective in the 20th Century', *History and Philosophy of the Life Sciences* 31(3–4) (2009): 355–76.
14. Michael Bresalier, Angela Cassidy and Abigail Woods, 'One Health in History', in *One Health: The Theory and Practice of Integrated Health Approaches*, ed. Jakob Zinsstag et al. (Wallingford, Oxfordshire: CABI, 2015), 1–15.
15. Abigail Woods and Stephen Matthews, '"Little, If at All, Removed from the Illiterate Farrier or Cow-Leech": The English Veterinary Surgeon, c.1860–1885, and the Campaign for Veterinary Reform', *Medical History* 54(1) (January 2010): 29–54.
16. Brassley, 'Murrains to Mad Cows'; Paul Brassley, 'Wartime Productivity and Innovation, 1939–1945', in *The Front Line of Freedom: British Farming in the Second World War* (Exeter: British Agricultural History Society, 2006); Woods, 'A Historical Synopsis of Farm Animal Disease and Public Policy in Twentieth Century Britain'.
17. Anne Hardy, 'Professional Advantage and Public Health: British Veterinarians and State Veterinary Services, 1865–1939', *20 Century British History* 14(1) (January 2003): 1–23; Anne Hardy, 'John Bull's Beef: Meat Hygiene and Veterinary Public Health in England in the Twentieth Century', *Review of Agricultural and Environmental Studies—Revue d'Etudes en Agriculture et Environnement* 91(4) (2010): 369–92; Woods and Matthews, 'Little, If at All, Removed from the Illiterate Farrier or Cow-Leech'.
18. James Wilsdon, 'The Past, Present and Future of the Chief Scientific Advisor', *European Journal of Risk Regulation* 5(03) (September 2014): 293–99.
19. Abigail Woods, 'From Practical Men to Scientific Experts: British Veterinary Surgeons and the Development of Government Scientific Expertise, c. 1878–1919', *History of Science* (2013), 457–80.
20. While CVL was run by MAFF, Pirbright was run by the Agricultural Research Council (now BBSRC), in line with the wider organisation of agricultural research institutes during the twentieth century—see Colin Thirtle, Paolo Palladino and Jenifer Piesse, 'On the Organisation of Agricultural Research in the United Kingdom, 1945–1994: A Quantitative

Description and Appraisal of Recent Reforms', *Research Policy* 26(4–5) (December 1997): 557–76; Parker, Miles. 'The Rothschild Report (1971) and the Purpose of Government-Funded R&D—a Personal Account'. Palgrave Communications 2 (2 August 2016): 16053. https://doi.org/10.1057/palcomms.2016.53.

21. Woods, 'A Historical Synopsis of Farm Animal Disease and Public Policy in Twentieth Century Britain'; Woods, 'From Practical Men to Scientific Experts'.
22. Christoph Gradmann, 'Robert Koch and the Invention of the Carrier State: Tropical Medicine, Veterinary Infections and Epidemiology around 1900', *Studies in History and Philosophy of Biological and Biomedical Sciences* 41(3) (September 2010): 232–40.
23. Woods, *A Manufactured Plague*, 95.
24. Convery, Ian, Maggie Mort, Cathy Bailey, and Josephine Baxter, 'The Health and Social Consequences of the 2001 Foot & Mouth Disease Epidemic in North Cumbria', *Animal Disease and Human Trauma* (Palgrave Macmillan, 2008), 1–153; Woods, *A Manufactured Plague*, 131–51; Martin Döring and Brigitte Nerlich, *The Social and Cultural Impact of Foot and Mouth Disease in the UK in 2001: Experiences and Analyses* (Manchester: Manchester University Press, 2009); we will return to the 2001 FMD outbreak in Chap. 6.
25. William A. Maloney, Grant Jordan and Andrew M. McLaughlin, 'Interest Groups and Public Policy: The Insider/Outsider Model Revisited', *Journal of Public Policy* 14(1) (1994): 17–38.
26. Naylor et al., 'The "Good Farmer"'; Wilkie, *Livestock/Deadstock.*
27. Law and Mol, 'The Actor Enacted'; Lewis Holloway and Christopher Bear, 'Bovine and Human Becomings in Histories of Dairy Technologies: Robotic Milking Systems and Remaking Animal and Human Subjectivity', *BJHS Themes* 2 (January 2017): 215–34; Rees, 'Animal Agents?'
28. Colter Ellis, 'The Symbiotic Ideology: Stewardship, Husbandry, and Dominion in Beef Production', *Rural Sociology* 78(4) (1 December 2013): 429–49; Naylor et al., 'The "Good Farmer"'; Claudia Baldwin, Tanzi Smith and Chris Jacobson, 'Love of the Land: Social–Ecological Connectivity of Rural Landholders', *Journal of Rural Studies* 51 (2017): 37–52; Sarah L. Crowley, Steve Hinchliffe and Robbie A. McDonald, 'Killing Squirrels: Exploring Motivations and Practices of Lethal Wildlife Management', *Environment and Planning E: Nature and Space* 1(1–2) (2018): 120–43.
29. Wilkie, *Livestock/Deadstock*; Colter Ellis, 'Boundary Labor and the Production of Emotionless Commodities: The Case of Beef Production', *Sociological Quarterly* 55(1) (January 2014): 92–118.
30. Law, 'Care and Killing'; J. Law and I. Moser, 'Contexts and Culling', *Science, Technology & Human Values* 37(4) (December 2011): 332–54;

Qurat UlAin et al., 'Is a "Good Death" at the Time of Animal Slaughter an Essentially Contested Concept?' *Animals* 7(12) (14 December 2017): 99.

31. Steve Pile, '"A Load of Bloody Idiots": Somerset Dairy Farmers' View of Their Political World', *Political Geography Quarterly* 10(4) (October 1991): 405–21; Shortall et al., 'True Cowmen and Commercial Farmers'.
32. Frank Butcher, 'TB time-bomb under a county's dairy farmers: 'It happened to me and it could happen again''. Farmer's Weekly, 22 June 1971, 51. In NA MAF 109/294, item 9.
33. Mort et al., 'The Health and Social Consequences of the 2001 Foot & Mouth Disease Epidemic in North Cumbria'; Convery et al., 'Death in the Wrong Place?'; Döring and Nerlich, *The Social and Cultural Impact of Foot and Mouth Disease in the UK in 2001.*
34. G. Enticott and F. Vanclay, 'Scripts, Animal Health and Biosecurity: The Moral Accountability of Farmers' Talk about Animal Health Risks', *Health, Risk & Society* 13(4) (June 2011): 293–309; G. Enticott, 'Techniques of Neutralising Wildlife Crime in Rural England and Wales', *Journal of Rural Studies* 27(2) (April 2011): 200–8.
35. Woods, 'Patterns of Animal Disease'.
36. William Beinart and Karen Brown, *African Local Knowledge & Livestock Health: Diseases & Treatments in South Africa* (Woodbridge: Boydell & Brewer Ltd., 2013); Alex M. Nading, 'Humans, Animals, and Health: From Ecology to Entanglement', *Environment and Society: Advances in Research* 4(1) (December 2013): 60–78; Karen Brown, 'Environmental and Veterinary History—Some Themes and Suggested Ways Forward', *Environment and History* 20(4) (November 2014): 547–59; Delia Grace, 'Zoonoses of Poverty: Measuring and Managing the Multiple Burdens of Zoonoses and Poverty', in *Zoonoses—Infections Affecting Humans and Animals: Focus on Public Health Aspects* (Dordrecht: Springer Netherlands, 2015), 1127–37.
37. Woods, 'A Historical Synopsis of Farm Animal Disease and Public Policy in Twentieth Century Britain'.
38. G. Enticott, 'Relational Distance, Neoliberalism and the Regulation of Animal Health', *Geoforum* 52 (March 2014): 42–50; Maye et al., 'Animal Disease and Narratives of Nature'.
39. Michael P. Duffy, 'The Rothschild Experience: Health Science Policy and Society in Britain', *Science, Technology & Human Values* 11(1) (1986): 68–78; Parker, 'The Rothschild Report (1971) and the Purpose of Government-Funded R&D'.
40. N. A. Phillips, J. Bridgeman and M. Ferguson-Smith, 'The Inquiry into BSE and Variant CJD in the United Kingdom' (London: HMSO, 2000), sec. annex 1; G. Enticott et al., 'The Changing Role of Veterinary Expertise in the Food Chain', *Philosophical Transactions of the Royal Society of London. Series B, Biological Sciences* 366(1573) (July 2011):

1955–65; Woods, 'A Historical Synopsis of Farm Animal Disease and Public Policy in Twentieth Century Britain.'

41. Pearce, Pugh and Ritchie, *Animal Health*, 342.
42. Muirhead, 'Bovine Tuberculosis in Wild Badgers in South Gloucestershire'; Muirhead, Gallagher and Burn, 'Tuberculosis in Wild Badgers in Gloucestershire: Epidemiology'; Gallagher, Muirhead and Burn, 'Tuberculosis in Wild Badger (*Meles Meles*) in Gloucestershire—Pathology'.
43. MAFF, 'Bovine Tuberculosis in Badgers. Report by the Ministry of Agriculture, Fisheries and Food', sec. app. 6; MAFF, 'Bovine Tuberculosis in Badgers. Second Report by the Ministry of Agriculture, Fisheries and Food' (London: Ministry of Agriculture, Fisheries & Food: HMSO, December 1977), sec. app. 5.
44. MAFF, 'Bovine Tuberculosis in Badgers. Third Report by the Ministry of Agriculture, Fisheries and Food' (London: Ministry of Agriculture, Fisheries & Food: HMSO, July 1979), 17.
45. Gallagher and Nelson, 'Cause of Ill Health and Natural Death in Badgers in Gloucestershire'.
46. Brown, 'Animal Health 1974: Report of the Chief Veterinary Officer', 53; T. W. Little, K. J. Burn and P. Stuart, 'Virulence for Calves of Tubercle Bacilli Isolated from Badgers', *Veterinary Record* 96(24) (1975): 533; MAFF, 'Bovine Tuberculosis in Badgers. Report by the Ministry of Agriculture, Fisheries and Food'.
47. MAFF, 'Bovine Tuberculosis in Badgers. Third Report by the Ministry of Agriculture, Fisheries and Food', 13; Little, Naylor and Wilesmith, 'Laboratory Study of Mycobacterium Bovis Infection in Badgers and Calves'; Overy and Tansey, *A History of Bovine TB c.1965–c. 2000*, 14–15.
48. MAFF, 'Bovine Tuberculosis in Badgers. Report by the Ministry of Agriculture, Fisheries and Food', 7.
49. MAFF, 'Bovine Tuberculosis in Badgers. Third Report by the Ministry of Agriculture, Fisheries and Food', 15.
50. MAFF, 'Bovine Tuberculosis in Badgers. Third Report by the Ministry of Agriculture, Fisheries and Food' (London: Ministry of Agriculture, Fisheries & Food: HMSO, July 1979), 10.
51. MAFF, 'Bovine Tuberculosis in Badgers. Report by the Ministry of Agriculture, Fisheries and Food', 1; Overy and Tansey, *A History of Bovine TB c.1965–c. 2000*, 36–38, 41–42. For citizen science, see e.g. Rick Bonney et al., 'Next Steps for Citizen Science', *Science* 343(6178) (2014): 1436–37. For a recent return to the badger survey, see Jessica Phoenix, 'Local Understandings of Bovine Tuberculosis (Working Title)' (PhD, University of Lancaster, in prep.); Elsa Sandoval Barron et al., 'A Study of Tuberculosis in Road Traffic-Killed Badgers on the Edge of the British Bovine TB Epidemic Area', *Scientific Reports* 8(1) (6 December 2018): 17206.

52. H. V. Thompson, 'Note LP/N 3868C to Richard Clark, 17 July 1974', NA MAF 109/383, item 154.
53. E. Dennis, 'Memo to I. Prest: Badgers/Bovine TB in Dorset', 24 July 1975, NA FT 41/91; H. V. Thompson, 'Memo to D.W.M. Herbert: Badgers and Tuberculosis in Cattle', 20 January 1975, NA MAF 109/384, item 30.
54. MAFF, 'Bovine Tuberculosis in Badgers. Report by the Ministry of Agriculture, Fisheries and Food', 3.
55. Clifton-Hadley et al., 'The Occurrence of Mycobacterium Bovis Infection in Cattle in and around an Area Subject to Extensive Badger (Meles Meles) Control', 181.
56. MAFF, 'Bovine Tuberculosis in Badgers. Third Report by the Ministry of Agriculture, Fisheries and Food', 4–5.
57. Clifton-Hadley et al., 'The Occurrence of Mycobacterium Bovis Infection in Cattle in and around an Area Subject to Extensive Badger (Meles Meles) Control'.
58. MAFF, *Press Release: Consultative Panel on Badgers and Tuberculosis, September 24 1975* (MAFF: London, 1975).
59. For further details on the development and use of Cymag in mammalian pest control, see Sect. 4.1.
60. MAFF, 'Bovine Tuberculosis in Badgers. Report by the Ministry of Agriculture, Fisheries and Food', 4.
61. MAFF, 'Bovine Tuberculosis in Badgers. Report by the Ministry of Agriculture, Fisheries and Food'; MAFF, 'Bovine Tuberculosis in Badgers. Second Report by the Ministry of Agriculture, Fisheries and Food'; MAFF, 'Bovine Tuberculosis in Badgers. Third Report by the Ministry of Agriculture, Fisheries and Food'.
62. H. W. Rees, 'Animal Health 1980: Report of the Chief Veterinary Officer' (London: Ministry of Agriculture, Fisheries and Food, 1980).
63. MAFF, 'Bovine Tuberculosis in Badgers. Third Report by the Ministry of Agriculture, Fisheries and Food', 3, 12.
64. J. F. D. Frazer, 'In Confidence: Badgers and Bovine TB Investigation', 8 September 1971, NA FT 41/88; I. Presst (Deputy Director), 'Badgers', 6 March 1974, NA FT/41/89.
65. Anon., 'Ministry Slammed Over "Needless" Badger Slaughter', *Gloucester Citizen*, 29 May 1977, 1; Ian Beales, 'How Much Longer Must this Blitz on Badgers Go On?' *Western Daily Press*, 14 Feb. 1979, 1.
66. See Chap. 5, also Thirtle, Palladino and Piesse, 'On the Organisation of Agricultural Research in the United Kingdom, 1945–1994', 565–66; Woods, 'From Cruelty to Welfare'; Sayer, 'Animal Machines'.
67. E. Clarkson, 'Badger gassing: just a job for two men, expendable mercenaries', *The Guardian*, 5 September 1979, 8; see also Zuckerman, 'Badgers, Cattle and Tuberculosis', 7.

68. MAFF, *Press Release: Badgers and Bovine Tuberculosis*, 25 September 1979 (MAFF: London).
69. Ibid.
70. Woods, *A Manufactured Plague*, 123; Pemberton and Worboys, *Mad Dogs and Englishmen*, 175–76; John Sheail, '"Torrey Canyon": The Political Dimension', *Journal of Contemporary History* 42(3) (2007): 485–504.
71. P. Mountbatten, 'Letter to Solly Zuckerman', 29 April 1974, ZUEA S2 PUB 425.
72. S. L. Zuckerman, 'Letter to HRH Duke of Edinburgh', 14 May 1974, ZUEA, S2 PUB 425.
73. For an overview of Zuckerman's life and research see P. L. Krohn, 'Solly Zuckerman Baron Zuckerman, of Burnham Thorpe, O.M., K.C.B', *Biogr. Mems Fell. R. Soc.* 41 (1995): 576–98.
74. Zuckerman, 'Badgers, Cattle and Tuberculosis', 103–7.
75. Zuckerman, 'Badgers, Cattle and Tuberculosis', 47.
76. Rees, 'Animal Health 1980', 1–2.; H. Clayton, 'Killing of tubercular badgers by gas to be resumed', *The Times*, 31 October 1980, 1.
77. D. Johnson, 'Badger the suspect in cattle epidemic', *The Guardian*, 27 October 1980.
78. Anon., 'RUN, BADGER, RUN The scientists are after you!' *Daily Express*, 31 October 1980, 15.
79. W. Newlands, 'Boycott goes to bat for the badger', *Daily Mail*, 10 December 1980, 38.
80. Stephen Harris, 'Badgers and TB', *Nature* 288 (11 December 1980): 532.
81. Anon., 'Scientists badger Lord Zuckerman over gassing', *New Scientist*, 4 December 1960, 619.
82. S. L. Zuckerman, 'OPINION: THE BADGER AND TB CONTROVERSY', *Sunday Times*, 4 January 1981, 12; *Nature* and S. L. Zuckerman, 'The Great Badger Debate', *Nature* 289(5799) (19 February 1981): 628–30.
83. See the letters pages of *Nature* vol. 289, issues 5794–5800; vol. 292, issue 5819; also M. Kaplan, 'Keep badgering', *New Scientist*, 10 January 1985.
84. E. Grice and O. Gillie, 'Badgers May Be Innocent, OK?' *Sunday Times*, 27 December 1980; P. Oldfield, 'Badgered to Death', *Guardian*, 15 May 1981, 15; P. Drabble, 'Brock is Innocent, OK? Gassing Badgers is Wrong', *Observer Magazine*, 27 September 1981, 33–39; A. Waugh, 'When top people are killed', *Sunday Telegraph*, 22 November 1981. All clippings in ZUEA S2 PUB 425.
85. A. Goodman, 'Letter to Lord Zuckerman', 26 November 1981. ZUA, S2 PUB 425, folder '1980–1985 press cuttings'.

86. RSPCA Wild Animals Advisory Committee, 'Badgers and Bovine Tuberculosis : The Case for Further Investigation' (Horsham: Royal Society for the Prevention of Cruelty to Animals, 1979), British Library. NA MAF 459/8, items 1–25.
87. J. Edginton and R. Lynch, 'THE TOXICITY OF HYDROGEN CYANIDE BY INHALATION TO FERRETS AND BADGERS' (Salisbury: Chemical Defense Establishment, Porton Down, 1982), in NA MAF 459/8. For ferrets as model organisms, see Michael Bresalier, 'Neutralizing Flu: "Immunological Devices" and the Making of a Virus Disease', in *Crafting Immunity: Working Histories of Clinical Immunology*, ed. Kenton Kroker, Jennifer Keelan and Pauline Mazumdar (Farnham: Ashgate, 2008), 107–45.
88. Edginton and Lynch, 'THE TOXICITY OF HYDROGEN CYANIDE BY INHALATION TO FERRETS AND BADGERS', 9–10; anon., 'CONFIDENTIAL: BADGERS AND TB—METHODS OF BADGER CONTROL', 2 June 1982, NA MAF 459/8, item 20.
89. Anon., 'NOTE OF A MEETING HELD AT 10.30am ON TUESDAY 1ST JUNE 1982 TO DISCUSS THE CHEMICAL ESTABLISHMENT'S REPORT ON EXPERIMENTS INTO THE TOXICITY OF HYDROGEN CYANIDE BY INHALATION TO FERRETS AND BADGERS', 1 June 1982, NA MAF 459/8, item 17.
90. Anon., 'NOTE OF A MEETING ...', 1 June 1982, NA MAF 459/8, item 17.
91. Anon., 'CONFIDENTIAL: THE TOXICITY OF HYDROGEN CYANIDE. MINUTES OF A MEETING', 15 June 1982, NA MAF 459/10, item 22.
92. Ibid.
93. J. Hepburn, 'CONFIDENTIAL. BADGERS AND TB—METHODS OF BADGER CONTROL', 23 June 1982, NA MAF 459/10, item 26, 3.
94. P. Walker, 'Letter to Lord Zuckerman: TB in Badgers', ZUEA, S2 PUB 425; MAFF 1 July 1982; *PRESS NOTICE, 1 JULY 1982 MINISTER'S STATEMENT* (MAFF: London); CONSULTATIVE PANEL ON BADGERS AND TUBERCULOSIS: Minutes of 23rd Meeting of the Panel, 23 July 1982, NA MAF 459/8, item 59.
95. J. Hepburn, 'CONFIDENTIAL. BADGERS AND TB—METHODS OF BADGER CONTROL', 23 June 1982, NA MAF 459/10, item 26, 6.
96. S. Young, 'Badger Poison Gas War Halted', *Daily Mirror*, 2 July 1982, 9; D. Johnson, 'Cyanide killing of badgers halted', *The Guardian*, 2 July 1982, 24; C. White, 'Badger gassing halted after "cruelty" warning', *Daily Mail*, 2 July 1982, 11.
97. Anon., 'SO CRUEL', *Daily Mirror*, 4 July 1982. In ZUEA Z2 PUB 425, folder '1982–1985, Press cuttings in year order only'.
98. A. Waugh, 'Auberon Waugh's Diary', *Private Eye* 525, 29 January 1982.

99. S. L. Zuckerman, 'Letter to Sir Robert Armstrong', 12 January 1981, ZUEA S2 PUB 425.
100. Anonymous letter dated 1 November 1980, ZUEA, S2 PUB 425, see also 'Nut Letters' folder in S2 PUB 425.
101. 'Mrs. Murray' is badger protection activist Ruth Murray, discussed in Chap. 2 and again in Chap. 5.
102. R. Armstrong, 'Note to Solly Zuckerman', 6 January 1981, ZUEA, S2 PUB 425.
103. P. Walker, 'Letter to Lord Zuckerman', 8 January 1981, ZUEA, S2 PUB 425.
104. S. L. Zuckerman, 'Note to Peter Walker', 19 January 1981, ZUEA, Z2 PUB 425.
105. Krohn, 'Solly Zuckerman Baron Zuckerman, of Burnham Thorpe, O.M., K.C.B', 587–88.
106. S. L. Zuckerman, 'Letter to Peter Walker', 13 February 1981, ZUEA, Z2 PUB 425.
107. P. Walker, 'Letter to Lord Zuckerman', 27 February 1981, ZUEA, Z2 PUB 425.
108. This included Zuckerman's work on various science-policy reviews, the creation of the UK Government's Department of the Environment and the Natural Environment Research Council, early advocacy for concerns about global warming, and the influential School of Environmental Sciences at the University of East Anglia. See Krohn, 'Solly Zuckerman Baron Zuckerman, of Burnham Thorpe, O.M., K.C.B.'; Jon Agar, '"Future Forecast—Changeable and Probably Getting Worse": The UK Government's Early Response to Anthropogenic Climate Change', *Twentieth Century British History* 26(4) (December 2015): 602–28; Clark, 'Pesticides, Pollution and the UK's Silent Spring, 1963–64'.
109. Krohn, 'Solly Zuckerman Baron Zuckerman, of Burnham Thorpe, O.M., K.C.B.'
110. Krohn, 'Solly Zuckerman Baron Zuckerman, of Burnham Thorpe, O.M., K.C.B.', 587.
111. S. L. Zuckerman, 'Note to Peter Walker', 28 September 1981, ZUEA, Z2 PUB 425, folder '1980–1985 press cuttings'.
112. Zuckerman, 'Badgers, Cattle and Tuberculosis', para. 36.; S. L. Zuckerman, 'Letter to Peter Walker', 28 September 1981, ZUEA S2 PUB 425.
113. Jonathan Burt, 'Solly Zuckerman: The Making of a Primatological Career in Britain, 1925–1945', *Studies in History and Philosophy of Biological and Biomedical Sciences* 37(2) (June 2006): 295–310; Robert G. W. Kirk, 'Between the Clinic and the Laboratory: Ethology and Pharmacology in the Work of Michael Robin Alexander Chance, c.1946–1964', *Medical History* 53(4) (October 2009): 513–36.

114. S. L. Zuckerman, 'Letter to J.R.R. Jeffers, Head of Institute of Terrestrial Ecology', 28 February 1981, ZUEA S2PUB 425.
115. S. L. Zuckerman, 'Letter to Sir Herman Bondi', 27 February 1981, ZUEA S2PUB 425.
116. S. L. Zuckerman, 'Letter to Sir Herman Bondi', 23 March 1981, ZUEA S2PUB 425.
117. S. L. Zuckerman, 'Letter to Sir Herman Bondi', 23 March 1981, ZUEA S2PUB 425.
118. *Nature* and Zuckerman, 'The Great Badger Debate', 630.
119. Zuckerman, 'Badgers, Cattle and Tuberculosis', 9–10.
120. The gendered dimension of these debates has not escaped me, and will be discussed in Sect. 5.4.
121. Zuckerman, 'Badgers, Cattle and Tuberculosis', 71–78.
122. Agar, 'What Happened in the Sixties?'; Agar, 'Transition: Sea Change in the Long 1960s'.
123. E. N. Wright, 'Confidential: Badger Control Operations—Implications of switching from gassing to trapping', 11 June 1982, NA MAF 459/8, item 27; MAFF, 'Press Notice: Minister's Statement to the Consultative Panel', 1 July 1982, NA MAF 459/8, item 50; MAFF, 'Bovine Tuberculosis in Badgers. Seventh Report by the Ministry of Agriculture, Fisheries and Food' (London: Ministry of Agriculture, Fisheries & Food: HMSO, August 1983), 2.
124. MAFF, Bovine Tuberculosis in Badgers. Seventh Report, 2–3; MAFF, 'Bovine Tuberculosis in Badgers. Eighth Report by the Ministry of Agriculture, Fisheries and Food' (London: Ministry of Agriculture, Fisheries & Food: HMSO, August 1984), 2; Dunnet, Jones and McInerney, 'Badgers and Bovine Tuberculosis', 6.
125. Zuckerman, 'Badgers, Cattle and Tuberculosis', para. 48.
126. MAFF, 'Bovine Tuberculosis in Badgers. Sixth Report by the Ministry of Agriculture, Fisheries and Food' (London: Ministry of Agriculture, Fisheries & Food: HMSO, August 1982), 22–28; 'MAFF Consultative Panel on Badgers and bTB, minute of meeting', 23 July 1982, NA MAF 459/8, item 59.
127. Stuart and Wilesmith, 'Tuberculosis in Badgers'; C. L. Cheeseman, J. W. Wilesmith and F. A. Stuart, 'Tuberculosis—The Disease and Its Epidemiology in the Badger, A Review', *Epidemiology and Infection* 103(1) (August 1989): 113–25; Clifton-Hadley et al., 'The Occurrence of Mycobacterium Bovis Infection in Cattle in and around an Area Subject to Extensive Badger (Meles Meles) Control'.
128. P. A. Barrow, 'Aspects of the Epidemiology of Bovine Tuberculosis in Badgers and Cattle. II. The Development and Use of a Typing System for Mycobacterium Bovis', *The Journal of Hygiene* 86(3) (1981): 247–57; P. A. Barrow and J. Gallagher, 'Aspects of the Epidemiology of Bovine

Tuberculosis in Badgers and Cattle. I. The Prevalence of Infection in Two Wild Animal Populations in South-West England', *The Journal of Hygiene* 86(3) (1981): 237–45.

129. MAFF Wildlife Unit, *The Thornbury Study Area: 1989 survey* (MAFF: London, private collection); see also Clifton-Hadley et al., 'The Occurrence of Mycobacterium Bovis Infection in Cattle in and around an Area Subject to Extensive Badger (Meles Meles) Control'.
130. See, e.g. MAFF, 'A review of bovine tuberculosis in Great Britain' (MAFF: London, September 1984), in ZUEA, S2PUB 425.
131. A. C. L. Brown, 'Animal Health 1972: Report of the Chief Veterinary Officer' (London: Ministry of Agriculture, Fisheries and Food, 1972), 56–57.
132. A. C. L. Brown, 'Animal Health 1973: Report of the Chief Veterinary Officer' (London: Ministry of Agriculture, Fisheries and Food, 1973), 62–64. For the wider history of computing across Whitehall, see Jon Agar, *The Government Machine: A Revolutionary History of the Computer* (Cambridge, MA: MIT Press, 2003). For brucellosis, see Karen Sayer, 'Brucellosis in Fact and Fiction: The Story of a Zoonosis', *Veterinary History* 18 (2016): 165–83.
133. See, e.g. Zuckerman, 'Badgers, Cattle and Tuberculosis', paras 69–75; Barrow, 'Aspects of the Epidemiology of Bovine Tuberculosis in Badgers and Cattle. II. The Development and Use of a Typing System for Mycobacterium Bovis'; Barrow and Gallagher, 'Aspects of the Epidemiology of Bovine Tuberculosis in Badgers and Cattle. I. The Prevalence of Infection in Two Wild Animal Populations in South-West England'.
134. Wilesmith became head of the VLA's epidemiology department in 1986 and subsequently led MAFF's investigations into BSE. Anon., 'Zuckerman Review: Meeting with senior veterinary staff of the Ministry', 24 April 1980, ZUEA S2 PUB 155; J. W. Wilesmith, 'A case-control study of M. bovis in cattle herds in relation to badger sett density', MAFF, 1980, ZUEA S2 PUB 115.
135. MAFF, 'Bovine Tuberculosis in Badgers. Eighth Report by the Ministry of Agriculture, Fisheries and Food', 9; H. W. Rees, 'Animal Health 1984: Report of the Chief Veterinary Officer' (London: Ministry of Agriculture, Fisheries and Food, 1984), 57–58; H. W. Rees, 'Animal Health 1986: Report of the Chief Veterinary Officer' (London: Ministry of Agriculture, Fisheries and Food, 1986), 65–66.
136. H. W. Rees, 'Animal Health 1985: Report of the Chief Veterinary Officer' (London: Ministry of Agriculture, Fisheries and Food, 1985), 57–58. For wider trends across UK government, see Agar, *The Government Machine*, 367–89.

137. For the culture and media of computing enthusiasts during the 1980s, see Tom Lean, *Electronic Dreams: How 1980s Britain Learned to Love the Computer* (London: Bloomsbury Academic, 2016).
138. Interview with Roger Sainsbury, 21/05/2015.
139. Interview with Roger Sainsbury, 21/05/2015.
140. NA MAF 430 series; for further information see http://discovery.nationalarchives.gov.uk/details/r/C16050.
141. Steere-Williams, 'Performing State Medicine during Its "Frustrating" Years', 98.
142. Jacob Steere-Williams, 'The Perfect Food and the Filth Disease: Milk-Borne Typhoid and Epidemiological Practice in Late Victorian Britain', *Journal of the History of Medicine and Allied Sciences* 65(4) (October 2014): 519.
143. Kari S. McLeod, 'Our Sense of Snow: The Myth of John Snow in Medical Geography', *Social Science & Medicine* 50(7–8) (April 2000): 923–35; Tom Koch, *Disease Maps: Epidemics on the Ground* (Chicago: University of Chicago Press, 2011).
144. Waddington, *The Bovine Scourge*; Peter J. Atkins, *Liquid Materialities: A History of Milk, Science and the Law* (Farnham: Ashgate, 2010); Olmstead and Rhodes, *Arresting Contagion*; Atkins, *A History of Uncertainty*.
145. Muirhead, 'Bovine Tuberculosis in Wild Badgers in South Gloucestershire'; Richards et al., 'Inquiry into Bovine TB in West Cornwall'; Muirhead, Gallagher and Burn, 'Tuberculosis in Wild Badgers in Gloucestershire: Epidemiology'.
146. Tom Koch and Kenneth Denike, 'Certainty, Uncertainty, and the Spatiality of Disease: A West Nile Virus Example', *Stochastic Environmental Research and Risk Assessment* 21(5) (August 2007): 523–31; Koch, *Disease Maps*.
147. A. Lebrecht, 'Stage 2 report: proposals for changes in functions of the Animal Health and Veterinary Group of MAFF', unpublished document, presented as evidence to Phillips, Bridgeman and Ferguson-Smith, 'The Inquiry into BSE and Variant CJD in the United Kingdom', 108. For MAFF's reorganisations during the 1980s and 1990s, see Paul Ingram, 'THE UNITED KINGDOM EXPERIENCE IN THE PRIVATIZATION OF EXTENSION', in *Public and Private Roles in Agricultural Development: Proceedings of the Twelfth Agricultural Sector Symposium*, ed. J. R. Anderson and C. de Haan (Washington, DC: World Bank Publications, 1988); Thirtle, Palladino and Piesse, 'On the Organisation of Agricultural Research in the United Kingdom, 1945–1994', 566–67; Phillips, Bridgeman and Ferguson-Smith, 'The Inquiry into BSE and Variant CJD in the United Kingdom', 85–112.
148. Dunnet, Jones and McInerney, 'Badgers and Bovine Tuberculosis', 17.

149. Dunnet, Jones and McInerney, 'Badgers and Bovine Tuberculosis', 12–13, 18.
150. Dunnet, Jones and McInerney, 'Badgers and Bovine Tuberculosis', 22–25.
151. A. P. Power, B. G. A. Watts and Fisheries and Food, Great Britain, Ministry of Agriculture, *The Badger Control Policy: An Economic Assessment* (London: Ministry of Agriculture, Fisheries & Food: HMSO, 1987).
152. Dunnet, Jones and McInerney, 'Badgers and Bovine Tuberculosis', 33.
153. A. C. L. Brown, 'Animal Health 1977: Report of the Chief Veterinary Officer' (London: Ministry of Agriculture, Fisheries and Food, 1977), 59–60.
154. Rees, 'Animal Health 1984: Report of the Chief Veterinary Officer', 49–50; Rees, 'Animal Health 1985: Report of the Chief Veterinary Officer', 3.
155. Dunnet, Jones and McInerney, 'Badgers and Bovine Tuberculosis', 28, 38.
156. Dunnet, Jones and McInerney, 'Badgers and Bovine Tuberculosis', 38–39.
157. MAFF, *Press Notice, April 7, 1986 Government Will Act Immediately on the Dunnet Report's Main Findings on Badger Control* (MAFF: London, 1986).
158. MAFF, 'Bovine Tuberculosis in Badgers. Eleventh Report by the Ministry of Agriculture, Fisheries and Food' (London: Ministry of Agriculture, Fisheries & Food: HMSO, August 1987), 5–13.
159. MAFF, 'Bovine Tuberculosis in Badgers. Fourteenth Report by the Ministry of Agriculture, Fisheries and Food' (London: Ministry of Agriculture, Fisheries & Food: HMSO, July 1990), 4–5.
160. H. W. Rees, 'Animal Health 1987: Report of the Chief Veterinary Officer' (London: Ministry of Agriculture, Fisheries and Food, 1987), 13; J. W. Wilesmith et al., 'Bovine Spongiform Encephalopathy: Epidemiological Studies', *The Veterinary Record* 123(25) (December 1988): 638–44.
161. Miller, 'Risk, Science and Policy'; Phillips, Bridgeman and Ferguson-Smith, 'The Inquiry into BSE and Variant CJD in the United Kingdom'; Kiheung Kim, *The Social Construction of Disease: From Scrapie to Prion* (New York: Routledge, 2006).
162. Steere-Williams, 'Performing State Medicine during Its "Frustrating" Years'.

4

Badger and Pest Control Science

The discovery of tuberculous badgers in the early 1970s required Ministry for Agriculture, Fisheries and Food's (MAFF) animal health researchers, veterinarians and policymakers to rapidly form new working partnerships in and outside of government. As recounted in Chap. 2, the first of these were colleagues within MAFF—the scientists and field officers of the Infestation Control Division (ICD). ICD was responsible for researching and controlling pest animals and other organisms which destroyed crops and stored food, threatening agricultural productivity and what we now describe as 'food security'.[1] For these reasons, even though ICD officers were co-located with veterinarians in MAFF's regional offices, they were usually involved with arable rather than livestock farming. Like the State Veterinary Service (SVS), ICD comprised a partnership of scientists in centralised research facilities—the Pest Infestation Control Laboratory (PICL)—and field-based Pests Officers located across the country. ICD was responsible for coordinating government 'pest control'—killing or preventing animals like rodents, birds and insects from eating, contaminating or damaging crops and food supplies. Unlike MAFF's veterinarians, ICD already knew badgers: as designated government experts on awkward animals, it was their job to decide which were officially 'pests' and what to do about them. From the late 1950s, ICD had received a steady stream of complaint letters about 'badger trouble'. When ICD investigated these complaints, they often found them to be overstated, and learned that badgers were very difficult to remove, leading them to conclude that the animals should be left alone whenever possible. Therefore, when MAFF Veterinary Officer Roger Muirhead started finding tuberculous badgers in Gloucestershire, he immediately turned to his local counterparts in ICD for help. This initiated a contested but enduring partnership between the SVS and ICD. When MAFF launched their expanded bTB research programme in 1975, it was under the aegis of ICD that a new field station devoted to studying badger ecology and behaviour was established. The new group deployed state-of-the-art field biology techniques and collaborated extensively with colleagues outside of MAFF to find, follow and make sense of the traces left behind by badgers. Despite the ongoing upheavals of government reorganisation and privatisation, the field ecology group thrived, and still exists as part of the National Centre for Wildlife Management, within Defra's Animal and Plant Health Agency (APHA). The badger communities living in and around this site have now been involved with biological research (including intermittent TV appearances) for over forty years.

This chapter will tell the story of how badgers and 'pest control science' came to play surprisingly significant roles in the professionalisation of biology and natural history in Britain during the late twentieth century. It will explore how the work of ICD and PICL was bound up with key developments in field biology, disease ecology and animal welfare science at this time. As PICL scientists investigated whether and how to 'control' pest animals while minimising suffering, they developed cross-disciplinary collaborative networks, building new theoretical and empirical knowledge via applied problems such as crop damage and wildlife disease. As they engaged with badger/bTB, ICD scientists and officers drew upon prior knowledge as well as that of new partners in animal health, academia and conservation: in the process they formed a new epistemic community oriented around *disease ecology*.[2] Ideas about the 'cultures of care' that form as people work together will be used to help us understand the knowledge and working practices of these scientists, just as has already been done with animal health in Chap. 3.[3]

These ideas—of *good care* for humans and animals; of *good science*, which builds reliable knowledge via ethical research practices; and of *good choices* made under economic constraints—have been weighed against one another differently by the various actors involved in badger/bTB. Research on scientific care has investigated the emotional labour of caring for and with colleagues, as well as the continually negotiated necessities of care for human and animal research participants.[4] Scientists working with animals have often found it necessary to standardise and distance themselves from their research 'subjects', while also caring for and connecting with those self-same animals.[5] During the 1950s the newly emerging field of animal welfare science sought to understand this paradox and develop guidance for good ethical practice for other laboratory researchers. Along the way, they developed the idea that good care for animals constituted a core aspect of 'good science'.[6] While such research has often involved productive and harmonious collaborations between scientists and veterinarians, the overall cultures of care developed by each group do differ. While both prioritise minimising animal suffering over preserving life, for scientists the pursuit of knowledge is an end in itself, at times justifying the 'sacrifice' and suffering of animals in ways which would not be countenanced in other contexts.[7] In research involving clinical (human) medicine, veterinary practice and biomedical science, these contrasts are revealed as animal subjects find themselves occupying multiple, often contradictory roles, particularly as logics of care, suffering, death and knowledge are weighed up during working practice on a day-to-day basis.[8]

While the literature on scientific care has tended to focus on the work of laboratory scientists, field biologists have also faced similar dilemmas as they conduct their research about animals, plants and wider environments. The tensions between knowledge, care, life and costs play out differently as these biologists dealt with the additional ethical and logistical complexities of working with wild animals, in the far less controllable spaces of field science. This chapter will explore how the scientists of PICL helped develop new working practices and ethical 'best practice' for researching and controlling wild animals in farms, forests and beyond. By the time that government vets were making connections between badgers and bTB, ICD already had well-formed ideas about badgers; about the possibilities for controlling infectious diseases in wildlife; and about ethical practice in field biology, which immediately informed MAFF's decision-making. While the research collaboration between ICD and the SVS proved to be highly productive, over the course of the 1970s and 1980s the scientific and ethical worldviews of the two groups diverged. As the controversy entered its second decade, MAFF's ecologists helped to forge a new consensus amongst field biologists, conservationists, animal advocates and politicians across party lines. While those involved with badger/bTB knew a great deal more about the problem than they had in 1971, bTB rates in cattle were steadily climbing. This coalition of disease ecology scientists, badger protection advocates and sympathetic politicians argued that the problem needed to be investigated through a 'proper experiment' directly testing the effects of badger culling on bTB in cattle.

4.1 Ecological Science and the State

To understand ICD's approach to badger/bTB, we need to put them into the broader contexts of relations between the British state and the sciences of agriculture, animals and environments in the second half of the twentieth century. As we have already seen, veterinarians benefited from state concerns over the productivity of livestock farming, initially during the late nineteenth century, then in the interwar period when they took on scientific roles. Following the Second World War, these and broader agricultural productivity agendas were boosted by the creation of international organisations for improving human health, animal health and food supplies. Doctors, veterinarians and scientists from many disciplines benefited from knock-on effects at the national level, directly from increased research funding and indirectly via the creation of new policies designed to further these goals. Examples included the creation of new strains of plants and animals; the development of new technologies for planting, harvesting and processing crops; and the creation of new chemical fertilisers and pesticides.[9] Across the British countryside, food production, the work of farmers and the lives of plants, animals and people were utterly transformed as the agricultural system intensified and modernised. The UK state also became more involved in the protection and conservation of wildlife, landscapes and forests at this time, creating new policy and organisational and legal structures in the process.[10] The emergence of what environmental historian Matthew Kelly and colleagues have characterised as the post-war 'nature state' brought to the fore the idea that natural environments and wildlife were limited resources to be protected. It also generated new tensions between the state's interventionist role in conservation and its equally interventionist role in boosting agricultural production and the wider economy.[11] In Chap. 5 we will explore the intertwined worlds of governmental, non-governmental and public actors committed to protecting animals and the natural environment (including badgers). This chapter will focus instead on those scientists charged by government with investigating wildlife not to protect them, but instead to prevent them interfering with human activities and interests—the animals we call 'pests'.

Over the past two centuries, the life sciences have transformed themselves—from descriptive, 'natural history' practices of observing, collecting and classifying organisms (conducted by a wide range of people)—into today's theoretically driven and specialised biological sciences (mostly conducted by paid professionals).[12] As the sciences professionalised through the twentieth century, new laboratory-based biosciences such as genetics and molecular biology built up their reputations by contrasting themselves as modern and scientific against 'old-fashioned' natural history. Similarly, evolutionary biologists built their professional legitimacy by generating new theoretical insights—and contrasting this with the descriptive practices of natural history.[13] Field sciences such as animal behaviour, ecology and agricultural science have found it even more difficult to establish their legitimacy. Building reliable knowledge outside of the easily controlled conditions of the laboratory poses particular challenges, particularly for experimental design, and so field scientists have developed new methodological and statistical tools designed to help them establish cause and effect in the wider world.[14] While field scientists have adopted a plethora of new technologies, their work is still fundamentally bound up with older techniques of collection, observation and deep engagement with wildlife and landscape.[15] They can struggle to be regarded as fully 'scientific', with knock-on effects to their ability to gain funding. As such, relationships between 'professional' and 'lay' scientists have been more porous than in other areas of biology, with sites such as natural history museums creating essential spaces for interaction.[16] This porosity continues into the present day, where field biology is a richly productive site for citizen science and other forms of participatory research.[17]

These tensions have been particularly manifest in the history of ecology: 'the study of organisms in relation to their [changing] environment'.[18] Ecologists are interested in conserving stable ecological systems, but also in the dynamics of *change* in these systems, including the roles played by humans. As such, the influence of ecological thinking upon contemporary environmental politics and policy has been profound.[19] The history of ecology tells a broader story of under-resourced yet canny scientists conducting applied research which helped them further their own theoretical and disciplinary agendas. Ecologists have also gained state support for their research by appealing to more immediate anthropocentric interests such as political advantage, economic gain and state national interests. In the USA, this became apparent during the Cold War, when ecological research was supported by the need to better understand the impacts of nuclear fallout on humans, animals and environments, including a drive to improve surveillance technologies (satellites and radio tracking). In Canada, ecologists carved out roles in fisheries research, helping with the recovery of collapsed populations following overfishing.[20] Ecologists interested in relationships between pathogens and their hosts found congenial homes working in public health, tropical medicine and parasitology—an important space for collaborating with doctors and veterinarians.[21] Ecologists have been able to provide governments with this kind of 'useful knowledge' in part because of their ability to build reliable knowledge in the wider world: in turn governments have provided resources and professional legitimacy.[22] Through the twentieth century ecologists have been involved with the constitution of the 'nature state', but also, when it suited them, the 'warfare state',[23] while in the UK the 'agricultural state' has also been central to the development of the discipline.[24] We will now explore how, as part of this agenda, British ecologists have benefited from state interactions with awkward animals (pests) in general and badgers in particular.

4.2 MAFF's Ecologists: Pest (Infestation) Control Laboratories

The mutual constitution of British ecology and policy has its roots in the 1920s, when plant ecologist Arthur Tansley convinced government that field biologists could contribute to national productivity via improving scientific understandings of forestry and agriculture.[25] While these connections with plant ecologists have been extensively investigated, the mammal ecologist Charles Elton was also a key player. Elton combined ideas from zoology, evolutionary biology, epidemiology, plant ecology and mathematics to create new insights into mammal populations, establishing the Bureau of Animal Population at Oxford University in 1932. Elton's group was the source of many foundational concepts in modern ecological science, including the term 'ecosystem'; the niche concept (the role that an organism occupies within an ecosystem) and the idea of 'invasive species'.[26] From the start, Elton gained funding for his research group by applying their ideas to practical problems such as game management, forestry and pest control, while elaborating and building empirical support for their theoretical ideas. During the Second World War the Bureau supported the war effort by focusing on questions of controlling mammal pests—principally rats, mice and rabbits—and preventing damage to food supplies, successfully lobbying government for funding. In 1939 the government established two in-house research laboratories devoted to the problems of pest control. The Pest Infestation Laboratory (PIL) in Slough, founded by a group of entomologists, agricultural scientists and plant ecologists at Imperial College London specialised in invertebrate and fungal infestations of crops and food supplies: following the war PIL was run by the Agricultural Research Council (ARC).[27] The Infestation Control Laboratory (ICL) specialised in pest control of rodents and other vertebrates: following the war ICL was taken into MAFF and was initially co-located with the SVS on the outskirts of London. As with animal health, government interest in pest control extended across research and policy: to this end they also established a Directorate of Infestation Control in 1943, employing a regional network of field officers.[28]

MAFF soon consolidated pest control research and policy into a single Infestation Control Division (ICD). New legislation supported this agenda, with Parliament passing the Agriculture Act (1947) and the Prevention of Damage by Pests Act (1949), creating a legal framework making it not just allowable but compulsory for landowners to take action against certain species.[29] Following the war Charles Elton's research group returned its attention to fundamental ecological research, passing on their responsibilities for pest control research to MAFF's ICL. As part of this transition, Harry V. Thompson, one of Elton's postdocs, was recruited by MAFF.[30] While he was initially engaged as one of many scientific officers at ICL, Thompson soon established his own research group continuing the Bureau's wartime work.[31] By 1959, the group had grown and diverged into specialist 'Rodent Research' and 'Land Pests and Birds' departments: the latter was relocated to a new field station further out of London.[32] Like the SVS, ICD was deeply affected by successive waves of government institutional change and restructuring, initially associated with the 1971 Rothschild report (as described in Chap. 3). Given that concerns had already been raised about the responsiveness of government research to the needs of policy and business, as well as over duplication of activities,[33] ICL and PIL were an obvious target for consolidation. It was decided to transfer most of PIL's 'applied' research on invertebrate pests from ARC into MAFF, merging it with ICL to create a new Pest Infestation Control Laboratory (PICL).[34] During the 1970s PICL was moved into a new umbrella organisation—the Agricultural Development and Advisory Service (ADAS), which would oversee the SVS and bring the rest of MAFF's non-veterinary researchers into a single Agricultural Science Service.[35] The importance of PICL at the time is indicated by the public information booklet in Fig. 4.1, which summarised its status and

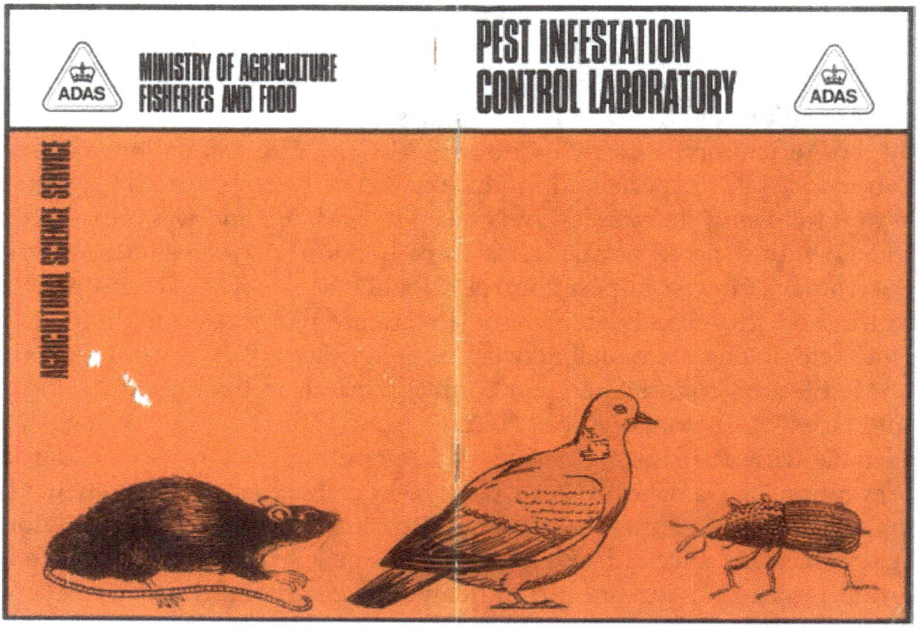

Fig. 4.1 PICL public information leaflet. Source: Pest Infestation Control Laboratories (1975)[37]

role as a government research institute, alongside peers such as the Central Veterinary Laboratory (CVL) and the National Institute of Agricultural Botany (NIAB).[36]

By the early 1970s, PICL comprised five research departments (Biology; Chemistry; Insecticides and Storage; Land Pests and Birds; and Rodents). It produced biennial reports for MAFF detailing all their research, policy and collaborative activities, including a list of journal publications.[38] Like the SVS, ICD's work was built upon strong partnerships between laboratory scientists and field officers, described as follows: 'they play an important part in identifying problems and in the application of research results, as well as by taking part in some of the Laboratory's research projects'.[39] Unlike the SVS, which persisted as a distinctly veterinary body until well into the 2000s, ICD underwent further rounds of reorganisation, during which it lost its institutional identity. The various departments of PICL were further merged into the Agricultural Science Service, and the reports became shorter, focusing on concrete, applicable research findings, without referencing journal publications.[40] While the research continued, ICD disappeared from MAFF records and field-based pest control services appear to have been privatised during the early 1980s. In 1987, the various laboratories and institutes of the Agricultural Science Service (now *sans* the veterinarians) were rebranded as the Central Science Laboratory (CSL).[41] These processes of institutional reorganisation and privatisation have continued: in 2009, CSL was merged with plant health and food research to form the Food and Environment Research Agency (FERA). In 2014, some parts of FERA were privatised, while the rest was merged back into veterinary services and animal health policy to create the APHA.

Thompson's 'Land Pests' group (formally established in 1959) was responsible for dealing with all non-rodent awkward mammal and bird species. This agenda was deeply entangled with another of Elton's core interests: the problem of invasive species. Policy decisions about what should be done to control which animals were largely contingent upon economic circumstance, often in combination with the strength of public feeling.[42] However, policy was also formed using PICL's expert advice: in the case of animals like rats and mice this was on how best to control them, but for other species this was on whether to take any action at all. Researchers assessed the damage the animals in question were causing, to human assets (e.g. crops), but also to ecosystems and landscapes. In the 1930s, when Elton made the case to government for applied ecological research, he had also convinced them that animals introduced from other countries were highly likely to be pests, leading to new legislation and early state attempts at eradicating muskrats.[43] Elton's case was based upon the argument that rats, mice and rabbits posed particularly severe threats to the national food supply because they were from other countries and were out of balance with the 'native' ecology of Britain. While Elton later popularised invasion biology to great effect, MAFF's scientists and field officers quietly got on with applying it in agricultural policy.[44] Between the 1930s and the 1990s, MAFF's ecologists directed many eradication campaigns, although only two—the muskrats and a later, long-term campaign to remove coypu (large aquatic rodents)—were successful.[45] The scientists also researched the ecology and behaviour of a wider menagerie of introduced species, including rabbits, hamsters, porcupines and deer.[46] ICD's expertise in lab and field placed them as key arbiters in whether the UK state officially classified an animal as a 'pest'—a decision with serious consequences for the animals in question.

In 1953, an international epidemic of myxomatosis (a highly infectious, painful and lethal viral disease of rabbits) reached the UK. The history of myxomatosis in Britain demonstrates ICD's multiple roles as policy adviser, participant in international research networks and arbiter of wildlife–human relations in British society. It would also profoundly shape many of the decisions MAFF would take when responding to tuberculous badgers twenty years later. Contrary to popular belief, Ministry officials did not introduce myxomatosis to Britain on purpose, even making an initial, unsuccessful attempt at containing the outbreak. Harry Thompson, 'MAFF's rabbit specialist' was one of the first government officials on the scene when reports of rabbits dying in Kent appeared.[47] While some saw myxomatosis as a convenient way of getting rid of a damaging pest, the unsightly and clearly painful symptoms also led to widespread concerns about the animals' suffering and demands for disease control for 'humanitarian' reasons.[48] In Australia the virus had been deliberately introduced—as a method of pest control, in a country where invasive rabbits were causing acute environmental and agricultural damage. This created an ideal opportunity for scientists there, including Francis Ratcliffe (another alumni of Elton's Bureau) and the virologist Frank Fenner, to study the ecology of pathogens in the wider environment. The Australian scientists found that, despite their intention to wield the pathogen as a biological weapon, the myxoma virus and rabbits had other ideas, adapting to each other's presence and creating less lethal versions of the disease. Myxomatosis in Australia was furthering scientific understandings of the co-evolution of viruses with their hosts, building careers in disease ecology, and contributing to broader cultural narratives of infectious disease and biological warfare in the Cold War era.[49]

In Britain, the arrival of myxomatosis was also seen by scientists as 'an extraordinary opportunity for fundamental ecological research'—academics with relevant interests rapidly obtained government funding, while MAFF further invested in ICD.[50] Scientists investigated the ecology and behaviour of rabbits, transmission, effects upon agriculture and landscapes, and methods for 'rabbit control'. Frank Fenner visited the UK and met with MAFF's scientists, creating a long-standing international collaboration.[51] Thompson and his colleagues rapidly concluded that it would not be possible to contain the spread of myxomatosis and argued that the consequent decimation of rabbits would be good for agriculture, meriting further research. Responding to public concerns over animal welfare, they presented a simple, standardised technique for killing infected rabbits—'gassing' them underground via the application of a new product called 'Cymag' (sodium cyanide powder, which generates hydrogen cyanide gas on contact with moisture in the air).[52] This made it possible for MAFF to fashion a policy acceptable to all sides of the debate. A 'Myxomatosis Advisory Committee' was appointed (comprising key experts and organisations), which consulted with all interests involved in the rabbit debate. The Committee concluded that myxomatosis could not be 'stamped out' and should instead be left to run its course. They recommended a policy of 'mopping up': culling surviving rabbits, further reducing their numbers and thereby addressing the pest problem.[53] Government acted swiftly, passing a second 'Pests Act' in 1954, creating legal requirements for landowners to cull rabbits and providing subsidies for gassing equipment to do so. While a resulting network of 'rabbit clearance societies' was established with enthusiasm, ultimately neither rabbits nor myxoma were eradicated.

Myxomatosis created further resources and legitimacy for ICL's research at a time when post-war productivity agendas were losing their immediate urgency. It advanced Harry Thompson's career, expanding his department within MAFF and making his scientific reputation—the group published a series of several high-profile journal articles about myxomatosis[54] and two major monographs on the ecology and behaviour of rabbits.[55] As Thompson's career blossomed, he worked with British mammal biologists to form the Mammal Society of the British Isles, still an important meeting space for professional and 'amateur' field biologists. The founder members included Thompson, Harry Southern (also of Elton's group at Oxford), ex-ICL colleague Peter Crowcroft, toxicologist Alistair Worden and badger naturalist Ernest Neal.[56] This foundational group links PICL directly into British networks of mammal ecology and natural history. It also reveals a more unexpected connection—with the Universities Federation for Animal Welfare (UFAW), a science-based campaign group. As well as being an enthusiastic naturalist, Alistair Worden was a significant figure in laboratory animal research. He founded the Huntingdon Research Centre (now Huntington Life Sciences) in Cambridge and was editor of the first edition of UFAW's highly influential *Handbook*, providing guidance for ethical research practice in animal research.[57] While UFAW are best known for their work with laboratory scientists, they were also involved with farm animal welfare and pest control from early in their existence.[58] Between them, myxomatosis and the founding of the Mammal Society made the connections between ecology, ethology, natural history and the new science of animal welfare directly traceable, if not more widely understood.[59]

The rapid presentation of Cymag as a policy solution for myxomatosis was made possible due to a longer collaborative history dating back to the 1920s, when debates over the social role of the rabbit in Britain (whether they should be regarded as an affordable source of food and fur or a serious agricultural pest) had come to the fore. Animal protection campaigners had argued that the 'gin trap' (a spring-loaded trap which catches an animal's leg in steel jaws)—widely used on rabbits—was cruel and campaigned for the devices to be made illegal.[60] Between the 1920s and the 1950s campaigners made several unsuccessful attempts to restrict the use of gin traps, and while they were abandoned by many during the war years, it was not until 1954 that the devices were finally outlawed.[61] During the 1930s UFAW funded a collaboration between scientists in ICL, at Oxford University and in the chemical industry to research alternatives to the gin trap. Building on broader developments in research on using cyanide compounds in mining, pest control and chemical weapons, they developed and tested new technologies for poisoning mammals underground.[62] This included Cymag, which killed rabbits quickly with minimal suffering. For animal welfare agendas this was the primary criteria for 'humane' methods of killing, meaning that UFAW and the RSPCA put the broader political context to one side and rapidly approved and recommended the new product to government.[63] Responding to wider debates about wildlife welfare and the politics of hunting, the Home Office appointed a committee in 1949 (chaired by barrister John Scott Henderson) to enquire into 'Cruelty to Wild Animals'. The group drew upon UFAW's research evidence to condemn the use of gin traps and concluded that Cymag was the most 'humanitarian' technique for controlling underground pests.[64] UFAW's broader strategy for improving animal welfare across laboratory, farm and wildlife contexts involved working in and with social and policy structures enacting human–animal relations, rather than challenging them from the outside. When engaging debates over rabbits and myxomatosis, they effectively used agricultural productivity agendas to make a case for 'humane' rabbit control. Together UFAW and ICL facilitated collaborative research exchanges which created new knowledge, built scientific careers and brokered policy solutions which were widely acceptable while also furthering the agenda of outlawing the gin trap.

The connections between UFAW, ICL and Elton's Bureau preceded even these collaborations. Before joining MAFF or Elton's group, as an undergraduate student at University College London, Harry Thompson had been mentored by Charles Hume, the founder of UFAW. Animal welfare was a lifelong commitment for Thompson: following the rabbit research at Oxford, he joined UFAW's scientific advisory group in 1947 and was a member of UFAW Council during the 1960s and again in the 1980s. After his retirement from MAFF, Thompson took up the position of President of UFAW from 1986 to 1996, continuing as President Emeritus until his death in 2004.[65] In this role, Thompson wrote of the 'moral obligation and human responsibility towards animals; not only those species which have been bred and reared to be of service to man, but also those which have been affected by man's environmental modifications'.[66] In his view, people should be morally committed to improving and taking responsibility for animal welfare precisely *because of* humanity's power over non-human animals and the natural world—just as when farmers talk of 'stewardship' care.[67] This is typical of the culture of care that developed out of—and in turn drove—ICD and UFAW's approach to pest control research and policy from the post-war years onwards. This culture was fundamentally anthropocentric and deeply pragmatic, but as the other lives of many of these scientists (as natural history 'enthusiasts') suggests, was also aesthetically and morally committed to improving the lives of non-humans for their own sake.

4.3 Defining and Redefining the Badger

In the National Archives, there is a folder entitled *Badgers—proposals for control* (MAF 131/70), dated 1959–1967, but including data going back to 1948. This folder is one of several created by ICD to keep records of exchanges between PICL's scientists, regional Pests Officers, colleagues in other ministries and members of the public—all about badgers. As we have seen, while the primary purpose of ICD was to further agricultural productivity by improving pest control, this made them arbiters of which animals should—and should not—be classified as 'pests'. To this end, after the war MAFF published two lavishly illustrated public information booklets, *Wild Birds and the Land* and *Wild Mammals and the Land*, through which they tried to convey to public audiences which creatures the Ministry considered to be 'harmful' and which were 'beneficial' to agriculture.[68] The latter volume declared the badger to be beneficial, highlighting its role in 'destroying pests of various kinds' and condemned the 'unjust persecution that had been its lot for centuries'.[69] This view would have been informed by the scientists of ICD, as can be seen in their badger files, consisting of internal and external debates over the behaviour of badgers and what (if anything) government should do about it. From the late 1950s, ICD recorded reports of 'damage by badgers', often following public complaints. These included accounts of badgers damaging grain and vegetable crops; predating poultry, piglets and even lambs; undermining riverbanks and breaking down fencing.[70] Upon investigation, ICD officers often found that that such cases were overstated, or implicated other animals such as foxes. Given this information, the fact that badgers were native to the UK, and that they were in the habit of hunting rabbits (a key invasive target), ICD scientists decided that that badgers should not be regarded as pests.[71] They did acknowledge that in exceptional cases so-called 'rogue' badgers could cause problems: this was a commonly held view amongst field biologists. The 'old rogue badger' was described by R. J. King of the Forestry Commission as follows: 'an old badger, usually an old boar, turned out of his sett by young pairing cubs, may become a rogue and may make many enemies among neighbouring poultry and sheep farmers'.[72] Under these circumstances, ICL scientists explored what action should be taken, particularly once it emerged that some regional Pests Officers were using Cymag on badgers even though this was illegal.[73] Options including the use of strong-smelling repellents and using excavators to remove entire setts were explored, but found to be either ineffective or laborious and expensive. The alternatives were not promising: 'digging out and killing by violence—usually impracticable; snaring—legal but cruel; shooting on emergence from the set—required much patience and is complicated by dusk or darkness'.[74] By the late 1960s, ICD had settled upon the last of these options, based upon the assumptions that the law could not be changed, and shooting would only need to be deployed under the exceptional circumstances of a 'rogue' animal.[75] In general, ICD's advice was to leave badgers alone, emphasising the positive attributes of the animals: they reminded members of the public that gassing was illegal.

Policy scholar Wyn Grant has argued that MAFF officers held this 'benevolent view' of badgers partly because of a lack of knowledge, but also because of British cultural constructions of the creatures as 'a cherished species endowed with elements of magic and mystery'.[76] While ICD scientists were well aware that relatively little was known about badgers—hence their frequent requests for detailed information from field officers—a close examination of their correspondence reveals their motivations to be more complex and pragmatic than simple sentimentality. It was during the 1960s that badgers became, in the words of environmental historian Robert Lambert, 'a mammal of interest',[77] not only to ICD, but also to animal protection campaigners, mass media and, judging by the increasing volume of reports and letters in the ICD files, to landowners, farmers and other members of the public. By the mid-1960s, the Home Office was consulting with ICD in response to burgeoning badger protection campaigns. As we will explore in the next chapter, this decade saw the reopening and further renegotiation of the long history of conflict in Britain between humans about badgers as well as between humans and badgers. As such, the adoption of the 'old rogue badger' by ICD officers (and a consequently limited control policy) can also be understood as an elegant way of steering a relatively neutral policy course between increasingly visible pro- and anti-badger interests. The idea of the 'rogue' animal had been applied to many other wild animals, so would have had broader currency with conservationists and wider publics.[78]

By the time that tuberculous badgers were documented in the early 1970s, ICD already had considerable and much-needed expertise—in disease ecology, from dealing with myxomatosis—and from negotiating Britain's long-standing but newly reignited badger debate. They appear to have initially experienced the rapidly unfolding bTB situation as an extension of routine pest control work with the animals—the news from Gloucestershire is filed amongst complaint letters about badger damage, which continued throughout the 1970s and beyond.[79] Some members of the public clearly also interpreted the news in these terms, as seen in the following letter to ICD from a resident of Dursley, Gloucestershire—within a few miles of the first tuberculous badger.

> I'm usually very fond of animals, but not badgers. So destructive, waste of time to plants, real loss. So if you can come & fish them out [unclear]—TB. I hope which is serious as you say for Cattle. We are in a farming district—cattle, sheep, pigs, etc. Thinking you can do something soon to ease our anxiety.[80]

All this would have contributed to ICD's initially sceptical reaction to the news from their veterinary colleagues, even though they were then persuaded. PICL's overall approach to bTB was fundamentally shaped by their past experiences—of the badger debate, of myxomatosis and of creating caring practices for working with wildlife.

Woodchester Park. In 1975 MAFF launched their new approach to badger/bTB, comprising a state-led culling policy, a new Consultative Panel including all parties in policy processes, and a major research programme involving both the SVS and ICD. PICL's report of 1974–1976 gives an excellent insight into the institution's perspective on the events recounted in Chap. 2:

> The badger, which has often been the subject of persecution, is a popular member of our wild fauna and it was unfortunate when, in 1971, it was shown to harbour bovine tuberculosis ... Although some naturalists have cast doubt on the findings and have possibly quite reasonably suggested that there may be other associations, the evidence is convincing and the Laboratory has co-operated with the Ministry's Veterinary Services in undertaking control measures. This has required the inauguration of a new research programme, and importantly there has been a need for the establishment of good public relations. All the work done so far has been in the Ministry's South Western region and the brunt of this activity has fallen on the Regional Pests Officer, RJ Clark and the Chief Regional Officer, K Harrison Jones, who have greatly helped beyond the Laboratory. It is impossible also to over-estimate the contribution to good public relations made by HV Thompson, the late Charles Armour and CA Swan, to none of whom had badger control been a particularly welcome occupation.[81]

Despite this ambivalence, PICL benefited from MAFF's interest in badgers, as well as more widely from the increased resources directed into agricultural research following the Rothschild report.[82] This had resulted in the recruitment or promotion of SVS staff: mostly researchers with some experience but who had not yet made their names, including specialists in wildlife pathology (Gallagher), veterinary epidemiology (Wilesmith) and field epidemiology (Sainsbury). There was a parallel expansion in ICD, including the recruitment of field officers to implement the culls, and researchers who could devote their whole attention to badgers. Thompson and his allies in the Nature Conservation Council (NCC) had lobbied for the recruitment of Hans Kruuk, a badger ecologist then working for NCC's Institute of Terrestrial Ecology.[83] While this effort was not successful, Kruuk's field assistant Peter Mallinson was persuaded to join MAFF, to work with Chris Cheeseman, a PICL researcher who had just received his doctorate for studies of mammal plague in Uganda and a small group of assistants. Initially engaged on a three-year contract, the new PICL field team immediately started studying the badger 'clearance trials' in Thornbury and elsewhere, while looking for a field study site in the South West.

Given PICL's involvement with international research networks and Harry Thompson's own links with UFAW and the Mammal Society, MAFF's immediate enrolment of schoolteacher Ernest Neal—recounted in Chap. 2—makes much more sense. Neal was a co-founder of the Mammal Society and by 1971 was known as the UK national expert on badgers—an animal which, unlike birds, primates, big cats or rodents, had received relatively little attention from professional biologists. Following his contributions to MAFF's investigations into bTB, Neal served on the Ministry's Badger Consultative Panel for fifteen years, acting as a key 'knowledge broker' connecting policy, agricultural science, field biology, conservation and badger protection.[84] While Neal and Thompson were by this time fully established experts of some renown, the young field biologists recruited by MAFF were coming into a discipline being transformed by technological and theoretical changes. The period between the 1950s and 1980s saw huge advances in the abilities of scientists to observe, theorise and understand wild animals in the field. These included developments in photography, film-making, tracking and computing technologies;[85] the adoption of mathematical modelling; theoretical developments such as sociobiology and behavioural ecology; improved understandings of animals' own motivations, and changes in field research practice.[86] By the early 1970s, PICL's research had already contributed to these developments, particularly in population biology, pest control science and disease ecology, but more was on the way. PICL's new badger ecology research team was forming at an exciting time.

After a short search, the new group settled upon a field site near Woodchester Park—an abandoned Victorian mansion-folly in Gloucestershire—to conduct their new studies of badger ecology and behaviour. A field studies centre had been run at Woodchester by science teachers Miriam and Roger Kelly since the 1950s, making it a well-established site for doing field biology research.[87] The Kellys' local knowledge, resources and connections with field biology were instrumental to the quick and successful establishment of the new MAFF station:

> He [Kelly] was the perfect person really to sort of liaise with. And when I said what we were doing, he was firstly very suspicious of me, of you know somebody from the government. When he saw I was bona fide and had no axe to grind and no sort of preconceived ideas, just wanted a place where I

> could quietly get on with the job, he got really very enthusiastic and really helpful, very co-operative. And in fact, wanted us to go there. He said 'A lot of universities come here, we do field courses, you could have students attached to your projects and you know collaborate with them.' He was right, it was perfect in that respect.[88]

Drawing on this local knowledge, MAFF researchers immediately started following and observing the resident badgers and mapping their territories in what PICL reports described as 'a typical Cotswold valley', with the mansion in the centre, surrounded by steeply wooded hillsides.[89] The core study area ran around the edge of the valley, covering about 11 km^2 and involved around twenty-five social groups—an unusually high density (see Figs. 4.2 and 4.3). The site is more or less unchanged, meaning

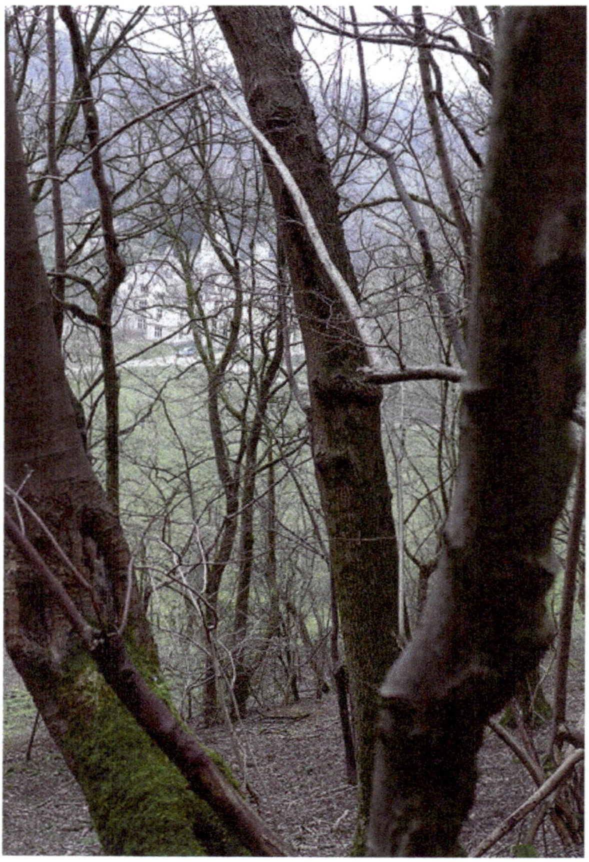

Fig. 4.2 Woodchester Mansion, viewed from the side of the valley (photo—author's own)

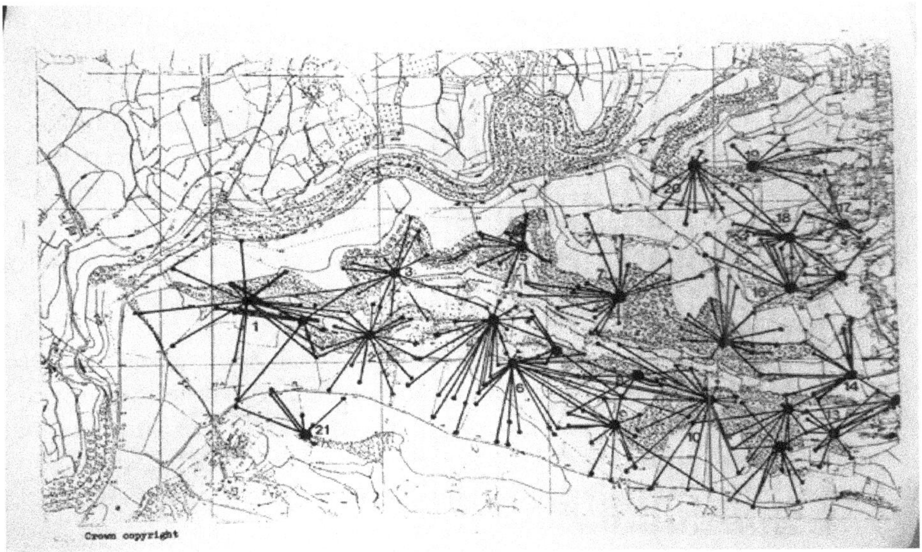

Fig. 4.3 Mapping badger communities. Source: MAFF (1977, appendix 7)

that the badgers of Woodchester have now been continually involved with scientific research for over forty years.[90]

Initially the group were based in a caravan parked down by the mansion, before moving into a nearby site which eventually acquired its own permanent offices, laboratories and veterinary clinical facilities. To follow badgers more effectively, the scientists initially focused on the practicalities of working with a large, strong, nocturnal and notoriously elusive wild animal in the field. The PICL scientists worked with UFAW and their veterinary counterparts in the SVS to find the best anaesthetics for badgers and explored how to effectively restrain and catch the animals using hand nets and snares. They also adapted an earlier design—developed by UFAW member and badger campaigner Ruth Murray—to create a cage-trap for use in the field.[91] The trap was tested by UFAW in 1974, and while it was considered to be impractical for policy, it was used by researchers to catch and release the animals without harming them.[92] Much of this work was done in partnership with veterinarian John Gallagher and the SVS officers in Gloucestershire, who provided expertise and resources for conducting clinical diagnoses, sampling and post-mortems, as well as the laboratory skills and resources to culture and identify *M. bovis* from the badger traces taken from animals in the field.[93] Elsewhere in the South West,

PICL continued collaborating with SVS on the badger clearance trials, at one point excavating and mapping an entire badger sett. Even equipped with the newly legalised tool of gassing, it proved to be hard work to fully remove badgers: one sett in Thornbury had to be gassed and blocked nineteen times during a single year, while the extensive use of repellents such as creosote failed to prevent new animals from reopening others.[94] Badgers' resistance to human attempts to get rid of them, and their tendency to move around and recolonise emptied setts would have already been familiar to ICD officers.[95] Given these difficulties, field tests were conducted on the dispersal of cyanide into badger setts. While the researchers found that Cymag was working and all the animals in these tests were killed, concentrations of cyanide in the furthest 'blind tunnels' were low. They therefore recommended the reapplication of 'larger quantities' of Cymag powder in difficult cases.[96] The clearance trials and routine culls involved surveying 'the locations of infected badgers and cattle and positions of sets and other badger traces', adding to a growing body of data informing the work of PICL and SVS scientists alike.[97]

The PICL scientists at Woodchester concentrated on researching the 'range size, movement, and population density of badgers in connection with their role in the transmission of tuberculosis to cattle'.[98] They surveyed the area, adopting new field biology techniques to observe and understand the badger communities they encountered. They also drew upon, collaborated with and contributed to networks of British mammologists, starting with the vital experience Mallinson had brought from his earlier fieldwork with Hans Kruuk. Kruuk was another member of Oxford field biology networks, having trained with Niko Tinbergen during the 1960s, making his name researching hyenas.[99] Kruuk had already started studying badgers in Wytham Woods (also the site of Elton's fieldwork), investigating how food density affected badger behaviour. A second Oxford biologist, David Macdonald, collaborated with the Woodchester researchers on adapting newly available 'telemetry' (remote data collection) equipment, making it possible to follow animal movements more precisely than ever before.[100] Finally, MAFF scientists worked with Stephen Harris, a lecturer at the University of Bristol, on further field techniques.[101] This collaboration continued into the 1980s, as Harris took over the Mammal Society's National Badger Survey from Ernest Neal, eventually replacing him on MAFF's Consultative Panel.[102] The PICL researchers adapted Kruuk's technique of 'bait-marking' (mixing coloured plastic pellets into food, which is then distributed across a group's territory as the animals eventually excrete it), which was deployed to map the badger social groups on the site. This was combined with telemetry: the PICL scientists designed and built their own radio tracking equipment suitable for use with recalcitrant badgers.[103] These techniques were combined with tagging and close field observations to produce intricate maps of the Woodchester badgers' territories, enabling comparisons to be made over time, space and species (see Fig. 4.3).

It was not long after establishing the Woodchester field station that the spreading problem of *M. bovis* became dramatically apparent via the traces it left on the bodies and behaviour of local badgers. In May 1977, a BBC Natural History Unit outside broadcast team visited the site to film *Badger Watch*, a pioneering programme in which the animals were filmed at night and broadcast 'live' to the nation, with expert commentary from MAFF researchers and external naturalists including Ernest Neal.[104] While the broadcast programme showed badgers pottering about their home range and peacefully feeding, behind the scenes a much darker drama was unfolding, as the following internal memo recounts:

> On 6th May a badger died at one of the entrances to the beech-tree set upon which the television series was centred. Although this occurred 3 days before the first of the transmissions the BBC staff were in fact on the site for about 2 weeks before and knew of the finding of this carcase. The occurrence was filmed by the BBC.

A second animal died the following week, and soon after the film crew left the whole social group was 'eliminated' by ICD officers using cage-trapping.[105] The Consultative Panel was immediately notified, and the developments were discussed at their next meeting. While MAFF did discuss the *Badger Watch* deaths in their next annual 'TB in Badgers' report, the footage was never broadcast, apparently by the mutual consent of all parties.[106]

Given the mass audience of *Badger Watch* and its subsequent role as a minor milestone in wildlife film history, it is tempting to speculate what impact the film of sick and dead wild badgers might have had on wider public debates. The deaths brought a new immediacy to the Woodchester group's research, particularly as more animals were found suffering from advanced TB that summer: over the following eight years the researchers estimated that approximately 10% of badger deaths in the area were due to *M. bovis* infection.[107] The researchers followed and observed several other infected badgers, finding their movements to be erratic, more wide ranging and encroaching more on farmed space than healthy animals. It looked rather like the 'old rogue badger' of the 1950s might turn out to be tuberculous.[108] These events provided a further opportunity to study a long-standing problem in badger control: the tendency of the animals to 'recolonise' emptied setts.[109] Scientists in and outside of MAFF had recognised this phenomenon from early on, with wildlife and farming groups also expressing concerns that uninfected badgers moving into 'contaminated' setts cleared by culling could spread disease.[110] When the arrival of *M. bovis* became known locally, the PICL research was supported by their nearest farming neighbour, even when his own cattle became infected. Despite this, SVS staff argued that all the badgers in the area should be culled—effectively ending the field ecology research at Woodchester. Therefore MAFF conducted an internal review of PICL's badger research programme.[111] Harry Thompson defended the work, arguing that MAFF would

> lose the advantage of over four years' work in identifying and understanding the resident badgers. To propose a move could also underestimate the very real problems of finding another site where the work would meet with an equivalent degree of understanding and security.[112]

This latter point was particularly important, as by this time MAFF was facing widespread criticism for its culling policy and even the clearances at Woodchester had been beset by 'interference' from members of the public destroying traps and snares.[113]

Consolidating Field Ecology in MAFF. As discussed in Chap. 3, instead of calming the growing criticisms of MAFF's culling policy as anticipated, the Zuckerman report opened up a wider public controversy over badger/bTB in the early 1980s. The harshest scientific critiques of the report's conclusions had come from the Mammal Society and academic biologists and ecologists, including Kruuk, Macdonald and Harris. Given Zuckerman's long-standing negative opinions of field biology, his dismissal of their submitted evidence and the ensuing hostile public, dispute between Zuckerman and the ecologists makes more sense.[114] Despite this, Zuckerman spoke highly of the Woodchester scientists and supported PICL's badger research, recommending the expansion of the work in his report. He appears to have been unaware of (or unwilling to acknowledge) the deep interpenetration of professional field biology with 'natural history'; the theoretical and practical connections between field ecology, epidemiology and animal welfare that had been forged by myxomatosis; or the developing collaborations between PICL and academics like Harris. It seems that Zuckerman had not only missed a 'sea-change' in science–society relationships (as evidenced by his surprise at the public controversy), but also within his own discipline of zoology.[115]

Zuckerman's support helped PICL win the internal MAFF debate over Woodchester, keeping the field stations open. Following this triumph Thompson laid out an ambitious new research agenda. This was fourfold: continuation of the long-term field research at Woodchester; joint SVS/PICL studies of the epidemiology of bTB in badgers; development of a test for the disease in living badgers; and finally, an experimental study. Thompson argued that 'it is necessary to compare "undisturbed" areas (where TB infected badgers are not killed) with "disturbed" areas (where infected badgers are killed, i.e. the general statutory control areas)'. He also proposed two rounds of comparison: between Woodchester and the surrounding area; and between new 'undisturbed' and full clearance areas in Cornwall. In effect, Thompson was arguing that MAFF's culling policies be suspended in places, to create experimental 'controls' against which these interventions could be compared.[116] While the first three research proposals were approved by MAFF, the idea of 'undisturbed' comparison areas was vehemently opposed by SVS officers (citing the concerns of farmers) and was quietly dropped.[117] The 1982 finding that badgers were unusually resistant to cyanide poisoning further reinforced the utility of PICL's research for MAFF. While the Porton Down scientists had argued that MAFF's policy of gassing badgers was 'inhumane', policymakers urgently sought the opinion of PICL's scientists before deciding what to do. PICL scientists were summoned to Porton to confidentially view a recorded film of the cyanide experiments:

> … the gas was sort of introduced and they started to get really agitated. And then they really got upset, really distressed, you could see that they were distressed, they were retching and vomiting and actually kekkering with a call that I recognised as a distress call … I just said [to MAFF superiors]: 'All of those assurances that you have given … about the humaneness of gassing have just gone out the window.'[118]

It was following this consultation that the decision was made to suspend gassing, whereupon PICL's earlier explorations of how to catch and kill badgers came into their own, enabling a rapid mobilisation of the alternative technology of cage-trapping. A new procedure was developed involving setting traps (checking them regularly to prevent undue stress and suffering), then dispatching trapped badgers quickly with a shot to the head. This was codified by MAFF in a *Badger Control Manual* by 1983 and remains a standard procedure for Defra today.[119] These developments once more underlined the importance of PICL's field ecologists to MAFF and secured the future of the Woodchester research programme.

As we have already seen, the PICL/SVS collaborative research on badger/bTB epidemiology was highly productive, giving rise to a string of joint publications.[120] While it took a lot of work to remove badgers from a 'clearance trial' area such as Thornburgh and keep them out, the effort appeared to be paying off. BTB incidence in cattle was dropping in these areas, particularly when compared to ad hoc 'fire brigade' culling, and SVS argued that these interventions were proving to be successful.[121] Unlike Thompson's fourth proposal, the removal trials started as policy interventions: as such, comparisons were made after the fact, meaning that other, uncontrolled factors may have affected the outcomes. In line with traditions of human public health research, where direct experiments (e.g. testing the effects of smoking) would not be considered, MAFF's veterinarians argued that suspending bTB controls would be similarly unethical and unacceptable to farmers, whose cooperation was essential. Instead, they took the view that associations between their interventions and drops in bTB could be established statistically, as is long-standing practice in much epidemiological research. Despite these disciplinary differences, the findings were used by a group of theoretical ecologists—members of the 'Silwood Circle' of Imperial College London—working on new mathematical models of relationships between pathogens, hosts and methods of disease control.[122] This body of work had already led modellers and field biologists to argue that in the case of rabies (which also transmits between humans, wild and domestic animals) vaccination was more effective than culling. Core to this argument was the idea that culling disrupts the social and territorial systems of wild animals, creating unstable populations that move around more and potentially spread disease.[123] The modelling of bTB suggested similar dynamics might be at work, and that (as seen in the clearance trials), badger culling would have to be systematically and repeatedly applied for a long time to have much effect.

The badger field research continued through the 1980s and 1990s, further benefiting from the 1986 Dunnet review and becoming increasingly sophisticated as the group grew and developed new skills—particularly in clinical veterinary procedures such as anaesthesia and taking biological samples. Woodchester became the centre of a wide research network, involving veterinary epidemiology, ecology, mathematical modelling, field biology and newer biomedical technologies such as DNA analysis. In the late 1980s and early 1990s MAFF's pest control researchers became part of a new government 'executive agency' of the CSL.[124] Despite ongoing reorganisations and semi-privatisation of government research, the Woodchester group flourished, as their connections with university scientists enabled them to participate in co-supervision and research proposals, bringing them income from sources beyond MAFF. While the modelling suggested that MAFF's traditional approach to 'stamping out' disease might not work so well when wildlife was involved, the empirical evidence was drawn from observations, statistical correlations, single interventions such as the clearance trials, and veterinary field experience. A consensus was forming across the ecologists and their allies in animal welfare and conservation that a new approach to bTB research was needed: one involving the kind of direct experimental comparison that first NCC and then ICD had advocated for many years. Crucially, this not only involved establishing 'undisturbed' areas to act as a control condition, but also applying a randomised experimental design (widely used across the agricultural and clinical sciences) to the problem.[125] Their position was summarised by Harry Thompson in 1990:

> At the urging of the Consultative Panel on Badgers and Tuberculosis, of which UFAW is a member, authority is now being sought to carry out a proper, randomized trial to compare the effects of TB in cattle, of control of badgers versus no control, on farms where a cattle TB breakdown is attributed to the presence of the disease in badgers—not before time, it could be said.[126]

When the Thatcher government fell in 1990, the change in administration initially made little difference to badger/bTB, where MAFF's policies continued as before. Over the previous few years, the unfolding BSE crisis had demanded the lion's share of MAFF's time, resources and attention, leaving bTB neglected by policymakers, politicians and scientists alike. Following the re-election of the Conservatives in 1992, government approaches to badger/bTB began to change. The 1973 Badgers Act was revised and extended, offering the animals more extensive legal protections than before. MAFF's new farming minister (Nicholas Soames) took a direct interest in the problem, visiting Woodchester, organising a scientific symposium, and instituting a new programme of research re-exploring the possibility of controlling bTB with vaccination. Soames was advised of the need for experimental interventions, and provisional plans were made for field trials to test a new 'live' blood test for bTB in badgers.[127] In the wake of this renewed interest, both ecological and veterinary research on bTB continued to thrive, with scientists now finding themselves able to consolidate their ideas and publish their long-term studies.[128] However, the results of this work were disappointing for politicians and policymakers expecting new solutions, with the anticipated test and new vaccine research failing to deliver. On 23 July 1996, the beleaguered Agriculture Minister (John Gummer) announced a new 'Independent Scientific Review of TB in Cattle and Badgers', to be chaired by behavioural ecologist Professor John Krebs. Less than a year later, the Conservatives lost the 1997 General Election, and Krebs's team reported their findings (including the recommendation that badger culling be tested using a controlled experiment) to a newly elected Labour government in June 1997.[129]

4.4 Managing Badgers through Scientific Care

In this chapter, we have explored the development of a new epistemic community around badger/bTB. While this can be broadly characterised as *disease ecology*, as we have seen with all these epistemic communities, it involves scientists from multiple disciplines alongside 'lay' naturalists working with badgers. This grouping centred upon a counterpart to the SVS, ICD, responsible for researching and managing wild animals making 'pests' of themselves. ICD originated in the ability of ecologists to reorient their work towards wartime and post-war agricultural productivity agendas, initially gaining funding from funding and then moving scientists into government positions, establishing new groups dedicated to 'pest control'. The scientists of ICD maintained close links with academic colleagues, drawing upon and contributing to critical developments in population ecology at this time. PICL scientists also contributed to the emerging science of animal welfare, collaborating with the scientific campaign group UFAW to create new 'cultures of care' for wildlife biology and pest control. PICL were also at the forefront of attempts to control and understand the international epizootic of myxomatosis when it reached the UK in the 1950s, contributing to scientific understandings of disease ecology during these decades. PICL's scientific care for wildlife and their role as government arbiters over awkward animals was seen in action during the 1960s, when badgers became a 'mammal of interest' to farmers and animal protection campaigners. While the former accused the animals of predating livestock and damaging crops, the latter argued that badgers were instead victims of human persecution and cruelty. As with the earlier wildlife conflict over rabbits and myxomatosis, ICD investigated these claims and brokered a policy compromise in which the animals were not regarded to be pests but did not merit special protection either.

When the news emerged of tuberculous badgers in the early 1970s, Britain's long-standing badger debate was reignited and PICL scientists were rapidly called upon to help their veterinary counterparts investigate the situation. Once the scale of the problem became clear, MAFF commissioned a major research programme involving both SVS and ICD, and PICL opened a new field station at Woodchester Park devoted to researching the ecology of badgers and bTB. Over the next ten years, PICL scientists developed 'humane' techniques for working with wild badgers, research which proved its worth to MAFF when it found that the animals were unusually resistant to cyanide 'gassing'. PICL's approach to scientific research and care was central to the formation of bTB control policies throughout this period, and they were repeatedly consulted on how to cull badgers with minimal impacts on animal suffering and wider public opinion. Unlike the (domestic) animal health-oriented SVS, PICL scientists were primarily motivated by a desire to build *reliable knowledge* motivated by and feeding into agricultural policy. Like their counterparts building animal welfare science in the laboratory, for these scientists *good care* for the wild animals they worked with was an intrinsic part of their practices of *good science*.[130] Developed in collaboration with laboratory colleagues and organisations such as UFAW, this version of *good care* was similar to the cultures of care of government animal health, prioritising populations over individuals, lack of suffering over preserving life, and integrating anthropocentric priorities in relation to boosting food production and minimising economic losses. As we will explore in the next chapter, the logics of care developed by conservationists and animal protection campaigners would become increasingly at odds with those held by MAFF's veterinarians and research scientists from the 1960s onwards.

PICL's early field investigations of badger movements, behaviour and ecology involved similar techniques (of mapping) and ideas (relating to the spatial movement of animals and pathogens) to those employed by their colleagues in animal health. However, as MAFF's veterinary and ecological research programmes proceeded, expanded and became increasingly sophisticated, their epistemologies—frameworks for researching and understanding—badger/bTB gradually diverged. Veterinary epidemiologists in the SVS interpreted the outcomes of badger clearance trials in terms of public health 'natural experiments', arguing that these interventions led to long-term reductions in the incidence of bTB in cattle. ICD's field officers and scientists were instead alerted to the sustained effort required to clear badgers and prevent 'recolonisation', following the traces of the animals as they established and re-established group territories. Ecologists and field biologists saw the single interventions as scientifically inadequate, as it was not possible to directly compare the effects of badger culling with fully 'undisturbed' areas. By the 1990s, ecologists in and outside of government had formed a consensus with allies in UFAW, conservation bodies and naturalists that a controlled experiment testing the effects of badger culling on bTB rates in cattle was necessary. Following the fallout from the BSE crisis, and the collapse of the 'live test' trial in the early 1990s, the new disease ecology epistemic community was able to successfully lobby ministers that a new approach to the science of badger/bTB was needed. This resulted in the appointment of the Krebs review team in 1996 and ultimately in the commissioning of the Randomised Badger Culling trial by Tony Blair's incoming New Labour government in 1998. The Krebs report opened a new chapter in the history of the badger/bTB controversy, which we will investigate in the final part of this book.

Notes

1. Rob Fish, Matt Lobley and Michael Winter, 'A License to Produce? Farmer Interpretations of the New Food Security Agenda', *Journal of Rural Studies* 29 (March 2012): 40–49.
2. Meyer and Molyneux-Hodgson, 'Introduction: The Dynamics of Epistemic Communities'; Dunlop, 'Epistemic Communities'.
3. Mol, Moser and Pols, *Care in Practice*; Davies et al., 'Science, Culture, and Care in Laboratory Animal Research'.

4. For emotional care as scientific practice, see e.g. Kerr and Garforth, 'Affective Practices, Care and Bioscience'.
5. Arnold B. Arluke, Lynda Birke and Mike Michael, *The Sacrifice: How Scientific Experiments Transform Animals and People* (West Lafayette, IN: Perdue University Press, 2007); Haraway, *When Species Meet*; Thom van Dooren, 'A Day with Crows—Rarity, Nativity and the Violent-Care of Conservation', *Animal Studies Journal* 4(2) (2015): 1–28; E. Giraud and G. Hollin, 'Care, Laboratory Beagles and Affective Utopia', *Theory, Culture and Society* 33(4) (July 2016): 27–49; Greenhough and Roe, 'Exploring the Role of Animal Technologists in Implementing the 3Rs'.
6. Robert G. W. Kirk, 'A Brave New Animal for a Brave New World: The British Laboratory Animals Bureau and the Constitution of International Standards of Laboratory Animal Production and Use, circa 1947–1968', *Isis: An International Review Devoted to the History of Science and Its Cultural Influences* 101(1) (March 2010): 62–94; Tone Druglitrø and Robert G. W. Kirk, 'Building Transnational Bodies: Norway and the International Development of Laboratory Animal Science, ca. 1956–1980', *Science in Context* 27(2) (April 2014): 333–57; Davies et al., 'Science, Culture, and Care in Laboratory Animal Research'; Druglitrø, '"Skilled Care" and the Making of Good Science'.
7. On 'sacrifice' in science, see Arluke, Birke and Michael, *The Sacrifice.*
8. Mette N. Svendsen and Lene Koch, 'Potentializing the Research Piglet in Experimental Neonatal Research', *Current Anthropology* 54(S7) (October 2013): S118–28; Mie S. Dam and Mette N. Svendsen, 'Treating Pigs: Balancing Standardisation and Individual Treatments in Translational Neonatology Research', *BioSocieties* 13(2) (2018): 349–67.
9. Alison Bashford, *Global Population: History, Geopolitics, and Life on Earth* (New York: Columbia University Press, 2014); Michael Bresalier, 'From Healthy Cows to Healthy Humans: Integrated Approaches to World Hunger, c.1930–1965', in *Animals and the Shaping of Modern Medicine: One Health and Its Histories*, ed. Abigail Woods et al. (Cham, Switzerland: Palgrave Macmillan; Springer International, 2018), 119–60.
10. Sheail, *Nature in Trust*; John Martin, *The Development of Modern Agriculture: British Farming since 1931* (Basingstoke: Palgrave Macmillan, 2000); Brassley, 'Wartime Productivity and Innovation, 1939–1945'.
11. Wilko Graf von Hardenberg et al., eds, *The Nature State: Rethinking the History of Conservation* (Abingdon: Routledge, 2017); Matthew Kelly, 'Conventional Thinking and the Fragile Birth of the Nature State in Post-War Britain', in *The Nature State: Rethinking the History of Conservation*, ed. Wilko Graf von Hardenberg et al. (Abingdon: Routledge, 2017), 114–34.
12. Nyhart, *Modern Nature.*

13. Vassiliki Betty Smocovitis, *Unifying Biology: The Evolutionary Synthesis and Evolutionary Biology* (Princeton: Princeton University Press, 1996).
14. Richard W. Burkhardt, 'Ethology, Natural History, the Life Sciences, and the Problem of Place', *Journal of the History of Biology* 32(3) (1999): 489–508; C. R. Henke, 'Making a Place for Science: The Field Trial', *Social Studies of Science* 30(4) (2000): 483–511; Robert E. Kohler, *Landscapes and Labscapes: Exploring the Lab–Field Border in Biology* (Chicago: University of Chicago Press, 2002); Graeme Robert Beale, 'Tinbergian Practice, Themes and Variations : The Field and Laboratory Methods and Practice of the Animal Behaviour Research Group under Nikolaas Tinbergen at Oxford University' (PhD, University of Edinburgh, 2008).
15. E.g. J. Lorimer, 'Counting Corncrakes: The Affective Science of the UK Corncrake Census', *Social Studies of Science* 38(3) (2008): 377–405.
16. Meyer, 'Caring for Weak Ties'; Mary E. Sunderland, 'Modernizing Natural History: Berkeley's Museum of Vertebrate Zoology in Transition', *Journal of the History of Biology* (September 2012).
17. Hauke Riesch and Clive Potter, 'Citizen Science as Seen by Scientists: Methodological, Epistemological and Ethical Dimensions', *Public Understanding of Science* 23(1) (January 2014): 107–20. For more on the history of citizen science, see Sally Shuttleworth, 'Old Weather: Citizen Scientists in the 19th and 21st Centuries', *Science Museum Group Journal* 3(3) (March 2015).
18. Peter Crowcroft—a member of Elton's group—provides this working definition. While the term is of course contested, the study of dynamic change in ecological systems is foundational for British research traditions in particular. Peter Crowcroft, *Elton's Ecologists: A History of the Bureau of Animal Population* (Chicago: University of Chicago Press, 1991), ix–xx.
19. Neil Carter, 'Greening the Mainstream: Party Politics and the Environment', *Environmental Politics* 22(1) (1 February 2013): 73–94.
20. Stephen Bocking, *Ecologists and Environmental Politics: A History of Contemporary Ecology* (New Haven: Yale University Press, 1997); Etienne Benson, *Wired Wilderness: Technologies of Tracking and the Making of Modern Wildlife* (Baltimore: Johns Hopkins University Press, 2010); Stephen Bocking, 'Nature on the Home Front: British Ecologists' Advocacy for Science and Conservation', *Environment and History* 18(2) (May 2012): 261–81; Jacob Darwin Hamblin, *Arming Mother Nature: The Birth of Catastrophic Environmentalism* (Oxford: Oxford University Press, 2013).
21. Warwick Anderson, 'Natural Histories of Infectious Disease: Ecological Vision in Twentieth-Century Biomedical Science', *Osiris* 19 (2004): 39–61; Mark Honigsbaum, '"Tipping the Balance": Karl Friedrich Meyer,

Latent Infections, and the Birth of Modern Ideas of Disease Ecology', *Journal of the History of Biology* (November 2015); Jones, 'Population Cycles, Disease, and Networks of Ecological Knowledge'; Rachel Mason Dentinger, 'Patterns of Infection and Patterns of Evolution: How a Malaria Parasite Brought "Monkeys and Man" Closer Together in the 1960s', *Journal of the History of Biology* 49(2) (April 2016): 359–95; Pierre-Olivier Méthot and Rachel Mason Dentinger, 'Ecology and Infection: Studying Host-Parasite Interactions at the Interface of Biology and Medicine', *Journal of the History of Biology* 49(2) (April 2016): 231–40.

22. For 'useful knowledge' see Joel Mokyr, *The Gifts of Athena: Historical Origins of the Knowledge Economy* (Princeton: Princeton University Press, 2002); Thomas Morel, Giuditta Parolini and Cesare Pastorino, eds, *The Making of Useful Knowledge* (Berlin: Max Planck Institute for the History of Science, 2016).
23. David Edgerton, *Warfare State: Britain, 1920–1970* (Cambridge: Cambridge University Press, 2005); David Edgerton, *Britain's War Machine: Weapons, Resources, and Experts in the Second World War* (Oxford: Oxford University Press, 2011), chap. 6; Kelly, 'Conventional Thinking and the Fragile Birth of the Nature State in Post-War Britain'.
24. Bocking, *Ecologists and Environmental Politics*; Bocking, 'Nature on the Home Front'.
25. E.g. John Sheail, 'Nature Protection, Ecologists and the Farming Context: A U.K. Historical Context', *Journal of Rural Studies* 11(1) (1995): 79–88; Matless, *Landscape and Englishness*; Helen Tilley, *Africa as a Living Laboratory: Empire, Development, and the Problem of Scientific Knowledge, 1870–1950* (Chicago: University of Chicago Press, 2011).
26. Crowcroft, Elton's Ecologists, 2; Matthew K. Chew and Andrew L. Hamilton, 'The Rise and Fall of Biotic Nativeness: A Historical Perspective', in *Fifty Years of Invasion Ecology*, ed. David M. Richardson (Chichester, Sussex: John Wiley & Sons, Ltd, 2010), 35–47.
27. John Sheail, 'Wartime Rodent-Control in England and Wales', in *The Front Line of Freedom: British Farming in the Second World War*, ed. Brian Short, Charles Watkins, and John Martin (Exeter: British Agricultural History Society, 2006), 55–66; Daniel Simberloff, 'Charles Elton: Pioneer Conservation Biologist', *Environment and History* 18(2) (2012): 183–202; Karen Sayer, 'The "Modern" Management of Rats: British Agricultural Science in Farm and Field during the Twentieth Century', *BJHS Themes* (January 2017): 1–29.
28. Sheail, 'Wartime Rodent-Control in England and Wales', 57–59.

29. John Sheail, 'Government and the Management of an Alien Pest Species: A British Perspective', *Landscape Research* 28(1) (2003): 101–11; Sheail, 'Wartime Rodent-Control in England and Wales'; Sayer, 'The "Modern" Management of Rats', 19.
30. Crowcroft, *Elton's Ecologists*, 25, 43, 151; John Sheail, 'The Mink Menace: The Politics of Vertebrate Pest Control', *Rural History* 15(2) (2004): 4.
31. Crowcroft mentions that several other Bureau researchers joined Thompson at ICL, including himself for a time. Crowcroft, *Elton's Ecologists*, 43–44.
32. MAFF, 'Pest Infestation Control—Combining the Report of the Infestation Control Laboratory 1968–1970 and Pest Infestation Research 1970' (London: Ministry of Agriculture, Fisheries & Food: HMSO, 1973); Sayer, 'The "Modern" Management of Rats'.
33. Roger Williams, 'Some Political Aspects of the Rothschild Affair', *Science Studies* 3(1) (1973): 32–36; Thirtle, Palladino and Piesse, 'On the Organisation of Agricultural Research in the United Kingdom, 1945–1994', 564.
34. MAFF, 'Pest Infestation Control—Combining the Report of the Infestation Control Laboratory 1968–1970 and Pest Infestation Research 1970', vii–4; W. Henderson, 'Continued Growth', in *Agricultural Research 1931–1981: A History of the Agricultural Research Council and a Review of Developments in Agricultural Science during the Last Fifty Years* (London: Agricultural Research Council, 1981), 73–74; L. M. Gosling and S. J. Baker, 'The Eradication of Muskrat and Coypus from Britain', *Biological Journal of the Linnean Society* 38 (1989): 39–51.
35. Pest Infestation Control Laboratory, 'Pest Infestation Control Laboratory Report, 1974–1976' (London: HMSO, 1978).
36. For histories of other parts of the Agricultural Science Service, see, e.g. Thirtle, Palladino and Piesse, 'On the Organisation of Agricultural Research in the United Kingdom, 1945–1994'; Paolo Palladino, *Entomology, Ecology and Agriculture: The Making of Science Careers in North America, 1885–1985* (New York: Routledge, 2013); Dominic Berry, 'The Resisted Rise of Randomisation in Experimental Design: British Agricultural Science, c.1910–1930', *History and Philosophy of the Life Sciences* 37(3) (2015): 242–60; Giuditta Parolini, 'Charting the History of Agricultural Experiments', *History and Philosophy of the Life Sciences* 37(3) (2015): 231–41.
37. Pest Infestation Control Laboratory, 'Pest Infestation Control Leaflet' (London: HMSO, c. 1975).
38. Pest Infestation Control Laboratory, 'Pest Infestation Control Laboratory Report, 1971–1973' (London: HMSO, 1975), 3.

39. J. A. Freeman, 'Research in Progress at the Pest Infestation Control Laboratory', *EPPO Bulletin* 4(3) (1 September 1974): 291–294.
40. While the 'PICL' name was officially abandoned in the early 1980s, I will use it throughout this text to make the story easier to follow.
41. For guidance through MAFF's reorganisations during the 1980s and 1990s, see Ingram, 'THE UNITED KINGDOM EXPERIENCE IN THE PRIVATIZATION OF EXTENSION'; Thirtle, Palladino and Piesse, 'On the Organisation of Agricultural Research in the United Kingdom, 1945–1994', 566–67; Phillips, Bridgeman and Ferguson-Smith, 'The Inquiry into BSE and Variant CJD in the United Kingdom', 85–112; Food and Environment Research Agency. Central Science Laboratory: Our History (graphic) (16 September 2009), hosted by Wikipedia at: https://en.wikipedia.org/w/index.php?title=File:CSL_timeline.PNG&oldid=468477845.
42. See, e.g. John Sheail, 'The Management of an Animal Population: Changing Attitudes towards the Wild Rabbit in Britain', *Journal of Environmental Management* 33(2) (1991): 189–203; John Sheail, 'The Grey Squirrel (Sciurus Carolinensis)—A UK Historical Perspective on a Vertebrate Pest Species', *Journal of Environmental Management* 55(3) (March 1999): 145–56; Sheail, 'The Mink Menace'.
43. Crowcroft, *Elton's Ecologists*; Sheail, 'Government and the Management of an Alien Pest Species', 103.
44. While Matthew Chew describes Elton's ideas as 'plainly alarmist Cold War popularisation', the history of PICL and the Bureau of Animal Population demonstrates the deep roots of invasion biology in the inter-war period. Matthew K. Chew, 'A Picture Worth Forty-One Words: Charles Elton, Introduced Species and the 1936 Admiralty Map of British Empire Shipping', *The Journal of Transport History* 35(2) (2014): 226.
45. Gosling and Baker, 'The Eradication of Muskrat and Coypus from Britain'.
46. Simon J. Baker, 'Escaped Exotic Mammals in Britain', *Mammal Review* 20(2–3) (1 June 1990): 75–96.
47. Bartrip, *Myxomatosis*, 44–59.
48. Peter W. J. Bartrip, 'Myxomatosis in 1950s Britain', *Twentieth Century British History* 19(1) (2008): 83–105; Bartrip, *Myxomatosis*.
49. Frank Fenner, *Nature, Nurture and Chance: The Lives of Frank and Charles Fenner* (Canberra: ANU E Press, 2006); Anderson, 'Nowhere to Run, Rabbit'.
50. Sheail, 'The Management of an Animal Population', 200.
51. Fenner, *Nature, Nurture and Chance*, 87–88.
52. For a comprehensive description of the chemical properties and industrial uses of sodium cyanide, see Centres for Disease Control and Prevention,

'CDC—The Emergency Response Safety and Health Database: Systemic Agent: SODIUM CYANIDE—NIOSH', CDC—The Emergency Response Safety and Health Database, 27 September 2018. This chemically differentiates Cymag from its notorious cousin, Zyklon-B, the hydrogen cyanide product used by Nazi Germany to commit genocide during the Holocaust, developed in the 1920s. Scott Christianson, *Fatal Airs: The Deadly History and Apocalyptic Future of Lethal Gases That Threaten Our World* (Santa Barbara, CA: ABC-CLIO, 2010), 61–73. Cymag was banned in the UK in 2004—until then it was licenced for rodent control, but appears to have also been used to poison wildlife; Advisory Committee on Pesticides, 'Pesticide Poisoning of Animals in 2004: Investigations of Suspected Incidents in the United Kingdom' (London: Defra, 2005).

53. Bartrip, 'Myxomatosis in 1950s Britain', 78–94.
54. E.g. K. M. Backhouse and H. V. Thompson, 'Myxomatosis', *Nature* 176(4494) (1955): 1155–56; H. V. Thompson, 'The Rabbit Disease—Myxomatosis', *Annals of Applied Biology* 41(2) (1954): 358–66.
55. H. V. Thompson and A. N. Worden, *The Rabbit*, New Naturalists Monographs 13 (London: Collins, 1956); H. V. Thompson and Carolyn M. King, eds, *The European Rabbit: History and Biology of a Successful Colonizer* (Oxford: Oxford University Press, 1994).
56. Anon., 'The Mammal Society of the British Isles', *Nature* 173 (22 May 1954): 980.
57. A. N. Worden, ed., *The UFAW Handbook on the Care and Management of Laboratory Animals: With an Appendix on Statistical Analysis* (Baltimore: Williams and Wilkins, 1947). The UFAW Handbook is now in its 8th edition, covering a range of species and research contexts, including a chapter on wildlife authored by Defra biologists Julie M. Lane and Robbie A. McDonald, 'Welfare and "Best Practice" in Field Studies of Wildlife', in *The UFAW Handbook on the Care and Management of Laboratory and Other Research Animals*, ed. Robert Hubrecht and James Kirkwood (Chichester, Sussex: Wiley-Blackwell, 2010), 92–106.
58. Kirk, 'Between the Clinic and the Laboratory'; 'The Invention of the "Stressed Animal" and the Development of a Science of Animal Welfare, 1947–1986', *Animal Welfare* 1947 (2014): 86.
59. Kirk, 'Between the Clinic and the Laboratory'; Kirk, 'A Brave New Animal for a Brave New World'; Kirk, 'The Invention of the "Stressed Animal" and the Development of a Science of Animal Welfare, 1947–1986'; Kirk, 'Recovering the Principles of Humane Experimental Technique: The 3Rs and the Human Essence of Animal Research', *Science, Technology, & Human Values* 43(4) (2018): 622–48.
60. Bartrip, 'Myxomatosis in 1950s Britain'.

61. Bartrip, *Myxomatosis*, 36–43.
62. As suggested by the parallel invention of Zyklon-B around this time (also originally developed as a pesticide), historical research into the drivers, research practices, industrial applications and public marketing of these chemicals has revealed the deep interpenetration of agricultural pest control (primarily but not exclusively directed at insects), chemical warfare, (post)colonial control of human populations, and genocide. See Christianson, *Fatal Airs*; Edmund P. Russell, '"Speaking of Annihilation": Mobilizing for War against Human and Insect Enemies, 1914–1945', *The Journal of American History* 82(4) (1996): 1505–29; Edmund P. Russell, *War and Nature: Fighting Humans and Insects with Chemicals from World War I to Silent Spring* (Cambridge: Cambridge University Press, 2001); Lance van Sittert, 'Routinising Genocide: The Politics and Practice of Vermin Extermination in the Cape Province c.1889–1994', *Journal of Contemporary African Studies* 34(1) (2 January 2016): 111–28; Adam M. Romero, 'Commercializing Chemical Warfare: Citrus, Cyanide, and an Endless War', *Agriculture and Human Values* 33(1) (March 2016): 3–26.
63. Sheail, 'The Management of an Animal Population'; John Martin, 'The Wild Rabbit: Plague, Polices and Pestilence in England and Wales, 1931–1955', *Agricultural History Review* 58, no. 2 (2010): 255–76.
64. Scott Henderson was later cited by MAFF to support badger gassing in 1975, and by Zuckerman in 1980; Henderson, 'Report of the Committee on Cruelty to Wild Animals', Cmd 8266, June 1951'; Michael Tichelar, '"Putting Animals into Politics": The Labour Party and Hunting in the First Half of the Twentieth Century', *Rural History* 17(2) (October 2006): 213–34; Griffin, *Blood Sport*.
65. UFAW, 'Obituaries: Harry V. Thompson', *Universities Federation for Animal Welfare News-Sheet* (2004), 2.
66. H. V. Thompson, 'Animal Welfare and the Control of Vertebrates', in *Proceedings of the Fourteenth Vertebrate Pest Conference* (Vertebrate Pest Conference, Sacramento, California, 1990), 5.
67. See Sect. 3.1.
68. F. Howard Lancum, *Wild Birds and the Land*, MAFF Bulletin 140 (London: Ministry of Agriculture, Fisheries & Food: HMSO, 1948); F. Howard Lancum, *Wild Mammals and the Land*, MAFF Bulletin 150 (London: Ministry of Agriculture, Fisheries & Food: HMSO, 1951). Both volumes went through multiple reprints over the following decade and in 1959 MAFF reported having sold almost 100,000 copies of *Wild Birds* (Hansard, 26 January 1959, vol. 598).
69. Lancum, *Wild Mammals and the Land*, 13, 10.

70. A. V. Neal, 'Damage by Badgers in Rotherfield Area', 'Badger Control' report, 18 August 1959, NA MAF 131/70, item 16; M. Neve, 'Letter to C.J. Armour: Badgers', 18 March 1963, NA MAF 131/70, item 68; 'HPC Bi-monthly report. Welsh region', March/April 1961, NA MAF 131/70, item 39; D. Imrie, 'Round the Game Preserves' (extract from *The Shooting Times and Country Magazine*), 3 June 1960, NA MAF 131/70, item 14.
71. C. J. Armour, 'Letter to G.H. Hill re Badgers', 27 July 1960, NA MAF 131/70, item 19.
72. R. J. King, 'The Badger Gate', *Quarterly Journal of Forestry* 58(4) (1964): 318. See also Lancum, *Wild Mammals and the Land*, 13; F. Burden, 'Paper prepared by Mr. F. Burden MP', 23 June 1965' NA HO 285/39; W. E. Rivers, 'Letter to J.R. Austin, Esq, Federation of Rabbit Clearance Societies', 2 February 1967, NA MAF 109/381, item 4.
73. G. R. Hill, 'Circular Letter No. 59/7: Badger Control', 28 June 1959, NA MAF 131/70, item 7; Imrie, D. 'Round the Game Preserves', 3 June 1960, NA MAF 131/70, item 14.
74. Anon., 'Minutes of the Divisional Pests Officers Conference', 25–26 May 1960, NA MAF 131/70, item 10/2.
75. W. E. Rivers, 'Letter to J.R. Austin', 2 February 1967, NA MAF 109/381, item 4.
76. Grant, 'Intractable Policy Failure: The Case of Bovine TB and Badgers', 563.
77. Lambert, 'The Grey Seal in Britain', 50.
78. For example, similar debates about 'rogue' seals were taking place at around the same time; see Lambert, 'The Grey Seal in Britain', 456. Indeed, conservationists are still debating whether 'rogue' animals exist; see Mara J. Goldman, Joana Roque de Pinho and Jennifer Perry, 'Beyond Ritual and Economics: Maasai Lion Hunting and Conservation Politics', *Oryx* 47(4) (October 2013): 490–500; George J. F. Swan et al., 'Ecology of Problem Individuals and the Efficacy of Selective Wildlife Management', *Trends in Ecology & Evolution* 32(7) (July 2017): 518–30.
79. R. G. Symes, 'Badger Damage: Fact or Fiction?' in *Mammals as Pests*, ed. Rory Putman (London: Chapman and Hall, 1989), 196–206.
80. S. L. Woolridge, 'Letter', 11 April 1972. NA MAF 109/381, item 40a.
81. F. H. Jacob, 'Director's Introduction', in Pest Infestation Control Laboratory, 'Pest Infestation Control Laboratory Report, 1974–1976', 11.
82. Thirtle, Palladino and Piesse, 'On the Organisation of Agricultural Research in the United Kingdom, 1945–1994'.
83. J. M. Seymour, 'Memo: TB-Badgers', 30 August 1974, NA MAF 109/295, item 80; H. V. Thompson, 'Memo: TB-Badgers', 6 September

1974, NA MAF 109/295, item 82. For further background on ITE and the NCC's navigation of the post-Rothschild research and policy landscape, see John Sheail, 'The Management of Wildlife and Amenity: A UK Post-war Perspective', *Contemporary Record* 7(1) (1993): 44–65.

84. For Neal's service on the Badger Panel, see MAFF, 'Bovine Tuberculosis in Badgers. Fifteenth Report by the Ministry of Agriculture, Fisheries and Food' (London: Ministry of Agriculture, Fisheries & Food: HMSO, 1991), 6; for knowledge brokers, see Morgan Meyer, 'The Rise of the Knowledge Broker', *Science Communication* 32(1) (March 2010): 118–27.
85. Gail Davies, 'Science, Observation and Entertainment: Competing Visions of Postwar British Natural History Television, 1946–1967', *Cultural Geographies* 7(4) (2000): 432; Jon Agar, 'What Difference Did Computers Make?' *Social Studies of Science* 36(6) (December 2006): 869–907; Benson, *Wired Wilderness*; Gouyon, 'Science and Film-Making'.
86. For post-war ethology, see Burkhardt, *Patterns of Behavior*; for evolutionary biology, Mason Dentinger, 'Patterns of Infection and Patterns of Evolution'; Smocovitis, *Unifying Biology*; for ecology, Bocking, *Ecologists and Environmental Politics*; for sociobiology, behavioural ecology and modelling in the 1960s and 1970s I would suggest Paolo Palladino, 'Ecological Theory and Pest Control Practice: A Study of the Institutional and Conceptual Dimensions of a Scientific Debate', *Social Studies of Science* 20(2) (May 1990): 255–81; Beale, 'Tinbergian Practice, Themes and Variations'; Amanda Rees, *The Infanticide Controversy: Primatology and the Art of Field Science* (Chicago: University of Chicago Press, 2009).
87. For further information on the Woodchester site, see www.woodchestermansion.org.uk. The park is now managed by the National Trust and was designated an SSSI in 1987. For more information on the Kellys, see Duff Hart-Davis, 'Country Matters: Guardians of the Haunted House', *The Independent*, 11 June 1994; Liz Wright, 'Obituary: Miriam Kelly', *The Guardian*, 28 August 2008. For Woodchester as a site for field biology, see Roger Ransome, *Natural History of Hibernating Bats* (London: Christopher Helm Ltd./Mammal Society, 1990); D. W. Yalden and R. F. Shore, 'Yellow-Necked Mice Apodemus Flavicollis at Woodchester Park, 1968–1989', *Journal of Zoology* 224(2) (1 June 1991): 329–32.
88. Anonymous interview source, 13/05/15.
89. Pest Infestation Control Laboratory, 'Pest Infestation Control Laboratory Report, 1977–1979' (London: HMSO, 1981), 111.
90. The badgers at Oxford University's Wytham Woods field site just about claim priority here, as they have been working with field biologists since 1972: Christina D. Buesching et al., 'The Mammals of Wytham Woods',

in *Wytham Woods: Oxford's Ecological Laboratory* (Oxford: Oxford University Press, 2010), 187–89.

91. C. J. Armour, 'Letter re Swan Trap', 17 April 1974, NA MAF 109/383, item 60; Universities Federation for Animal Welfare, 'UFAW Annual Report, 1973–1974' (South Mimms: Universities Federation for Animal Welfare, 1974), 17; Universities Federation for Animal Welfare, 'UFAW Annual Report, 1974–1975' (South Mimms: Universities Federation for Animal Welfare, 1975), 11–12. For Ruth Murray's cage-trap, see Ruth R. Murray, 'Live Trapping of Badgers, Their Removal, Release and Rehabilitation in a New Area', *Mammal Review* 1(3) (1 September 1970): 86–92; for Murray herself, see Chap. 5.
92. Universities Federation for Animal Welfare, 'UFAW Annual Report, 1974–1975'; MAFF, 'Bovine Tuberculosis in Badgers. Report by the Ministry of Agriculture, Fisheries and Food'; C. L. Cheeseman and P. J. Mallinson, 'Radio Tracking in the Study of Bovine Tuberculosis in Badgers', in *A Handbook on Biotelemetry and Radio Tracking* (Oxford: Pergamon, 1980), 649–56. See also MAF 109/384, items 109–13.
93. See, e.g. C. L. Cheeseman et al., 'The Population Structure, Density and Prevalence of Tuberculosis (Mycobacterium Bovis) in Badgers (*Meles Meles*) from Four Areas in South-West England', *Journal of Applied Ecology* 18(3) (1981): 795–804.
94. MAFF, 'Bovine Tuberculosis in Badgers. Report by the Ministry of Agriculture, Fisheries and Food', 6; Pest Infestation Control Laboratory, 'Pest Infestation Control Laboratory Report, 1974–1976', 173–74.
95. See MAF 131/70; also in MAF 109/383, e.g. items 48, 104, 165.
96. MAFF, 'Bovine Tuberculosis in Badgers. Third Report by the Ministry of Agriculture, Fisheries and Food', 26.
97. Pest Infestation Control Laboratory, 'Pest Infestation Control Laboratory Report, 1974–1976', 174.
98. Ibid., 176.
99. Hans Kruuk, *The Spotted Hyena: A Study of Predation and Social Behavior* (Chicago: Chicago: University of Chicago Press, 1972); N. Tinbergen et al., 'Egg Shell Removal by the Black-Headed Gull, Larus Ridibundus L.; A Behaviour Component of Camouflage', *Behaviour* 19(1/2) (1962): 74–117.
100. David W. Macdonald, 'Radio-Tracking: Some Applications and Limitations', in *Animal Marking* (London: Palgrave, 1978), 192–204; Charles J. Amlaner and David W. MacDonald, eds, *A Handbook on Biotelemetry and Radio Tracking: Proceedings of an International Conference on Telemetry and Radio Tracking in Biology and Medicine, Oxford, 20–22 March 1979* (Oxford: Pergamon Press, 1980); Benson, *Wired Wilderness.*

101. Zuckerman, 'Badgers, Cattle and Tuberculosis'; C. L. Cheeseman and Stephen Harris, 'Methods of Marking Badgers (*Meles Meles*), Notes from the Mammal Society—No. 44', *Journal of Zoology* 197(2) (1 June 1982): 289–91.
102. C. L. Cheeseman et al., 'Comparison of Dispersal and Other Movements in Two Badger (*Meles Meles*) Populations', *Mammal Review* 18(1) (1 March 1988): 51–59; MAFF, 'Bovine Tuberculosis in Badgers. Fifteenth Report by the Ministry of Agriculture, Fisheries and Food', 6.
103. Cheeseman and Mallinson, 'Radio Tracking in the Study of Bovine Tuberculosis in Badgers', 68.
104. For more information see Peter Bale, 'Badger Watch', *The Radio Times* (BBC Television, 5 May 1977); Wildscreen, 'WildFilmHistory—Badger Watch (1977)', WildFilmHistory, 2008.
105. 'MAFF Consultative Panel on Badgers and TB: Badger Watch—BBC Television', June 1977. NA FT 41/92.
106. MAFF, 'Bovine Tuberculosis in Badgers. Second Report by the Ministry of Agriculture, Fisheries and Food', sec. appendix 7.
107. C. L. Cheeseman et al., 'Dynamics of Tuberculosis in a Naturally Infected Badger Population', *Mammal Review* 18(1) (1988): 61–72.
108. For descriptions of this behaviour, see C. L. Cheeseman and P. J. Mallinson, 'Behaviour of Badgers (*Meles Meles*) Infected with Bovine Tuberculosis', *Journal of Zoology* 194(2) (1 June 1981): 284–89.
109. *MAFF Badger Group Research Programme 1981. MAFF, Agricultural Science Service, Worplesdon Laboratory*, ZUEA S2 PUBS 4255.
110. A. Warne, 'Memo re Badger killing in Areas with bTB', May 1974, NA MAF 109/383, item 104; A. McDiarmid, 'Comments on report concerning TB in badgers', 12 January 1972, NA MAF 287/752, item 10; see also Eunice D. Overend, 'Badgers and TB—Does Gassing Spread the Disease?' *Oryx* 15(4) (August 1980): 338–40.
111. B. E. Camp, 'Memo re Zuckerman Review: Future Programme of Work at Woodchester Park', 29 May 1980. ZUEA S2PUBS 115, folder *Badger Report 1980 Minutes of Enquiry.*
112. 'Lord Zuckerman's visit to Woodchester Park', 26 March 1980; 'Lord Zuckerman's meeting with Mr. Curwen (Woodchester, Glos.)—27 March 1980'; 'Memo from B.E. Camp re Zuckerman Review: Future Programme of Work at Woodchester Park', 29 May 1980. All in ZUEA S2PUBS 115, folder *Badger Report 1980.*
113. 'MAFF Consultative Panel: Progress Report on Operational and Investigational Work in the SW Region, Sept–Dec 1979', in ZUEA S2PUBS 115, folder *Badger Report 1980.*
114. For Zuckerman's earlier hostile interactions with field ecology and ethology see Burt, 'Solly Zuckerman'; Kirk, 'Between the Clinic and the Laboratory'.

115. Agar, 'Transition'.
116. H. V. Thompson, 'Memorandum. Badgers, Cattle and Tuberculosis: Some Research Proposals', 30 January 1981. NA MAF 459/8, item 1.
117. J. W. Davies, 'Re: Badgers, Cattle and Tuberculosis: Some Research Proposals', 16 February 1981, NA MAF 459/8, item 2; 'Notes on a Meeting held at Tolworth Tower', 26 February 1981, NA MAF 459/8, item 4b.
118. Anonymous interview source, 13/05/15.
119. *MAFF Badger Control Manual and Code of Practice*, MAF 459/24; for Defra's most recent Best Practice guidelines, see Defra, 'Cage-Trapping and Dispatch of Badgers under Licence to Prevent the Spread of Bovine TB in Cattle', 26 August 2014.
120. Stuart and Wilesmith, 'Tuberculosis in Badgers'.
121. Clifton-Hadley et al., 'The Occurrence of Mycobacterium Bovis Infection in Cattle in and around an Area Subject to Extensive Badger (*Meles Meles*) Control', 191–92.
122. 'MAFF Badger Group Research Programme, Agricultural Science Service, Worplesdon Laboratory', ZUEA SS2PUB425, see also MAFF, 'Bovine Tuberculosis in Badgers. Sixth Report by the Ministry of Agriculture, Fisheries and Food'; R. M. Anderson and Robert M. May, 'Population Biology of Infectious Diseases: Part I', *Nature* 280(5721) (2 August 1979): 361–67; R. M. Anderson et al., 'Population Dynamics of Fox Rabies in Europe', *Nature* 289(5800) (26 February 1981): 765–71; R. M. Anderson and W. Trewhella, 'Population Dynamics of the Badger (*Meles Meles*) and the Epidemiology of Bovine Tuberculosis (Mycobacterium Bovis)', *Philosophical Transactions of the Royal Society B: Biological Sciences* 310(1145) (1985): 327–81. For further information on Roy Anderson, Bob May, John Krebs and the 'Silwood Circle' of ecologists, see Hannah Gay, *The Silwood Circle: A History of Ecology and the Making of Scientific Careers in Late Twentieth-Century Britain* (London: Imperial College Press, 2013), 151–64; 204–12.
123. David W. MacDonald, *Rabies and Wildlife: A Biologist's Perspective* (Oxford: Oxford University Press, 1980); Anderson et al., 'Population Dynamics of Fox Rabies in Europe'.
124. See footnote 39 for MAFF's ongoing processes of reorganisation and privatisation.
125. Berry, 'The Resisted Rise of Randomisation in Experimental Design'.
126. Thompson, 'Animal Welfare and the Control of Vertebrates', 6.
127. D. G. Newell and R. Glyn Hewinson, 'Control of Bovine Tuberculosis by Vaccination', *Veterinary Record* 136(18) (6 May 1995): 459–63; C. L. Cheeseman, 'Why a Badger Cull Won't Work', Badgergate, 9 June 2013; Overy and Tansey, *A History of Bovine TB c.1965–c. 2000*, 55: 59–60.

128. J. A. Brown, C. L. Cheeseman and S. Harris, 'Studies on the Spread of Bovine Tuberculosis from Badgers to Cattle', *Journal of Zoology* 227(4) (August 1992): 694–96; R. S. Clifton-Hadley, J. W. Wilesmith and F. A. Stuart, 'Mycobacterium-Bovis in the European Badger (*Meles Meles*)—Epidemiologic Findings in Tuberculous Badgers from a Naturally Infected Population', *Epidemiology and Infection* 111(1) (August 1993): 9–19; MAFF, 'Bovine Tuberculosis in Badgers. Seventeenth Report by the Ministry of Agriculture, Fisheries and Food' (London: Ministry of Agriculture, Fisheries & Food: HMSO, 1994), 13–18; Clifton-Hadley et al., 'The Occurrence of Mycobacterium Bovis Infection in Cattle in and around an Area Subject to Extensive Badger (*Meles Meles*) Control'.
129. Krebs et al., 'Bovine Tuberculosis in Cattle and Badgers'; Select Committee on Agriculture, 'House of Commons—Agriculture—Fifth Report' (London: House of Commons, 27 April 1999), sec. III. THE KREBS REPORT.
130. Druglitrø, '"Skilled Care" and the Making of Good Science'.

5

Badger Protection Campaigns

As we have already explored in Chap. 1, badgers have occupied an oddly significant role in British culture and politics since the late nineteenth century at least; and appear to have been involved in wildlife conflicts (conflicts between humans and animals and conflicts between humans about animals) for even longer.[1] This chapter will pick up the story of the Great British Badger Debate in the mid-1960s, when it was reignited by animal advocates drawing media, public and policy attention to the persecution, hunting and maiming of badgers due to their social role as 'vermin'. While campaigners made several attempts at obtaining new legal protections for the animals, it was not until after the discovery of tuberculous badgers that the Badgers Act was made law in 1973. This chapter will move the focus away from Ministry for Agriculture, Fisheries and Food's (MAFF) scientists and veterinarians to instead address the more diffuse epistemic community of *badger protection*. While these campaigners were less directly connected with policy, their deep knowledge of these awkward creatures and public influence made them invaluable partners for Ministry scientists and policymakers during the 1970s. Just as we have already done with *animal health* and *disease ecology*, to understand *badger protection* campaigners' responses to badger/bTB, we must place them in their broader historical contexts—this time of mid-twentieth-century natural history, environmental and animal politics. This chapter will explain how a diverse coalition of animal welfare NGOs, animal rescue activists, naturalists, field biologists, members of both Houses of Parliament, the Women's Institute and the *Daily Mirror* was built in support of the cause of badger protection. It will show how the process of building this coalition brought into closer alignment the previously separated concerns of conservation and animal protection. Along the way, it will illustrate the multiple cultures of care involved in badger protection and demonstrate how shifting relationships between them have led to dramatic and sometimes unforeseen policy change.

We have already explored how the shared goals of building reliable knowledge while 'humanely' researching and controlling wildlife and pests created close working relationships between the Mammal Society, MAFF's Pest Infestation Control Laboratory (PICL) and the Universities Federation for Animal Welfare (UFAW). In the absence of state economic constraints and with the protection and welfare of animals as their highest priority, non-governmental cultures of care around British wildlife have been considerably more variable. Debates over *who or what* should be cared for and *how* that care should be enacted have resulted in the interests of conservationists and animal advocates moving in and out of alignment over time and according to the issue at hand. By the mid-twentieth century, these tensions had created a distanced relationship between conservation and animal protection movements in Britain. As naturalists started to follow and learn from badgers in the wild, they became increasingly aware that other people were persecuting and killing these obscure beasts. These naturalists used their skills of observation and expression to convey the situation to others, create empathy for badgers and build new alliances, generating public and political pressure for protective legislation. Along the way, they started to change what it meant for a species to be 'threatened', bringing previously excluded concerns about animal suffering into conservation campaigning.

This chapter will document these changes as MAFF implemented a state-led culling policy, while investigating the poorly understood connection between badgers and bTB. The early consensus over gassing as the 'most effective and humane method of killing badgers'[2] turned out to be highly fragile and disintegrated over the 1970s. By the end of the decade, many more people were involved in badger protection, acting on the single issue but also as part of wider concerns about environmental politics. A flourishing of new badger protection groups, naturalists and animal welfare campaigners were reporting problems with gassing—which were initially dismissed and then vindicated by laboratory experiments, leading to the abandonment of the technique. These debates before and following the Zuckerman report had the effect of uniting conservation and animal welfare interests behind the cause of badger protection. During the 1980s, campaigners turned their attention back to their core concerns of badger persecution, leaving MAFF's scientists to investigate the increasingly complex science of badger/bTB, while policymakers tinkered with bTB policy. By the time that the forming epistemic community around disease ecology had forged the 1990s consensus that government needed to conduct a controlled experiment testing the effects of culling upon bTB rates in cattle, badger advocacy coalitions had shifted once more, leaving some in favour of the idea, while others vociferously opposed it. Following from our explorations of the 'cultures of care' of the animal health and disease ecology epistemic communities, we will now unpick the multiple modes of caring—about animals and environments—involved in campaigning about badgers.[3]

5.1 British Conservation and Animal Protection

Britain's 'badger debate' has generally turned upon whether the animals should be regarded as dangerous and awkward vermin (to be removed or destroyed), or charismatic wildlife (to be admired and protected). Before discussing the 1960s campaigns for badger protection, I will contextualise them into the longer history of the politics of animal care in Britain, showing how interests lobbying for the conservation of wildlife and landscapes have moved in and out of alignment with concerns about cruelty to animals over the past two hundred years. The century between the 1835 Cruelty to Animals Act (which prohibited bear and badger baiting) and the Second World War saw the beginnings of change in the social role of badgers, whereby the older, verminous Bad Badger was gradually eclipsed by the heroic and mysterious Good Badger. These changing cultural ideas were part of a larger set of social changes in human–animal relations in the UK, as campaigners mobilised over the killing and exploitation of wildlife from sport-shooting, natural history collecting and wider environmental damage; as well as cruelty to animals on several fronts including sport-fighting, vivisection and the abuse of pets and livestock.[4] It was during the nineteenth century that key British organisations campaigning for the protection and preservation of animals and landscape came into being. These included the Royal Society for Prevention of Cruelty to Animals (RSPCA) (1824), National Trust (1884) and the Royal Society for the Protection of Birds (RSPB) (1889), founded in a wider context of campaigning for social causes, including vegetarianism, temperance, the abolition of slavery and universal suffrage.[5] Concerns for non-humans initially centred upon cruelty to domestic animals (pets, livestock and experimental animals): it was after the RSPCA became involved in campaigns against hunting wild birds and egg collecting that attention turned to wildlife, resulting in the founding of the RSPB. The National Trust (for Places of Historic Interest or Natural Beauty) was primarily concerned with the preservation of land, including human artefacts (such as buildings) and non-human features (landscape but also plants and animals). While the RSPCA campaigned against stag hunting and hare coursing during the 1870s, its involvement in wildlife welfare remained limited.[6]

Over the decades spanning the end of the nineteenth and start of the twentieth century, significant gains were made in protecting wildlife—particularly birds—as part of the natural environment, as well as in preventing cruelty to domestic and laboratory animals. However, concerns about the suffering of wild mammals fell between the stools of these increasingly prominent lobbies. Key legislation such as the 1911 Protection of Animals Act was passed by Parliament partly because it only included 'captive and domestic animals', leaving hunting and cruelty to wildlife to continue unabated.[7] 1920s and 1930s campaigns against fox hunting and the use of spring-loaded 'gin traps' were not supported by the RSPCA or National Trust.[8] However, cultural and social attitudes towards wildlife did start to change, in a society primed by the ideas of Romanticism to increasingly think of nature as a source of sublime wonder, and wild animals as figures of sympathy—it was around this time that the most famous 'good badger' fiction, *Wind in the Willows*, was published. Following the National Trust's programmes of land acquisition, the Society for the Promotion of Nature Reserves (now known as the Wildlife Trusts) was founded in 1911, creating a more organised structure for the acquisition and legal protection of land.[9] Before and after the First World War, many poets and artists were inspired by British landscapes, and helped to rekindle concerns over the destructive potential of modernity to create human and animal suffering and damage wider environments.[10] While upper-class participation in fox hunting rose during the interwar years, middle- and lower-class hunting practices such as otter hunting and badger digging started to decline in popularity. Frustrated by limited progress, and by the RSPCA's disengagement from wildlife welfare, members of the RSCPA broke away to form the League against Cruel Sports (LACS) in 1924. While no further legislation was passed at this time, LACS did succeed in politicising the issue to the extent that hunting interests founded their own organisation to counter these campaigns.[11]

Following the Second World War, the parallel debates over agriculture, conservation, animal welfare and wildlife protection entered a new phase as the state took on a more prominent role in supporting scientific research and coordinating and implementing policy across the board. This shift took place alongside the post-war creation of international infrastructures for furthering social, medical, environmental and animal health policy. This included the creation of the United Nations and its agencies; and the further development of older NGOs beyond their Victorian philanthropic roots into the international, policy-facing institutions we see today.[12] In Britain, this renewed importance of the state was initially shaped by the demands of the war effort on multiple fronts, but then came to full fruition as part of post-war reconstruction, with the creation of state-led policy infrastructures, including the NHS, welfare state, state education and transport networks.[13] As we have seen in the previous chapters, veterinarians and ecologists alike benefited from wartime and post-war state agendas for boosting agricultural productivity, embedding their epistemic communities in government, gaining further resources to support their research and initiating new policies for controlling infectious diseases and agricultural pests. Ecologists deployed multiple strategies to make their research relevant to government and further their own agendas. As well as gaining support from the Ministry of Agriculture via pest control, ecologists also worked closely with conservationists to advance their shared long-term strategy of protecting wildlife and landscapes. A coalition of scientists, naturalists, journalists and civil servants worked together to convince government that conservation could help advance British interests by supporting national forestry and leisure industries.[14] The creation of the British 'nature state' was brought about via the creation of interconnected policy structures, new institutions and legislation, firstly regulating planning in 1947 and then protecting specific sites and landscapes (including the creation of National Parks) from development in 1949.[15] The protected land encompassed coastal, marshland, moor, meadow and forested landscapes, and brought in specific sites with unique features or rare species which had already been under the management of non-governmental bodies for some years. The legislation enabled the creation of the Nature Conservancy (renamed in the 1970s as the Nature Conservancy Council, NCC) as the world's first statutory conservation body, charged with the multiple roles of administering and physically maintaining protected land; providing scientific advice to government; and developing new scientific research to better understand the animal and plant communities living at these sites. Between government bodies and NGOs, the Nature State created new scientific, administrative and field practice jobs, as well as national and regional policy mechanisms for lay naturalists to feed into conservation governance.[16]

The previous chapter has explored how productivism supported the transformation of naturalists into professional pest control biologists. The establishment of government and non-governmental frameworks dedicated to the protection of landscape and wildlife created another route for naturalists to become professionals, this time as conservation scientists, policymakers, administrators and land managers. While historical narratives of the professionalisation of the biological sciences imply that the enthusiast-led natural history of the nineteenth century simply faded away, this was not really the case. Instead, professional conservation roles were developed and supported by ongoing working partnerships with 'lay' (i.e. without formal training or payment) naturalists, and a persisting blurring of the boundaries between the two.[17] As conservation campaigns gradually gained traction, natural history practices also shifted away from the catching, killing and collection of wild animals towards observation and recording in the field. In the UK, these changes in practice were further enabled first by the establishment of the National Parks and nature reserves as spaces of leisure, and second by changes in technology. The wider uptake of private motor vehicles made it possible for more people to visit and enjoy the countryside and encounter wild animals, up to and including safari parks by the 1960s.[18] This expanded ability to spend time in these 'wilder' spaces was further facilitated by developments in technologies of vision—binoculars and cameras—making it much easier to see and record wild animals than ever before. These changes created a new popular natural history, not only as amateur scientific practice and leisure pursuit, but also as new forms of mass media content enthusiastically consumed by naturalist audiences. This in turn drove a further wave of professionalisation of naturalists, this time into specialist natural history writers, journalists, broadcast media producers, directors, cameramen and presenters. In Britain, the creation of popular natural history in the media was initially driven by publishing, with widespread sales of field guides, semi-popular monographs and what we now call creative 'nature writing'.[19] Broadcast media followed, with the establishment of the BBC Natural History Unit in Bristol during the early 1950s and subsequent commissioning of natural history filmmaking by other channels.[20]

Further gains were also made in terms of the legislation and policy around wildlife welfare. Renewed attempts to outlaw fox hunting failed in 1949, in large part due to the need for the Labour government to maintain alliances with rural and agricultural interests. However, these pressures did bring about the Scott Henderson parliamentary enquiry into 'Cruelty to Wild Animals', which published its report in 1951.[21] Rather than directly addressing hunting, the report was framed in terms of 'pest control' and comprised a detailed assessment of the welfare implications of all techniques for killing wild animals in use at the time. While it supported the continuation of hunting (with four of the seven members connected to hunting interests), the report gave impetus to further research on humane pest control and the outlawing of the gin trap in 1954.[22] The Protection of Birds Act was also passed in 1954, providing a template for protective legislation against any person who 'kills, injures or takes' wild animals.[23] In the early 1960s campaigners turned their attention to problems of pollution, successfully lobbying for legislation for clean rivers and clean air in the 1950s; then capitalising on wider public concerns following the publication of Rachel Carson's *Silent Spring* (1964) to lobby for regulatory action on pesticides. 'Controversies over pollution and pesticides continued' persisted throughout the 1960s, contributing to widening political debates over environmental issues.[24] The co-production of state and NGO infrastructures for conservation with the creation of popular natural history in media had led to a further resurgence of lay field practice. This brought more people into contact with wildlife and wider environments, as naturalists explored field sites across the world as well in their own backyards. In turn, this increased the membership of conservation NGOs and boosted the working base of nature reserves and natural history societies with younger, newly enthusiastic volunteers, who were also becoming increasingly mobilised by new environmental social movements.[25]

5.2 Following, Understanding and Protecting Badgers

These rapid changes in conservation encompassing popular natural history, campaigning and state activity were all in progress as campaigning for badger protection in Britain got underway. The popular outputs of Ernest Neal—most notably his widely sold monograph *The Badger* (1948) and contributions to BBC programming—inspired other naturalists to start following and writing about badgers, making them increasingly visible to wider audiences.[26] Neal's career provides an excellent illustration of the interpenetrated nature of relationships between 'amateur' naturalists and 'professional' biologists in field biology and conservation, which to an extent continues into the present day.[27] Far from the elite networks of MAFF and the University of Oxford, Ernest Neal had carved out a very different space for himself in field biology. Coming from a relatively modest background, Neal supported himself by working through a zoology degree at Chelsea Polytechnic in London, and then took up a career teaching biology in the rural South West of England. He combined teaching with his passions for natural history and photography, and it was during fieldwork with students that he first encountered, photographed and then systematically studied wild badgers during the 1930s.[28] His 1948 book *The Badger* summarised this work and was chosen by the publisher Collins to be the first species-focused monograph to be published in its influential New Naturalist series. As the write-up of one of the first systematic field studies of any British mammal, *The Badger* was a significant scientific work as well as an exceptionally popular natural history book.[29] A pioneering nature photographer, Neal contributed to the early development of the BBC Natural History Unit, eventually appearing on over 100 television and radio programmes between 1952 and 1984, including *Badgers* (1954), in which the animals were first filmed at night, and *Badger Watch* (1977), a groundbreaking live broadcast.[30] He gained his PhD in 1960: a collaboration with physiologists at the London Hospital Medical School, investigating the unusual reproductive cycles of badgers, illustrating the breadth of his scientific engagements with the species.[31] By the 1970s his expert status was such that Neal was the first scientist to be consulted by MAFF about the implications of tuberculous badgers. He acted as a critical 'knowledge broker' between agricultural, conservation and animal protection networks, as well as between governmental, professional and lay scientific worlds.[32] As a founder member of the Mammal Society, Neal was instrumental to their decision to carry out a national survey of badger populations in 1963. The survey was implemented by a network of County Recorders (appointed by the Society) with the help of local 'enthusiasts' mapping out the setts in their area: this created networks fostering formation of the local groups which would eventually become today's Badger Trust.[33]

In 1955 the artist illustrator for Enid Blyton and nature writer Eileen Soper published *When Badgers Wake*, an evocative account of the badger families living near her home in Hertfordshire in the south of England.[34] Accompanied by a wealth of expressive and evocative drawings (Fig. 5.1), Soper wrote of her experiences of learning to follow badgers in the field, and of gaining the trust of the animals over the seasonal cycles of several years. She provided accounts of several episodes where badger groups had been harassed and killed, acts she laid at the door of neighbouring farmers. While some had been shot, Soper was adamant that people were also 'gassing' badgers, relating here the scene of devastation found at a sett she had been observing:

> Visiting the wood one clear spring morning, I found every set stopped. Gas had been used, and there was no sign that any badgers had lived to make their way out. To complete the scene of destruction, motor-cyclist riders had held tests over the sets, cutting up the ground till the wood was a quagmire.[35]

Soper's account is significant on several fronts. The timing (early 1950s) slightly precedes MAFF badger archives drawn upon in Chap. 4,

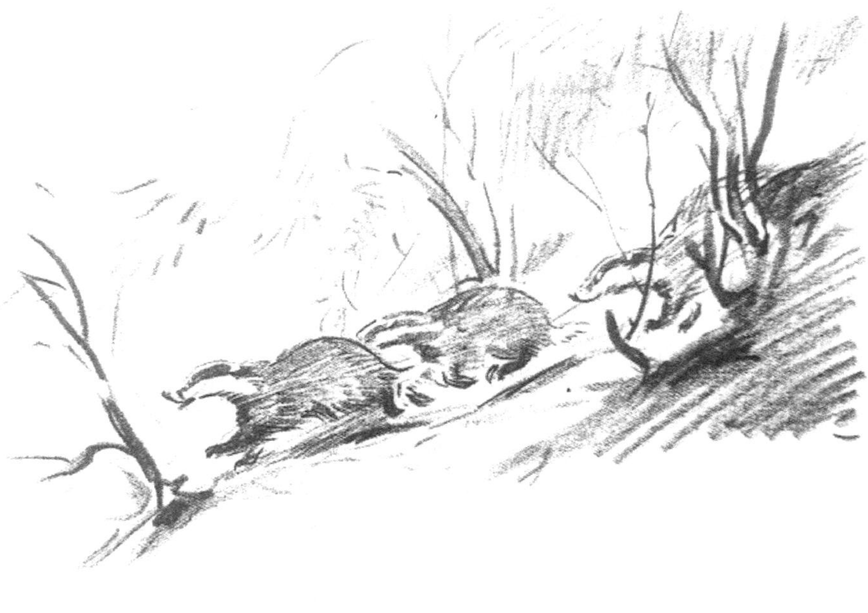

Fig. 5.1 Typical Soper illustration of badgers in action.[38] Source: Soper, *Eileen Soper's Book of Badgers* (51).

confirming that there was an intensification in wildlife conflicts with and about badgers around this time. As ICD officers had determined by this time, gassing badgers was illegal. However, they had found that it was being illicitly carried out, including on at least one occasion by their own field officers.[36] Soper also provided a measured discussion of why badger persecution was unjustified, the beneficial consequences of having the animals around and the possibility of 'rogue' individuals. This corresponds closely with the case being developed at this time by ICD—that badgers were not pests and should generally be left alone. Unlike government scientists she was free to empathise with 'her' badgers about the experience of human persecution and of being gassed: 'My thoughts turned to the badgers lying dead beside their cubs. It is not surprising that animals go in fear when they can die choked by something unseen and unheard in the den that was their only hope of security.'[37] While Soper was clearly well informed about the developing policy consensus, she had a very different view of the 'humaneness' and moral implications of killing badgers by gassing.

Eileen Soper was the earliest member of a network of amateur naturalists working with and writing about badgers during the 1950s, 1960s and 1970s (many of whom were in correspondence with each other and with Ernest Neal), inspired by and contributing to the popular natural history boom.[39] These included novelist and nature writer Norah Burke, who published *King Todd* in 1963: like Soper, Burke wrote about the natural history of badgers alongside a passionate denouncement of the cruelties of badger persecution.[40] Other naturalist-authors of successful badger books published during the 1970s included Jane Ratcliffe, a Cheshire housewife who started following badgers while practicing wildlife photography; journalist and BBC presenter Phil Drabble; the Labour Member of Parliament for Wentworth, Peter Hardy (sponsor of the 1973 Badgers Act); and retired navy captain Wickham Malins.[41]

The badger protection campaign stepped up a gear in the 1960s when Norah Burke's *King Todd* was published in 1963, attracting reviews and wider commentary, including from prominent naturalist and conservationist Richard Fitter.[42] In 1964 this debate reached a much wider audience when Devon dairy farmer Ruth Murray worked with John Pilger—an up-and-coming investigative reporter at the *Daily Mirror*—on a major expose about the horrors of badger digging (hunting) and baiting (fighting with dogs).[43] While Murray was often described as a naturalist, her involvement with badgers had initially come via breeding Daschund dogs, and was 'fostered against a combined farming and sporting background'.[44] While Murray was not an author or artist, she worked adeptly with media to draw wider public attention to her wildlife rescue work, and particularly to issues of badger persecution, ably assisted by her tamed orphaned female, Tikki (Fig. 5.2). By the mid-1960s, British politics of wildlife welfare was changing once more, as the LACS remobilised, the Hunt Saboteurs Association was founded, and a still resistant RSPCA was witnessing a resurgence of internal debates over whether to campaign against hunting.[45]

The *Mirror*'s expose and subsequent news campaign were excellently timed and had an immediate impact. Within two weeks the Conservative MP Frederick Burden (chair of the Parliamentary Animal Welfare Committee) had signalled his intention to draw up a Private Member's Bill extending specific legal protections to the badger.[46] The LACS started campaigning about badgers from 1965 onwards, running advertisements and providing commentary in further stories in the national press.[47] Naturalists including Ernest Neal wrote letters to newspapers and engaged in extensive correspondence with civil servants and MPs, arguing the case for legal protection.[48] Burden's Bill proposed outlawing badger hunting, but also creating a legal framework for the licenced control of 'rogue' animals, citing the 1951 Scott Henderson Committee.[49] The proposals were opposed by LACS as well as Burke, who argued that, 'In the hands of the ignorant, gas would promptly be used to exterminate badgers everywhere.'[50] Working with Ruth Murray and the Labour MP Donald Chapman, LACS proposed an alternative bill which would extend specific

Fig. 5.2 Ruth Murray and her pet badger Tikki. Source: *Daily/Sunday Mirror*, c. April 1970. Reproduced by permission of Trinity Mirror/Mirrorpix/Alamy Stock Photos

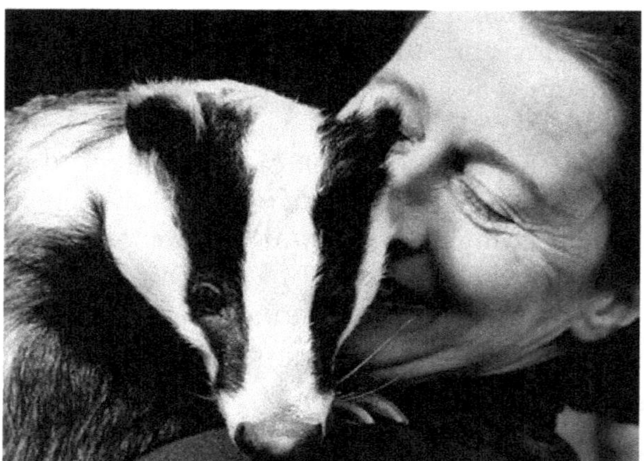

legal protection to badgers, building upon the earlier Protection of Animals (1911) and Birds (1954) Acts.[51] The scientists of PICL were consulted by colleagues in the Home Office, enabling them to disseminate their position on the 'helpfulness' of badgers and the illegality of (illicitly conducted) gassing, although they did not recommend going ahead with the proposed legislation.[52] The Home Office also consulted other government departments, including the Forestry Commission and NCC, reaching a consensus that while persecution was happening, the evidence that it was widespread was not strong enough, and that general legislation protecting all animals 'that are relatively harmless to economic interests' would be a better idea.[53] While neither the Burden nor the Chapman bills reached the stage of formal Parliamentary debate, badger protection acquired further advocates in both the Commons and Lords, including the naturalist and Labour MP Peter Hardy, and the 8th Earl of Arran—now best known for his championing of the decriminalisation of homosexuality in 1967.[54]

As well as following and observing badgers, Jane Ratcliffe had considerable expertise in not only rescuing the animals, but also in successfully returning them to the wild, 'translocating' individuals under threat. Via lectures, letters and membership of natural history societies, Ratcliffe convinced her fellow naturalists that badger persecution was a concern for them, leading to the formation of the earliest badger protection groups. She successfully mobilised her local WI behind her cause, putting forward a resolution eventually endorsed by the WI's AGM (representing about half a million women) in 1970. Ratcliffe lobbied civil servants and politicians via many letters, and like Murray, she took to the media, writing articles and giving interviews.[55] The campaign gathered support during 1971, as animal welfare groups and the Mammal Society organised symposia on the topic, while increasing numbers of conservation NGO's lent their support.[56] Once the issue had been raised from so many different angles, badger protection was increasingly and prominently covered across the national press—as an aspect of the wider blood-sports debate and as an issue in its own right (see Chap. 7, Fig. 7.1). By early 1972, further attempts were made at legislation: a wide-ranging bill proposed in the House of Lords by Lord Arran, based upon the earlier Chapman proposals; and a narrower, more pragmatic Private Members bill proposed in the Commons by Peter Hardy. Following extensive negotiations, Arran revised his proposals while Hardy dropped his, presenting Arran's Bill when it was brought to the Commons. The Badgers

Act was passed in July of 1973: bringing together specific protections for badgers with a legal framework for government to licence killing the animals.[57] As already explored in Chap. 2, the Badgers Act enabled MAFF's subsequent research and policy programmes. MAFF and Home Office officials had been opposed to the initial versions of Lord Arran's bill, but following the discovery of tuberculous badgers, they changed their position.[58] Jane Ratcliffe later noted that during 1972 the attitude of the Home Office, who until then had showed little interest, 'now became, at the least benevolently neutral, and almost verged on the helpful'.[59]

A final, critical shift within government took place within the NCC, responsible for scientific research and expert advice on environmental issues. Naturalists had been writing to NCC officers to voice their concerns about badgers since at least 1955, but NCC officers regarded the badger to be 'a relatively common animal', and therefore not a conservation concern. Correspondents were referred on to the RSPCA or UFAW.[60] Responding to reports of illegal badger gassing, NCC officers referred correspondents to MAFF's ICD. In 1965, the NCC remained unenthusiastic, replying to Norah Burke that they would only be interested in legislation to protect 'all mammals that are relatively harmless to economic interests', while stressing the need for 'selective control of badgers'.[61] The NCC maintained this stance, advising Home Office colleagues that badger protection was not required, and interpreting the early findings of Ernest Neal's badger survey to support their position, even though Neal himself disagreed.[62] However, once the NCC heard the news about bTB their attitude towards badgers changed, becoming much more protective. As well as expressing scepticism about the quality of MAFF's evidence, NCC officers were immediately concerned about the consequences for the animals once the news became public: 'The danger thereafter is that a widespread purge of Badgers will occur.'[63] In frequent contact with Harry Thompson of PICL, the NCC started lobbying to 'get involved with the steering of the research'.[64] While contributing to the early collaborative investigations explored in Chap. 2, the NCC was excluded from MAFF's formal 'Badger and Bovine TB' research programme. The strength of anxiety from officers about threats from farmers to form their own 'action groups' against badgers suggests that the NCC would by then have welcomed the proposed legislation (regulating and licencing culling).[65]

Between the mid-1950s and early 1970s, campaigners brought badger persecution to wider public attention and built an unlikely coalition on the animals' behalf, including tabloid journalists, the WI, naturalists, anti-blood-sports activists and politicians from both main parties. While the campaign initially gained ground, attempts to pass legislation foundered in a lack of cooperation from civil servants, and disagreements over whether and how government should act to control so-called 'rogue' badgers. The discovery of tuberculous badgers in Gloucestershire in 1971 acted as a catalyst, in which the urgent need to understand and act on a completely new problem also threatening badgers brought together wide-ranging ideals with pragmatic policy proposals, resulting in the passing of the Badgers Act in 1973. While the differences between the even wider range of actors involved with the new problem of badger/bTB did not disappear, this shared purpose created a spirit of collaboration which was to persist for the next few years. However, by the end of the 1970s, this coalition had dissolved, creating new fault lines of contention over badgers.

5.3 In Sickness and in Health? Caring for Tuberculous Badgers

As explored in Chap. 2, by 1975 MAFF had built a consensus around its new policy regime, in which the scientific uncertainties were investigated while the ministry implemented a 'humane' policy of gassing badgers in response to bTB in cattle. Naturalists and badger protection campaigners were integral to the formation of this consensus, as well as to MAFF's ability to understand the problem. Like the scientists of PICL, they had been following and learning about badgers for many decades prior to the animals' social transformation into disease vectors. Therefore, not only did Harry Thompson turn to his colleague Ernest Neal, but local ICD and SVS officers worked with the immediately available expertise of badger naturalists. The local 'badger recorder' of the Mammal Society, Arthur Killingley, helped MAFF officers with initial surveys in Gloucestershire, while the animal handling expertise of Jane Ratcliffe and Ruth Murray was drawn upon to help PICL scientists develop ethical practices for catching and killing the animals. Following the public disaster of the Scrubbet's Farm culling demonstration, badger advocates also agreed that gassing was a more acceptably humane culling technique than the previously deployed option of snaring. In turn, as we have seen, government officials in MAFF and the Home Office finally aligned themselves with the campaign for badger protection. This resulted in the passing of the dual-purpose Badgers Act in 1973, and an amendment to

Peter Hardy's Wild Creatures and Plants Protection Bill in 1975, legalising the use of Cymag on badgers. MAFF's new policies were initially supported by campaigners, with 'wildlife interests' formally contributing to the effort via the Consultative Panel, included Neal alongside representatives of bodies including the NCC, UFAW, the NFU and the Country Landowners Association. Soon after the new policy started to be implemented, this consensus started to fragment. Memories of illegal badger gassing resurfaced, alongside campaigners' fears that government bTB control would legitimise and encourage the still present threat of badger persecution. Following the lead of Ratcliffe and Murray, more badger groups were established, often growing out of local natural history societies and Wildlife Trusts.[66] Members of these groups studied the animals closely, providing more and more data about badger traces, while keeping a close eye on the activities of MAFF officers. They increasingly reported incidents where blocked, gassed setts had been dug out from the inside, and the reappearance of disoriented animals which had not been killed. Ruth Murray became even more critical of MAFF's policies, contesting the idea that badgers contracted bTB at all, and leading 'sit-in' protests against culling near her animal sanctuary on Dartmoor.[67]

In Somerset, a naturalist by the name of Eunice Overend (Fig. 5.3) was becoming involved in the issue. Like Ernest Neal, Overend had gained a biology degree, then worked as a teacher while continuing her studies of the natural history and geology of her area.[68] As well as writing her own monographs, Overend published several articles in the conservation journal *Oryx*, while her illustrations of badgers were used in others' publications. Her initial interventions in the debate drew upon her scientific training, whereby Overend argued that bTB in badgers was analogous to 'consumption' in humans, persisting in the body for many years before becoming 'active' and infectious, particularly when triggered by stress. Initially she supported MAFF's gassing policy but argued against the 'translocation' of persecuted animals (as practised by Ratcliffe and Murray) for this reason.[69] However, as MAFF's policy rolled out, Overend changed her mind. Having learned that this was no longer a localised problem, and observing the difficulties involved in fully clearing badgers from an area, she argued that culling policies were disrupting badger social groups. Prefiguring the 'perturbation' hypothesis of the ISG (see Chap. 6), she speculated that gassing was stressing the animals, making them move around more, their TB more active and spreading the disease.[70] Overend published a weekly natural history column in the Bristol-based

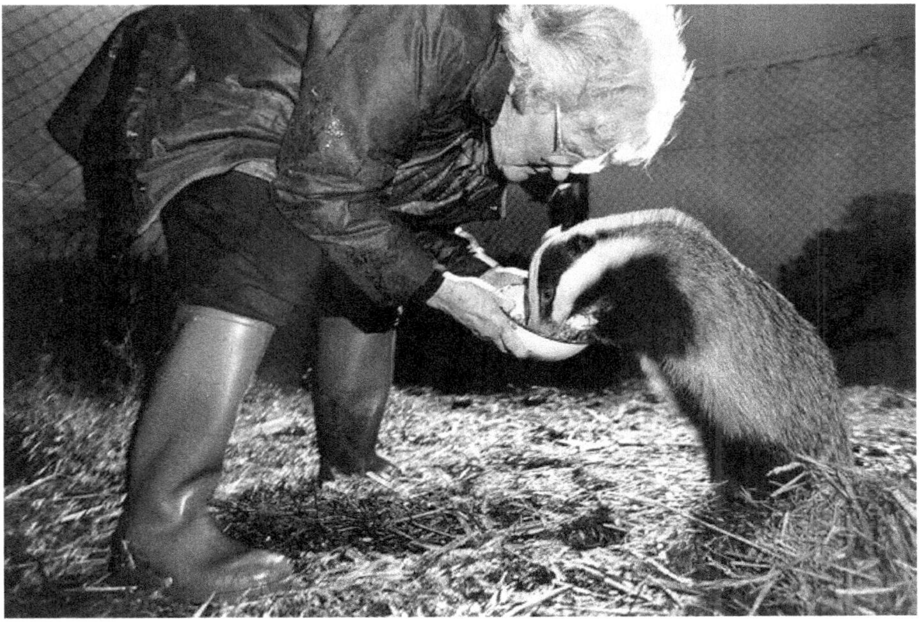

Fig. 5.3 Eunice Overend and unnamed badger, c. 1993. Photograph by Roger Bamber, reproduced by his permission with thanks

Western Daily Press, where she found an ally in the editor, Ian Beales, who launched a major anti-gassing campaign. Both Beales and Overend submitted evidence to the Zuckerman enquiry, which included a notorious meeting with Zuckerman where Overend brought along a dead badger as evidence of the persecution problem.[71]

These badger protection campaigns took place within and contributed to a wider context of accelerating shifts in animal and environment politics in Britain during the second half of the 1970s. As discussed over the previous two chapters, these changes broadly align with Agar's 'sea-change' in science–society relations, which involved increasing challenges of 'expert' views by 'lay' people and a new visibility for public controversy.[72]

After fifty years of internal controversy over wildlife welfare, in 1977 the RSPCA reformed its internal governance in favour of the society's membership, shortly afterwards adopting an anti-hunting stance and launching new campaigns.[73] Also, at the urging of members, the RSPCA conducted an internal review of the badger/bTB situation. The resulting report, published in 1979, continued to support MAFF's policy (including the link between bTB and badgers), but raised ethical and practical concerns about Cymag.[74] The RSPCA's lobbying of MAFF initiated the sequence of events which prompted Lord Zuckerman to recommend that the effects of cyanide on badgers be experimentally tested.[75] These changes in the RSPCA's position were driven by the emergence of newer, more radical forms of animal politics. Frustrated with the lack of progress achieved by 'traditional' campaigning methods and inspired by the tactics of anti-nuclear movements, activists had started directly disrupting hunts by misleading dogs, confronting hunters and generally getting in the way. These tactics were initiated in Devon in the late 1950s: the Hunt Saboteurs Association was founded by members of LACS in 1963, becoming active across the country by the mid-1970s. It was around this time that some radical hunt saboteurs abandoned non-violence, further forming new groups such as the Animal Liberation Front, committed to freeing animals held in laboratory science, factory and fur farming facilities.[76] The South West was rapidly becoming a 'hotspot' not just for bTB, but also for new forms of radical animal politics.

A similar change (from expert-led, semi-institutionalised campaigning towards citizen-led activism) was also taking place in conservation. Alongside the renewed enthusiasm for popular natural history and conservation volunteering, environmental politics as we recognise it today was also emerging. While international impetus came from the publication of *Silent Spring* (1964), the first Earth Day (1970), the founding of the UN Environment Programme (1972) and the initiation of the European Economic Community's (EEC) environmental policy programmes, British campaigns were also integral to this transition. The 1970s saw the founding of the British Green Party, the appearance of specialist environmental media and a plethora of 'grassroots' protest groups taking action on issues from nuclear energy to oil spills to mining to air pollution.[77] These changes were so profound that scholars of environmental politics refer to them as the transition between 'first' and 'second' waves of environmental protest—from conservation/protection to more radical and broader 'ecological environmentalism'.[78] Animal and environmental politics both saw the emergence of new philosophies overturning the anthropocentric arguments of earlier generations. The post-war consensus around 'animal welfare'—built by scientists working in laboratory biomedicine, UFAW, the RSPCA and MAFF's pest control researchers—was now being challenged. New zoocentric philosophies of 'animal rights' appeared, which argued that animal lives and freedoms should be protected for their own sake, rather than in the interests of people.[79] Similarly, the post-war conservation consensus—that government should protect natural resources and wildlife for anthropocentric reasons such as tourism or food production—was challenged by new 'eco-centric' philosophies arguing for the intrinsic value of the environment.[80] These shifts were reflected in the emergence of specialist environmental media: in Britain these ideas and concerns were also influenced by fictional portrayals reaching much wider audiences. The BBC's *Doomwatch* (1970–1972) used the device of a government science unit to explore environmental fears, while *Dr Who* storylines of this decade famously featured themes of environmental and nuclear destruction.[81] While these stories were primarily occupied with the disastrous consequences for humans of environmental damage, they also included themes of animal harm. Animal deaths acted as 'sentinels', warning of what was in store for humanity; while more complex stories critiqued traditional conservationism.[82] As British environmental and animal politics were undergoing similar processes of change, they were also converging.

The writing of Richard Adams expressed these developing concerns using children's fiction, deploying the long-standing form of the anthropomorphic animal story.[83] Like its nineteenth-century predecessor, *Black Beauty*, Adams's *Watership Down* (1972) used the voices of animal protagonists to draw attention to the cruelties inflicted upon animals by humans; like other, more grown-up animal tales such as Orwell's *Animal Farm* (1945), it introduced political elements into a dark tale of refugee rabbits. *Watership Down* is a long and complex book, with environmental destruction and animal persecution as central themes. Significantly for the badger/bTB debate, myxomatosis, gassing, snaring and hunting dogs all feature in the story, as agents of a uniformly hostile humanity.[84] Despite (or perhaps because of?) this grim content, *Watership Down* was a bestseller in the UK, and was made into a similarly popular animated film, which disturbs child and adult audiences alike to this day.[85] *Watership Down* had the effect of creating greater empathy for animals and drawing public attention to animal politics. Like Soper, Adams was an amateur naturalist who became increasingly disgusted at animal persecution and used his creativity to express these feelings and enrol others into his cause.[86] Through the 1970s, Adams used his position as a bestselling author to boost the visibility of animal politics, taking the position of President of the RSPCA from 1980 to 1982 (then resigning due to resistance to his campaigning stance).[87] While *Watership Down* was about rabbit myxomatosis, it reminded readers of the contested history of gassing at exactly the time that MAFF was introducing its usage in bTB control. This was in a wider context of campaigning that was rapidly joining the dots between 'pest control', chemical poisons, environmental damage, warfare and genocide.[88] In the film (released in 1978), a nightmarish sequence imagines (as Eileen Soper had) what it would be like to be gassed:

> 'Our warren ... destroyed.' 'Destroyed? How?' 'Men came ... filled in the burrows, couldn't get out. There was a strange sound ... hissing, the air turned bad, runs blocked with dead bodies ... we couldn't get out! Everything turned mad ... warren, us, boots, grass ... all pushed into the earth.'[89]

The consensus forged around MAFF's policy in 1975 had temporarily changed badgers' role from vermin/charismatic victim to that of the diseased, suffering animal patient, to be 'put out of its misery'. However, this was reliant upon an unstable congruence of the cultures of care involved with badger/bTB. As MAFF's culling policy was implemented this consensus crumbled, while as more people became involved, the badger's social role rapidly returned to that of victim, now additionally of 'The Men from the Ministry'.[90] Popular representations of environmental doom and persecuted animals combined with the first-hand accounts of naturalists, in a wider context of changing political and empathic relations with non-humans, to create a rapid backlash against culling.

Such negotiations—over how best to protect environments while also attending to the suffering and death of animals—were visible across British animal politics at the time. For example, during the late 1970s there was a parallel controversy over government culling of seals in the Scottish islands, carried out due to concerns over high seal populations and their impact on fish stocks. Resistance to seal culling started with naturalists closely following the animals themselves; and was built by shocking media coverage and unusual alliances, in this case between scientists, the World Wildlife Fund (WWF), Greenpeace, UFAW, the Seal Preservation Society and hunt saboteurs.[91] The seal culling debate rapidly shifted beyond the UK to an international focus: along the way it was mutually shaped by yet another animal controversy, about whaling. As with seals, whaling controversies involved rapidly shifting alliances between scientists, governments, food producers, and environmental and animal protection campaigners.[92] Environmental historian Robert Lambert argues that the seal protest movement would not have achieved its goals without 'the emergence of a new coalition of middle class protestors in Britain', comprising naturalists, animal welfare campaigners and 'people who on a weekend walk at the beach hope to see a seal, or just want to know that seals are out there doing well'.[93] Further evidence that relationships between British conservation and animal welfare agendas were changing comes from debates about otters. Like badgers, otters have symbolic resonances for British culture and landscapes: like badgers they were assigned conflicting social roles (pest/charismatic victim), like badgers they were hunted for sport, and like badgers they are known for asserting their own agency.[94] While the British otter debate has a longer history, it was during the 1960s that the plight of otters was brought to public attention via the empathic accounts of naturalists; and during the 1970s that conservationists and anti-hunting campaigners allied to gather evidence of the problem and lobby for change.[95] The conservationist and organic farming advocate Lord Peter Melchett described these changes as follows:

> The other change was global and was the gradual acceptance that they [conservationists] had to deal with animal welfare—it had been completely off-limits, they were nutcases, they were anti-hunting and shooting; they couldn't be spoken to. Completely different planet. But things like the campaign against whaling brought together WWF and the RSPCA and other groups such as Greenpeace and Friends of the Earth.[96]

While conservation and animal politics had converged, they had not aligned, as demonstrated by episodes such as the releases of American mink (an invasive species) from fur farms by animal liberation activists, and the assiduous attempts of conservationists and ICD officers to eradicate them.[97]

When Lord Zuckerman's 1980 review supported MAFF's position, the report provoked further public controversy and was fiercely contested by field biologists, naturalists and badger advocates. Despite dismissing campaigners' concerns over gassing, Zuckerman commissioned further research, which in turn undermined his and MAFF's position by finding that badgers were unusually resistant to cyanide poisoning. It was rapidly concluded that Cymag was not a humane way to cull badgers, forcing MAFF officers to rapidly explore other techniques. They drew upon early designs for a badger trap developed by Ruth Murray and previously shelved collaborative research between PICL and UFAW to develop a standardised trapping-then-shooting technique, in general use by 1982.

Meanwhile, the convergence of conservation, natural history, environmental and animal protection agendas had built into significant political pressure for change. The plethora of new naturalist and environmental groups that had sprung up over the previous decade allied with older scientific societies and conservation NGOs to form a new collective representative body, Wildlife Link, in 1979. They applied pressure on government and the NCC to formulate new, wide-ranging environmental protection legislation, contributing to the passing of the Wildlife and Countryside Act in 1981.[98] The Act included specific protections for a series of rare species; outlawed the use of snares, poisons and guns to kill a further list of animals; created further protections for landscapes; and formalised legislation around public rights of way.[99] Independently of the Zuckerman review process, the Act also significantly advanced the cause of badger protection by making it possible to prosecute those killing the animals without a licence. Following these developments, while MAFF's culling policy formally remained unchanged, the new trapping technique proved to still be more time consuming and expensive than gassing. Following the more critical Dunnett review, published in 1986, which drew MAFF's attention to these increased costs, badger culling was scaled back considerably.[100]

Following these victories, the heat went out of the public controversy, as evidenced by the decoupling of press coverage of badgers from that of bTB discussed in Chap. 7. Acknowledging the public exposure of the uncertainties around badger/bTB that the Zuckerman episode had exposed, MAFF further expanded their research programmes and the 1980s saw a fruitful period of collaborations between SVS and Agricultural Science Service researchers. Local badger groups continued to proliferate and in 1986 they formed the National Federation of Badger Groups (NFBG), broadly modelled on the organisation of the Wildlife Trusts. The NFBG refocused their attention on badger persecution, arguing that the existing legal framework still allowed for too many loopholes to prevent baiting and digging. NFBG and the Wildlife Trusts enrolled anti-hunting allies such as the LACS and Labour MPs in publicly lobbying Parliament over the need for further legal protections, adopting striking visual imagery to draw media attention (Fig. 5.4).[101] It was following the fall of Margaret Thatcher and the start of John Major's government that these campaigns paid off, with strengthened versions of the 1973 Badgers Act passing through Parliament in 1991 and 1992. While the legislation did not formally affect bTB policy, it created a further offence of disturbing the animals or their setts, putting

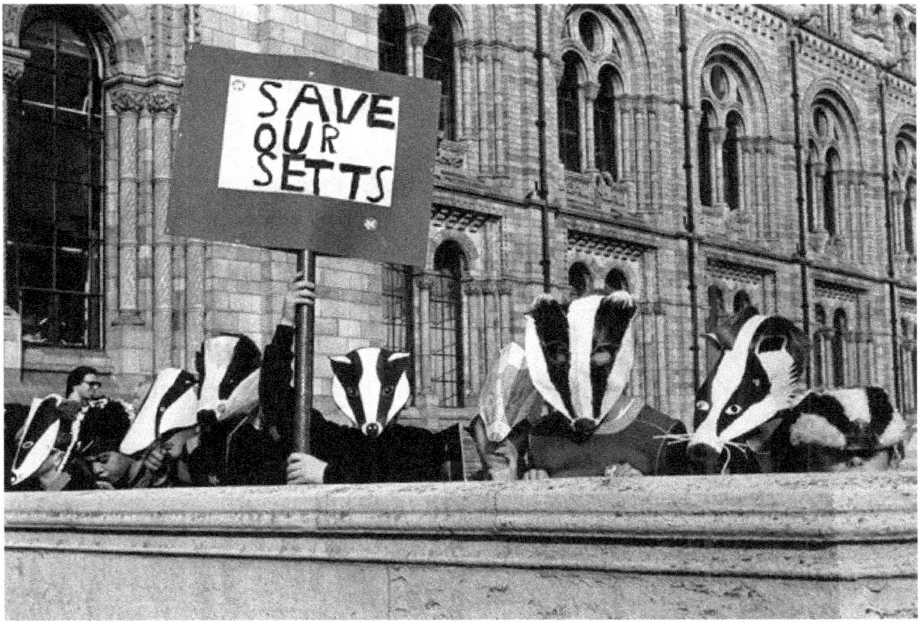

Fig. 5.4 Representatives of the UK Wildlife Trusts in Westminster, July 1990. Photographs supplied by Dr Gordon McGlone and reproduced with permission of the Wildlife Trusts

further barriers in the way of badger culling. In 1998, when the incoming Labour government rewarded ecologists' lobbying for government to undertake 'a proper experiment' on the effects of culling, the responses of badger advocates were mixed. While some welcomed the move, arguing that better evidence was needed to support policy, others, including the NFBG, were vociferously opposed to any further killing of badgers.[102] In the 1990s, the coalitions and cultures of care around badger protection, science and policy had shifted once again.

5.4 Care, Expertise and Gender in Badger Protection

The epistemic community forming around badger protection was deeply interpenetrated with animal health and particularly disease ecology, with key individuals such as Ernest Neal participating in all three and activists like Ruth Murray contributing to new knowledge about catching badgers.

Despite these interconnections, badger protection campaigners came into direct conflict with MAFF officers, scientists and veterinarians. One point of difference which has not yet been discussed is that of gender. While the government, veterinary and scientific stories of badger/bTB have been mostly male, in this chapter we have met many charismatic, strong-willed and highly intelligent women. This is a point of pride for present-day campaigners, who speak of 'three formidable ladies' in the badger protection movements of the past—Ruth Murray, Jane Ratcliffe and Eunice Overend.[103] In 2015, environmental journalist Patrick Barkham wrote candidly about Ratcliffe (his grandmother), describing the 'unconventional women' who 'changed our relationship with badgers for good'.[104] Barkham traces this lineage back to 1920s naturalist and hunter Frances Pitt, through Eileen Soper and Norah Burke, to Jane Ratcliffe and her mobilisation of the WI, Ruth Murray's confrontations with MAFF and Eunice Overend's questioning of culling.[105] Gender clearly played a role in these women's participation in the debate, particularly in interactions with journalists, who called them nicknames like Badger Woman and printed images of them cuddling badgers like babies.[106] It also surfaced in Lord Zuckerman's interactions with badger campaigners, before and after his report: as we have already seen, he had little respect for professional field biologists and ecologists, and even less for animal advocates.

In my view, to characterise this as a conflict between uncaring, patronising, male 'experts' and caring female lay activists (connected with animals and nature) would do all involved a considerable disservice. As we have seen, veterinarians and pest control scientists had well-developed cultures of care which helped them engage with the badger/bTB problem in a way that was consistent with their ethical working practices. Men such as Harry Thompson and Ernest Neal played significant roles in advocacy for badger welfare via their involvement in the Mammal Society and UFAW, while MPs and Lords were essential to the passing of protective legislation. While the badger protection movement was unusual in the number and prominence of women naturalists and campaigners, they were not alone. Ernest Neal's colleagues in the BBC, including Phil Drabble and the film-maker Eric Ashby, used their public positions to campaign passionately against badger gassing.[107] As the debate moved into the 1980s, naturalists such as Michael Clark, Martin Hancox and Richard Meyer became involved, sitting on the Consultative Panel, volunteering for the Mammal Society and writing new works of popular natural history, sharing their fascination for badgers.[108] The significance of women in the history of badger protection lies less in their presence or absence, but in their prominence—as charismatic advocates, network builders and trusted experts—and in the stories which campaigners tell now about their importance. This is part of a wider tradition of women in animal advocacy which goes back at least as far as the origins of British animal welfare societies in the 1820s and continues into the present day.[109]

While a full discussion of the complexities of gender, empathy and animal politics is far beyond the scope of this book, the gender dynamics of the epistemic community around badger advocacy at this time are so different that it would be remiss to ignore them. Why did women play such prominent roles here but not in the worlds of government veterinarians or pest control science? One part of the answer is obvious and relates to the broader story of professionalisation: while veterinary, scientific and civil service careers had started to open up to women by the 1960s and 1970s and was a matter of active struggle in wider society, this does not appear to have extended to government and academic veterinary and ecological experts.[110] Eunice Overend's biography provides a classic example of a woman struggling to access these professional networks: after gaining a biology degree from the University of Exeter, she was engaged by Sir Peter Scott to work as a curator at the pioneering Slimbridge nature reserve near Bristol. After a few years, she was forced to leave in order to help care for her sick mother in Frome, and then worked as a teacher while pursuing natural history studies in her spare time.[111] The filmmaker Maurice Tibbles described Overend admiringly as 'one of the last Victorian style naturalists': however, her biography suggests this may have been more through circumstance than choice.[112] There are further complexities around gender, animals and professionalisation: women's entry into many professions has often been enabled by them taking up 'caring' or 'empathic' (but also lower-status) specialisms such as small animal practice, or famously in the case of field biology, primatology.[113] While organisations like UFAW and the Mammal Society created crossover spaces where 'lay' naturalists and campaigners could collaborate with MAFF 'experts',[114] their participation was always highly contingent.

While this explains why women were absent from professional networks, it does not necessarily explain their presence and prominence in badger protection campaigning, or animal advocacy more generally, especially prior to the women's movements of the 1970s and 1980s. While it is tempting to reach for essentialist explanations involving women's emotionality and ability to connect with animals (and many have), better answers can be found by examining the intersections of gender, power, expertise and empathy. Badger protection campaigning developed within a long-standing British tradition of women's involvement in animal advocacy, whereby knowledge and networks have passed from one generation to another. As biology professionalised we can infer that, like Eunice Overend, more women were left in 'amateur' naturalist roles.[115] We know that the 'cultures of care' of animal welfare science constituted themselves as rational against the emotionality of animal advocates: it seems plausible that the same process was happening in the opposite direction.[116] Indeed, the vital skill of many of the campaigners discussed here has been their ability to mobilise their empathy for persecuted badgers, and to creatively communicate these feelings with wider audiences using writing, illustration, photography and film. While knowledge was important for badger advocates, just as it was to the pest control scientists, valid knowledge could be derived from a wider range of sources, including personal experience of working closely with animals.[117] This helps to explain the vociferous conflict between Lord Zuckerman and Ruth Murray—Murray had become an authoritative expert within the badger protection community and had argued for many years that badgers did not get bTB. Zuckerman, in his role as a government-appointed scientist and 'medical man', could not do otherwise than contest this and undermine the legitimacy of Murray's claims.

This analysis of gender and professionalisation can be further applied to help us understand the changing relationships between badger advocates, scientists and MAFF officers as bTB policy developed through the 1970s. To do this, we also need to bring in an idea from policy studies—the (fuzzy and contested) distinction between lobby/interest groups able to influence government decisions ('insiders') and those with relatively little leverage or power (outsiders)—the NFU is considered to be a classic 'insider'.[118] During the first few 'crisis' years, government knew very little about badgers and so enrolled help from people who did: naturalists and badger advocates including Neal, Murray and Ratcliffe. The partnership provided MAFF with critical scientific knowledge as well as on-the-ground experience of handling the animals; in turn the badger advocates received help in their long-term aim of passing badger protection laws. This explains how Ruth Murray was able to access the 1973 culling demonstration and obtain enough evidence to mount a legal case against MAFF. Following these events, Murray became an 'outsider'—there is no further evidence of collaborative research and she used the legal case to draw further media attention to badgers. While MAFF's 1975 policy programme attempted to maintain good relations with 'wildlife interests' via the Consultative Panel, the early consensus rapidly collapsed as problems with gassing became evident, alongside the Panel's lack of power to shape policy. Murray contested the link between badgers and bTB, refused to allow Ministry officials access to her animal sanctuary, where over 200 animals were being kept at one point, and refused to share information with allies, as Ernest Neal put it, 'for reasons of her own'.[119] While (Zuckerman aside) MAFF's archival correspondence is scrupulously polite about Ruth Murray, she was clearly not easy to work with. MAFF's epistemic communities rapidly grew 'apart from those clustered around' the issue of badger protection, to create the oppositional atmosphere that Zuckerman found himself mired in. Gender features in the inside–outside model for bTB precisely because the professionals dealing with the problem were mostly men, while more of the 'lay experts' (naturalists and badger advocates) were women. This gendered pattern of inside–outside influence (where the 'outsider's' status as a woman is used to further undermine her influence) has actually been seen before—in the early period of policy formation around bTB control during the early twentieth century.[120]

5.5 Cultures of Caring for and with Animals

In contrast to the animal health and disease ecology epistemic communities, explored in Chaps. 3 and 4, the badger protection epistemic community did not build a single culture of care around which their working practices could stabilise. Instead there were ongoing negotiations between several intersecting cultures of care, which I will now outline. First, we have *conservation care*, also manifested in popular natural history. Conservationists tend to be primarily concerned with care for populations, ecosystems and landscapes. Like MAFF's pest control scientists, they were also deeply concerned with 'good science', but ultimately gave a higher priority to protecting environments. While post-war conservationists made their case for government support via anthropocentric 'national interests', by the 1960s (unlike MAFF's ecologists or veterinarians), conservationists had become less concerned about economic or agricultural productivity—the 'logics of cost'. Balancing and compromising between these priorities often creates what Van Dooren has termed the 'violent care' of conservation—the willingness and sometimes enthusiasm to sacrifice the lives of individuals for the sake of populations, particularly valued species or ecosystems.[121] Examples would include conservationist support for the Scottish seal culls discussed above, or ongoing commitments to eradicate invasive species. Field experience and observation are critical components of conservation care. It was field-based accounts of problems with gassing, often coming from 'lay' naturalists, which were the primary driver of the collapse of the early 1970s culling consensus, and which were roundly dismissed (but ultimately vindicated) by the Zuckerman review. Second, there is *animal welfare care*, which critically informs laboratory animal science, and which we have already encountered through the pest control scientists and UFAW of the previous chapter. Like veterinarians, who played key roles in the formation of this culture, animal welfare actors prioritise preventing animal suffering over preserving life, making humane killing a critical priority. As we have seen, animal welfare tends to be expert-led and made 'good science' a priority through which 'skilled care' can be delivered and vice versa.[122] The 1951 Scott Henderson Committee on wildlife welfare was framed in these terms and was mobilised by MAFF to foster the early consensus on badger gassing. From the 1970s onwards, animal welfare partly constituted itself as 'good science' in opposition to what participants saw as the 'logics of the heart' of animal rights activists.[123]

This leads us to the third and most politically contentious of the cultures of care involved in badger protection—*animal rights care*. This decentres older anthropocentric reasons for caring about animals, meaning that logics of cost rapidly fade into the background and are sometimes actively challenged (for example when damaging property during protests). Instead, developing animal rights cultures tried to imagine, empathise with and act in the interests of animals themselves. The work of Eileen Soper and Richard Adams demonstrates attempts to make this leap: through writing and visual imagery, they invited the reader to imagine experiencing the world as an animal, albeit an anthropomorphised one, including their pain and fear. Animal rights' empathic stance means that a key goal of advocates is to prevent animal suffering, just as animal welfare does. However, unlike the ultimately anthropocentric stance of animal welfare (which sees humans as benevolently responsible for animals), animal rights seeks to create a moral equivalence between human and animal life. Therefore animals should be granted the same fundamental rights as humans, such as the right to freedom: hence 'animal liberation'. This equivalence extends to the right to life, as articulated in human medical ethics. It also lies at the heart of animal rights activists to move beyond non-violent protest into more radical acts such as animal releases, sabotage and at times symbolic or physical threats to their opponents.[124] During the 1970s, the broader culture of care around animal rights was constituting itself alongside the rapidly developing badger/bTB debate. While badger protection campaigners were initially focused on the suffering and killing of the animals during practices of baiting, hunting and digging, the rapid shift to anti-gassing refocused campaigns onto state-sponsored killing. As articulated by *Watership Down*, the cultural resonances of 'gassing' for a society where both World Wars and the Holocaust were still in living memory further drove resistance to MAFF's policies. Badger campaigning also changed in line with the turn to animal rights, moving from 'insider' tactics (network building, lobbying and letter writing, collaborations with MAFF) towards self-consciously 'outsider' actions (prosecuting the Farming Minister, emotive demonstrations). While we know that Ruth Murray worked with the LACS and that there were early public protests about badger gassing on Dartmoor, the co-location of anti-hunting and badger protection campaigning in the South West of England bears much more investigation (Fig. 5.5).

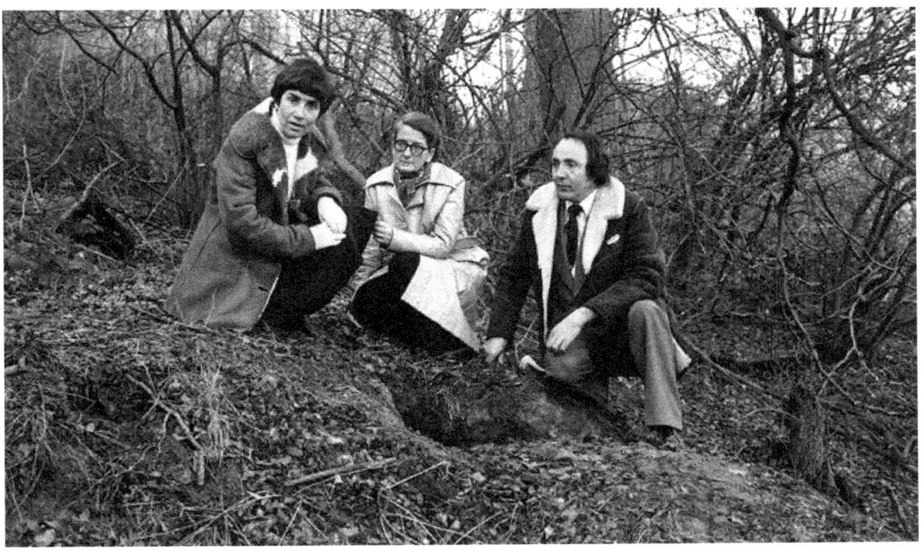

Fig. 5.5 Anti-badger gassing activists in the Cotswolds, 1976. Photograph by Jane Bown for *The Observer*, reproduced by permission of Guardian News and Media Ltd

The analysis laid out over Chaps. 3, 4 and 5—of the shifting social roles, traces and cultures of care around badger/TB—would be incomplete without a closer examination of the agency of these animals. How was the agency of badgers understood and depicted by those involved in researching, campaigning and advocating on their behalf? While *conservation care*, following the determined lead of Elton and the Nature State, was primarily driven by care for populations and ecosystems, it also involved a deep emotional, aesthetic and embodied interest in 'the field'. This comprised a deep appreciation of experiential knowledge of landscapes; the belief that to properly study wildlife, the naturalist must work with the contingency, freedom and agency of animals; and a pragmatic recognition of the violent, messy, unhuman nature of animal lives and deaths. Eunice Overend provided an excellent example of this culture of care, as seen in Fig. 5.3. Unlike the more popular trope of a human cuddling a badger, often a juvenile (Fig. 5.1), this photograph shows an active negotiation between human and animal. When asked about her involvement in 'badger protection' in a life history interview, her response was sharp: 'I wasn't doing it to protect badgers as such, 'cos they can easily protect themselves, you see. Just try catching one, you'll see! [laughs].'[125] Overend had a keen appreciation for the agency of these animals and had little patience for campaigners who sought to gain public sympathy by eliding badgers' less appealing traits. While *animal welfare care* is similarly pragmatic about animal life and death, the commitment to creating 'good science' and strong evidence to leverage policy change meant that overt recognitions of animal agency were not possible at the time, particularly in scientific articles and other formal documents. However, in practice, good relationships and emotional connections between researchers and animal participants can often be critical to new theoretical insights and rigorous findings.[126] This sometimes led to a contradictory approach to animal agency, as evidenced in the writings and other outputs of the pest control scientists. For example, Harry Thompson (head of the PICL Mammals group and later president of UFAW) wrote, 'The basic attraction of wild animals is the *aesthetic pleasure* to be derived from watching and hearing them pursuing their own affairs without interference' (my emphasis).[127] Pest control science seemed to formally practice *animal welfare care*, while also informally practicing *conservation care*. *Animal rights care*, which was emerging at this time, also seems to have had a deeply contradictory approach to animal agency. On the one hand, the underlying philosophical position is all about animal agency and the political attempt to gain recognition for animal rights. Similarly, the empathic stance of animal rights requires and creatively persuades people to imagine the agency and lived experiences of other animals. Campaigning for 'badger protection' in a way that caught the attention of mass media and such a diverse range of allies involved positioning of the animals as powerless victims, pretty much by definition without agency. The gendered media imagery of 'badger women' and depictions of the animals being cuddled by humans (Fig. 5.1) was highly effective in creating public sympathy and political momentum. However, these forms of representation, in which human campaigners 'speak for' animal victims, came at the expense of any recognition of badger agency, as well as the authority of the women.[128] This agency, manifested in badgers' insistence on defending themselves when attacked, eating awkward things and not staying where they were put, could therefore be easily linked to the older social role of the Bad Badger.

As we have traced through this chapter, between 1965 and 1995, the politics of care in badger advocacy has shifted back and forth, reflecting changes in what was known about badgers; in the three cultures of care explored through the middle section of this book; in relationships between science and society; and in broader political attitudes to animals and the environment. To summarise, over this period there were four key stages in the debate over badgers and bTB:

Stage One: Creating concern. Naturalists including Ernest Neal, Eileen Soper and Norah Burke drew media, public and political attention to badgers through their popular natural history research, writing and illustration, while campaigners Ruth Murray and Jane Ratcliffe built a diverse coalition of support for badger protection.

Stage Two: Tuberculous badgers. MAFF veterinarians' unanticipated discovery of tuberculous badgers in Gloucestershire connected the previously unrelated worlds of animal health policy and badger protection. It required Ministry officials to enrol the help of naturalists and badger advocates to urgently investigate the previously unknown phenomenon of tuberculous badgers. As the scale of the problem became apparent, MAFF formed a rapid consensus with policy 'insiders'—that rapid action was required in the form of badger culling, best delivered via gassing with Cymag.

Stage Three: Anti-gassing. Memories of 'gassing' (of people during the Holocaust, as well as of badgers being persecuted by humans) resurfaced and combined with naturalists' accounts that Cymag was not working properly in the new badger culling policy. This led to a rapid collapse of MAFF's policy consensus and protests, driven in part by the adjacent emergence of new social movements around environmental issues and animal rights. The controversy was then inflamed by the Zuckerman review, intended to be an 'objective look at the problem'.

Stage Four: Badger protection. Badger gassing was withdrawn following the vindication of campaigners' concerns by research at Porton Down. This victory, combined with wider wildlife protection legislation, resulted in a shift in focus in badger campaigning back to persecution and protection, with further gains during the early 1990s.

Through the 1960s and 1970s, animal advocates worked to create badger persecution as an issue of concern in the wider public sphere, building an extraordinarily diverse coalition in support of helping the animals. Considering the broader political, economic and cultural changes that Britain underwent during this period, it is now easier to see how Lord Zuckerman, product and producer of the post-war, expert-led science–state coalitions which gave rise to MAFF's initial approach to bTB, was so surprised by the fierce contestation of his review. Not only had the sciences of mammal field biology and ecology changed as they explored the complexities of wildlife disease ecology, but British societal attitudes to non-human animals and environments were undergoing radical change. I argue that these shifts were woven into what historian Jon Agar argues was a global 'sea-change' in the relationship between science and society over the 'long 1960s'. Crucial aspects of this change included the formation of the modern environmental sciences, a new public visibility for scientific disagreements, the rise of new social movements, and a change in the balance of power between 'experts' and 'lay' people.[129] This newly public iteration of Britain's long-standing 'badger debate' was driven by and contributed to major changes in how people imagined and related to animals, bringing about a new era of animal politics in the process.

Notes

1. Hill, 'Perspectives of "Conflict" at the Wildlife–Agriculture Boundary'; Crowley, Hinchliffe and McDonald, 'Conflict in Invasive Species Management'.
2. Scott Henderson, 'Report of the Committee on Cruelty to Wild Animals. Cmd 8266, June 1951', para. 327.

3. For epistemic communities see Meyer and Molyneux-Hodgson, 'Introduction'; Dunlop, 'Epistemic Communities'. For cultures of care see Davies et al., 'Science, Culture, and Care in Laboratory Animal Research'.
4. Cassidy, 'Badger–Human Conflict'.
5. RSPCA is the Royal Society for Protection of Animals, founded in 1824. RSPB is the Royal Society for the Protection of Birds, founded in 1889. For the early relationships between these organisations, see Sheail, *Nature in Trust*, chap. 1; Evans, *A History of Nature Conservation in Britain*, chap. 3; Griffin, *Blood Sport.*
6. Sheail, *Nature in Trust*, 11.
7. Griffin, *Blood Sport*, 174.
8. Griffin, *Blood Sport*, 174; Bartrip, *Myxomatosis*, 36–43.
9. Sheail, *Nature in Trust*, 58–67; Sands, *Wildlife in Trust*, 1–18.
10. Examples include the art of Paul Nash and Eric Ravillous; of particular relevance to badgers is Edward Thomas's poem 'The Combe' (1914); for early twentieth-century environmental aesthetics see Peter Coates, David Moon and Paul Warde, eds, *Local Places, Global Processes: Histories of Environmental Change in Britain and Beyond* (Oxford: Windgather Press, 2016).
11. Griffin, *Blood Sport*, 180–2; Daniel Allen, Charles Watkins and David Matless, '"An Incredibly Vile Sport": Campaigns against Otter Hunting in Britain, 1900–1939', *Rural History* 27(1) (April 2016): 79–101.
12. Matthew Hilton et al., *The Politics of Expertise: How NGOs Shaped Modern Britain* (Oxford: Oxford University Press, 2013); Glenda Sluga, *Internationalism in the Age of Nationalism* (University of Pennsylvania Press, 2013).
13. For broader debates around the establishment of the post-war British state, particularly relating to the welfare state and post-war military/scientific infrastructures, see Edgerton, *Warfare State.*
14. Sheail, *Nature in Trust*; Sheail, 'The Management of Wildlife and Amenity'; Evans, *A History of Nature Conservation in Britain.*
15. For the 'Nature State', see Hardenberg et al., *The Nature State.*
16. Sheail, *Nature in Trust*; Kelly, 'Conventional Thinking and the Fragile Birth of the Nature State in Post-War Britain'.
17. Meyer, 'Caring for Weak Ties'; Shuttleworth, 'Old Weather'.
18. Sean Nixon, 'Trouble at the National Trust: Post-War Recreation, the Benson Report and the Rebuilding of a Conservation Organization in the 1960s', *Twentieth Century British History* 26(4) (October 2015): 529–50; Andrew J. P. Flack, 'Lions Loose on a Gentleman's Lawn: Animality, Authenticity and Automobility in the Emergence of the English Safari Park', *Journal of Historical Geography* 54 (2016): 38–49.

19. Peter Marren, *The New Naturalists: Half a Century of British Natural History* (London: HarperCollins, 1995); Coates, Moon and Warde, *Local Places, Global Processes.*
20. Gregg Mitman, *Reel Nature: America's Romance with Wildlife on Film* (Cambridge, MA: Harvard University Press, 1999); Davies, 'Science, Observation and Entertainment'; Jean-Baptiste Gouyon, 'From Kearton to Attenborough: Fashioning the Telenaturalist's Identity', *History of Science* 49.1(162) (2011): 39–74; Gouyon, 'The BBC Natural History Unit'.
21. Tichelar, 'Putting Animals into Politics'.
22. The committee also included the biologist Peter Medawar, a member of UFAW, and Frances Pitt, a naturalist who wrote about badgers and was vice president of the pro-hunting Field Sports Society; see Griffin, *Blood Sport*; Bartrip, 'Myxomatosis in 1950s Britain'; Bartrip, *Myxomatosis*; Tichelar, 'Putting Animals into Politics', 227; Tichelar, *The History of Opposition to Blood Sports in Twentieth Century England*. The committee's report was later cited by the 2000 Burns Inquiry into Hunting with Dogs, which resulted in the banning of fox hunting in the UK; see Lord Burns et al., 'Report of Committee of Inquiry into Hunting with Dogs in England & Wales' (London: HMSO, 9 June 2000).
23. Evans, *A History of Nature Conservation in Britain*, 102–3.
24. Kroll, 'The "Silent Springs" of Rachel Carson'; Clark, 'Pesticides, Pollution and the UK's Silent Spring, 1963–1964'.
25. Sands, *Wildlife in Trust*, 49–68.
26. Neal, *The Badger*. Neal was not the first twentieth-century naturalist to follow badgers, although he was the first to study them systematically. A notable predecessor was Frances Pitt (1888–1964), photographer, illustrator, author and member of the Scott Henderson committee. See Frances Pitt, 'The Badger—A Creature of the Night', in *Woodland Creatures: Being Some Wild Life Studies* (London: G. Allen & Unwin Ltd, 1922), 11–35; Frances Pitt, *Diana, My Badger: Being the Story of Diana the Badger, her sister Jemima, and Squire Brock Whom Diana met in the Woods*, The Library of Animal Friends, 10 (London: Arrowsmith, 1929).
27. For expert–lay relationships in the field sciences, see, e.g. Meyer, 'Caring for Weak Ties'; Riesch and Potter, 'Citizen Science as Seen by Scientists'; Shuttleworth, 'Old Weather'.
28. Neal's autobiography is the best source of information on his life and work: Ernest G. Neal, *The Badger Man* (Ely: Providence Press, 1994).
29. For more on the *New Naturalists*, their role in British natural history and the significance of *The Badger*, see Marren, *The New Naturalists. The Badger* was published as a mass-print Pelican paperback in 1958, staying in print until 1977. When Collins dropped the title, Neal continued revis-

ing the work, eventually co-authoring with MAFF scientists: Ernest G. Neal and Chris Cheeseman, *Badgers* (London: A&D Poyser, 1996), 197. It is still cited by field biologists today, e.g. Judge et al., 'Abundance of Badgers (Meles Meles) in England and Wales'.

30. Peter Scott and Desmond Hawkins, 'Badgers', *The Radio Times* (BBC Television, 12 November 1954); Bale, 'Badger Watch'. See Neal, *The Badger Man*, 143–61; Marren, *The New Naturalists*; Gail Davies, 'Networks of Nature: Stories of Natural History Film-Making at the BBC' (PhD, University of London, 1998), 109–10; and BBC listings archive *Genome* http://genome.ch.bbc.co.uk/ for Neal's BBC contributions.
31. Neal, 'The National Badger Survey'; Neal, *The Badger Man*, 161–69.
32. For knowledge brokers, see Meyer, 'The Rise of the Knowledge Broker'.
33. Neal, 'The National Badger Survey'; E. D. Clements, Ernest G. Neal and D. W. Yalden, 'The National Badger Sett Survey', *Mammal Review* 18(1) (1 March 1988): 1–9; John R. Flowerdew, 'Advances in the Conservation of British Mammals, 1954–2004: 50 Years of Progress with The Mammal Society', *Mammal Review* 34(3) (July 2004): 169–210.
34. Eileen Alice Soper, *When Badgers Wake/Written and Illustrated by Eileen A. Soper* (London: Routledge & Kegan Paul, 1955); Eileen Alice Soper, *Eileen Soper's Book of Badgers* (London: Constable and Robinson, 1992), 7. See also Soper's personal diaries, published online at: https://badger-diaries.wordpress.com/.
35. Soper, *Eileen Soper's Book of Badgers*, 35.
36. See Sect. 4.3.
37. Soper, *Eileen Soper's Book of Badgers*, 35.
38. Soper, *Eileen Soper's Book of Badgers*, 51.
39. E.g. Edna Jane Ratcliffe, *Through the Badger Gate. The Story of Badgers, their Persecution and Protection, and of a Cub Reared and Returned to the Wild* (London: Bell, 1974), 8; Michael Clark, *Badgers/Michael Clark ; with Illustrations by the Author* (London: Whittet, 1988), 7–8; Soper, *When Badgers Wake*.
40. Norah Burke, *King Todd: The True Story of a Wild Badger; and of the Deer, Foxes, and Other Animals in the Forest Where He Lived/Illustrated by D.J. Watkins-Pitchford* (London: Putnam, 1963).
41. Wickham Malins, *Bully & the Badger: The Remarkable Story of a Badger Cub Fostered by a Bull Terrier and Eventually Returned to the Wild. With Drawings by Eileen A. Soper; Foreword by Ernest G. Neal* (London: Robert Yeatman, 1974); Ratcliffe, *Through the Badger Gate*; Peter Hardy, *A Lifetime of Badgers* (Newton Abbot: David and Charles, 1975); Phil Drabble, *No Badgers in My Wood; Illustrations by Eileen A. Soper* (London: Joseph, 1979).

42. Anon., 'Clearance Societies asked to spare the badger', *Guardian*, 8 February 1962, 6; R. Fitter, 'Beastly to Badgers', *Observer*, 28 July 1963, 26; R. Nye, 'In the night forest (book review)', *Guardian*, 29 November 1963, 14. Fitter was a key figure in British conservation, closely involved with the UK Council for Nature, the IUCN and the NGO Flora and Fauna International: Richard Fitter and Jacqui Morris, 'The Fauna and Flora Preservation Society—Conserving Wildlife for 90 Years', *Journal of Biological Education* 27(2) (1 June 1993): 103–6.
43. J. Pilger, 'The persecution of Badger Brock', *Daily Mirror*, 17 November 1964, 16–17. Pilger went on to make his name at the *Mirror* reporting on the Vietnam War and became a famous left-wing journalist, documentary maker and campaigner. After this story, Pilger largely focused on human politics.
44. Murray, 'Live Trapping of Badgers, Their Removal, Release and Rehabilitation in a New Area', 86. Daschunds (also known as sausage dogs) were traditionally bred for small-game and badger hunting—the name originates from the German for badger (*dachs*).
45. Griffin, *Blood Sport*, 192; anon., 'Fox-hunting "cruel, barbaric and degrading": Hecklers in full cry at RSPCA meeting', *Guardian*, 16 June 1960, 5; G. Moorhouse, 'The Hunt at Bay', *Guardian*, 30 December 1964, 5.
46. B. Tay, 'MP acts to end badger slaughter', *Daily Mirror*, 30 November 1964, 11.
47. Anon., 'The Horror of Badger Digging—League against Cruel Sports', *Daily Mail*, 18 December 1965, 12; anon., 'Support For Law against Badger "Digs"', *Daily Telegraph*, 18 January 1965, 17.
48. E. Neal, 'Protecting the Badger in Britain', *Times*, 19 April 1965, 10; N. Burke, 'EVIDENCE SHOWING WILD ANIMALS TO BE USEFUL ANIMALS. Letter to NCC', 7 December 1964, NA FT 1/59.
49. Henderson, 'Report of the Committee on Cruelty to Wild Animals', para. 327.
50. LACS, 'Letter: The Badger's Case for Protection'; N. Burke, 'Letter: Gas Risks', both *Daily Telegraph*, 17 February 1965.
51. D. Chapman, 'Letter to Right Hon Roy Jenkins re Bill for Protection of the Badger and enclosures', 6 Oct. 1966, NA HO 2085/40.
52. P. E. Baker (Home Office), 'Letter to H.V. Thompson', 16 July 1965 NA HO 285/39. Baker also wrote to P. F. Garthwaite of the Forestry Commission regarding their publications about 'rogue' badgers; King, 'The Badger Gate'.
53. M. Blackmore (NCC), 'Letter to Norah Burke', 2 February 1965, NA FT 1/59; see also H. V. Thompson (PICL), 'Letter to P. Beedle (HO)', 28 February 1966, NA HO 285/39.

54. Lord Arran started working on badger protection from 1966 (HL Deb 4 July 1966 vol. 275 c927), while Hardy was involved from 1970 (e.g. HC Deb 8 December 1970 vol. 808 c225).
55. Ratcliffe, *Through the Badger Gate*, 97–119.
56. Animal Defence Society Badger Symposium, 27 December 1971, in ZUEA S2 PUB 425; E. G. Neal (chair), *National Badger Survey Annual Conference*, 6–8 Oct. 1972, in NA FT 1/60; Anon., 'Licence to Kill Badgers Urged', *Daily Telegraph*, 29 November 1971, 10.
57. Accounts of the negotiations around the 1973 Badgers Act can be found in Ratcliffe, *Through the Badger Gate*, 111–19; Hardy, *A Lifetime of Badgers*, 137–40; Neal, *The Badger Man*, 215–17.
58. V. H. Bath, 'Memo: Badgers Bill', 4 December 1972; NA FT 1/60.
59. Ratcliffe, *Through the Badger Gate*, 114.
60. R. J. Elliot (NCC), 'Letter to Mrs. E.J. Wilson', 18 November 1955; I. Prest, 'Letter to Mrs. S. Thompson', 15 February 1963, both in NA FT 1/59.
61. M. Blackmore (NCC), 'Letter to Miss Norah Burke', 2 February 1965. NA FT 1/59.
62. J. F. D. Frazer, 'Memo: Minister's case—badger protection', 14 June 1971; E. G. Neal, 'Letter to Marcus Kimball, Working Party on Mammalian Predator Control', 12 July 1971. NA FT 1/59.
63. J. W. Blackwood (NCC), 'Note for the File: Badgers and Bovine TB Investigation', 27 August 1971, NA FT 41/88.
64. D. A. Cadwaller, 'Note for the File: Badgers and Bovine TB in Gloucestershire', 23 March 1972, NA FT 41/88.
65. D. A. Cadwaller, 'Memo, Badgers—West Penwith', 13 April 1973, NA FT41/88.
66. Ratcliffe, *Through the Badger Gate*, 105–10; Sands, *Wildlife in Trust*, 112.
67. Zuckerman, 'Badgers, Cattle and Tuberculosis', 9–10.
68. Elspeth Huxley, *Peter Scott: Painter and Naturalist* (London: Faber and Faber, 1993), 165; Eunice D. Overend, *Oral History Recording of an Interview with Eunice Overend*, oral history recording, home in Frome (Taunton, 2012), ADQP/1/2/45, Somerset Heritage Centre; Pauline Kidner, *Tribute to Eunice Overend by Pauline Kidner, Secret World Wildlife Rescue—Badger Trust Conference*, 2016; anon., 'Eunice Overend—Biology teacher and maverick wildlife campaigner', *The Times*, 10 January 2017, 52.
69. Eunice D. Overend, 'T.B. IN CATTLE AND BADGERS', November 23, 1975, *The Gazette (Dursley)*, in NA MAF 109/384, item 82; Eunice D. Overend, 'TB in British Badgers', *Oryx* 13(3) (February 1976): 240–42.

70. Overend, 'Badgers and TB—Does Gassing Spread the Disease?'; Robert W. Howard and Eunice D. Overend, *Badgers without Bias: An Objective Look at the Controversy about Tuberculosis in Badgers and Cattle/by Robert W. Howard; with Decorations by Eunice D. Overend* (Bristol: Abson in association with Avon Wildlife Trust, 1981); Overend, *Oral History Recording of an Interview with Eunice Overend.*
71. I. Beales, 'The watchdogs meet tomorrow, as the gassing goes on', 21 June 1979, *Western Daily Press*, in ZUEA S2 PUBS 425.
72. Agar, 'Transition'.
73. Griffin, *Blood Sport*, 192–93; Tichelar, *The History of Opposition to Blood Sports in Twentieth Century England*, 50–69.
74. RSPCA Wild Animals Advisory Committee, 'Badgers and Bovine Tuberculosis : The Case for Further Investigation'.
75. See Sec. 3.3.
76. Tichelar, *The History of Opposition to Blood Sports in Twentieth Century England*, 150.
77. Evans, *A History of Nature Conservation in Britain*, chap. 7; M. Bell and John Sheail, 'Experts, Publics and the Environment in the UK: Twentieth-Century Translations', *Journal of Historical Geography* 31(3) (2005): 496–512; Wilson, 'The British Environmental Movement', chap. 5.
78. A third wave, 'grassroots environmentalism', emerged in the 1990s—see Griggs and Howarth, 'Protest Movements, Environmental Activism and Environmentalism in the United Kingdom'.
79. Kean, *Animal Rights*; Garner, *Animals, Politics and Morality.*
80. Griggs and Howarth, 'Protest Movements, Environmental Activism and Environmentalism in the United Kingdom'.
81. Dolly Jorgensen, 'A Blueprint for Destruction: Eco-Activism in Doctor Who during the 1970s', *Ecozon@: European Journal of Literature, Culture and Environment* 3(2) (2012): 11–26; Wilson, 'The British Environmental Movement', 263–82; Lisa Garforth, *Green Utopias: Environmental Hope Before and After Nature* (Cambridge: Polity Press, 2017).
82. For animal 'sentinels' see Frédéric Keck, 'Feeding Sentinels: Logics of Care and Biosecurity in Farms and Labs', *BioSocieties* 10(2) (2015): 162–76; for *Dr Who* and conservation, see Jorgensen, 'A Blueprint for Destruction', 18–21.
83. Cosslett, *Talking Animals in British Children's Fiction, 1786–1914.*
84. Richard Adams, *Watership Down* (London: Rex Collings Ltd, 1972). His other books from this decade, *Shardik* (1974) and *The Plague Dogs* (1977), dealt with human slavery (and a totem bear) and dogs escaping from an animal research facility, respectively.
85. Amy Duncan, 'Channel 5 Horrifies Viewers by Showing Watership Down on Easter Sunday (Again)', *Metro*, 16 April 2017.

86. Alison Flood, 'Watership Down Author Richard Adams: I Just Can't Do Humans', *The Guardian*, 4 January 2015, sec. Books. For animals, empathy and creativity, see Barbara Hardy Beierl, 'The Sympathetic Imagination and the Human–Animal Bond: Fostering Empathy through Reading Imaginative Literature', *Anthrozoös* 21(3) (1 September 2008): 213–20; J. Keri Cronin, *Art for Animals: Visual Culture and Animal Advocacy, 1870–1914* (Pennsylvania: Pennsylvania State University Press, 2018).
87. Richard Adams, 'The Rights of Animals', *Daily Mirror*, 16 November 1978, p. 15; BBC, 'Obituary: Richard Adams', *BBC News Online*, 27 December 2016, sec. UK.
88. See Sect. 4.2 for a full discussion of these connections, alongside the development and usage of Cymag in pest control; see also e.g. Russell, 'Speaking of Annihilation'; Agar, 'Transition'; Christianson, *Fatal Airs*.
89. Martin Rosen, *Watership Down*, film (United Kingdom: Nepenthe Productions Ltd, 1978).
90. N. W. Littler, 'Badgers: how the men from the ministry may be wrong', *The Times*, 13 March 1978, 16. *The Men From the Ministry* was a satirical BBC radio series broadcast between 1962 and 1977, a precursor to the more famous TV satire *Yes Minister/Yes Prime Minister*.
91. Lambert, 'The Grey Seal in Britain', 459–63.
92. D. Graham Burnett, *The Sounding of the Whale: Science and Cetaceans in the Twentieth Century* (Chicago: University of Chicago Press, 2012).
93. Lambert, 'The Grey Seal in Britain', 460.
94. T. L. L. Goedeke and S. Rikoon, 'Otters as Actors: Scientific Controversy, Dynamism of Networks, and the Implications of Power in Ecological Restoration', *Social Studies of Science* 38(1) (February 2008): 111–32; Karen Victoria Lykke Syse, 'Otters as Symbols in the British Environmental Discourse', *Landscape Research* 38(4) (August 2013): 540–52; Allen, Watkins and Matless, 'An Incredibly Vile Sport'.
95. Evans, *A History of Nature Conservation in Britain*, 158–59. In the otter case the book converted to a film was *Ring of Bright Water* (1960, 1969).
96. Peter Robert Henry Mond Melchett and Louise Brodie, *Peter Melchett Interviewed by Louise Brodie*, British Library Oral Histories (London, 2010), British Library.
97. Sheail, 'The Mink Menace'.
98. Melchett and Brodie, *Peter Melchett Interviewed by Louise Brodie*.
99. Evans, *A History of Nature Conservation in Britain*, 180–91; Sands, *Wildlife in Trust*, 112–14.
100. J. Ardill, 'Ministry will cut badger killing', *Guardian*, 8 April 1986, 2; George M. Dunnet, David M. Jones, and John P McInerney, '*Badgers and Bovine Tuberculosis: Review of Policy*' (London: HMSO, 1986).
101. Overy and Tansey, *A History of Bovine TB c.1965–c. 2000*, 24–26.

102. Cassidy, '"Big Science" in the Field'; see also ch. 6.
103. Overy and Tansey, *A History of Bovine TB c.1965–c. 2000*, 31.
104. Barkham, *Badgerlands*, 110.
105. Barkham, *Badgerlands*, 109–29.
106. See, e.g. Mike Linley, 'Survival: Badger Woman' (Norwich: Anglia Television, 9 February 1995); J. Pilger, 'The persecution of Badger Brock', *Daily Mirror*, 17 November 1964, 16–17; G. Lakeman, 'Battle of the Badger Lady', *Daily Mirror*, 12 November 1980, 27.
107. Eric Ashby, 'At Home with Badgers', *Wildlife on One* (BBC Television, 13 April 1978); Drabble, *No Badgers in My Wood.*
108. Clark, *Badgers/Michael Clark*; Richard Meyer, *The Fate of the Badger Second Edition. New 30th Anniversary Edition 1986–2016*, 2nd edition (Cornwall: Fire-raven Writing, 2016).
109. Hilda Kean, 'The "Smooth Cool Men of Science": The Feminist and Socialist Response to Vivisection', *History Workshop Journal* 40 (1995): 16–38; Kean, *Animal Rights*; Emily Gaarder, *Women and the Animal Rights Movement* (New Brunswick, NJ: Rutgers University Press, 2011).
110. Where women do appear in the National Archives files, they tend to be assistants/secretaries, badger advocates and (exceptionally) senior civil servants such as Elizabeth Attridge, later Permanent Secretary for MAFF during the BSE crisis.
111. Overend, *Oral History Recording of an Interview with Eunice Overend.*
112. Anon., 'Obituary: Eunice Overend: Biology teacher and maverick wildlife campaigner who studied badger behaviour at the sanctuary she ran in Wiltshire', *The Times*, 10 January 2017, 52.
113. For 'lady vets' in the twentieth century, see Julie Hipperson, 'Professional Entrepreneurs: Women Veterinary Surgeons as Small Business Owners in Interwar Britain', *Social History of Medicine* 31(1) (1 February 2018): 122–39. For women in primatology, see Donna J. Haraway, *Primate Visions: Gender, Race, and Nature in the World of Modern Science* (London: Routledge, 1989); Rees, *The Infanticide Controversy.*
114. Meyer, 'Caring for Weak Ties'.
115. The biography of British naturalist Dr Mary Gilham provides a good example of such a marginalised female career trajectory in twentieth-century British natural history: Mary Gillham Archive Project, '"A Dedicated Naturalist", the Mary Gillham Archive Project', Peoples Collection Wales, 19 June 2017.
116. Druglitrø and Kirk, 'Building Transnational Bodies'.
117. Beale, 'Tinbergian Practice, Themes and Variations'; Lorimer, 'Counting Corncrakes'; Lys Alcayna-Stevens, 'Habituating Field Scientists', *Social Studies of Science* 46(6) (2016): 833–53; Philip Lowe et al., 'Expertise in

Rural Development: A Conceptual and Empirical Analysis', *World Development* 116 (1 April 2019): 28–37.

118. Maloney, Jordan and McLaughlin, 'Interest Groups and Public Policy'; Wyn Grant, *Pressure Groups and British Politics* (Basingstoke: Macmillan Education, 2000); M. Winter, 'Intersecting Departmental Responsibilities, Administrative Confusion and the Role of Science in Government: The Case of BSE', *Parliamentary Affairs* 49(4) (October 1996): 550–65.
119. Neal, *The Badger Man*, 216. R. Murray, 'Badger Protection Bill: Letter to Raymond F. Rowley, League against Cruel Sports', 25 October 1966, NA MAF131/70, item 125. For conflicts between Murray and other badger advocates, see 'Minutes of the 6th Meeting of the Consultative Panel', 17 February 1977, NA FT 41/92.
120. Peter J. Atkins, 'Lobbying and Resistance with Regard to Policy on Bovine Tuberculosis in Britain, 1900–1939: An Inside/Outside Model', in *Tuberculosis Then and Now: Perspectives on the History of an Infectious Disease* (Montreal: McGill-Queen's University Press, 2010), 197–220.
121. Van Dooren, 'A Day with Crows'; Crowley, Hinchliffe and McDonald, 'Conflict in Invasive Species Management'; Crowley, Hinchliffe and McDonald, 'Killing Squirrels'.
122. Davies et al., 'Science, Culture, and Care in Laboratory Animal Research'; Druglitrø, '"Skilled Care" and the Making of Good Science'.
123. Thompson, 'Animal Welfare and the Control of Vertebrates'; Druglitrø and Kirk, 'Building Transnational Bodies'; Druglitrø, '"Skilled Care" and the Making of Good Science'.
124. Garner, *Animals, Politics and Morality.*
125. Overend, *Oral History Recording of an Interview with Eunice Overend.*
126. Cassidy et al., 'Animal Roles and Traces in the History of Medicine, c.1880–1980'; Greenhough and Roe, 'Exploring the Role of Animal Technologists in Implementing the 3Rs'; Woods et al., *Animals and the Shaping of Modern Medicine.*
127. Thompson, 'Animal Welfare and the Control of Vertebrates', 5–7.
128. Donna Haraway has similarly argued that a major pitfall that many animal advocates fall into is 'speaking for', while forgetting, eliding or even suppressing the agency of the beings they are trying to help: Haraway, 'The Promises of Monsters'.
129. Agar, 'What Happened in the Sixties?'; Agar, 'Transition'.

PART III

Contestations of Badger and bTB

6

bTB Policy and RBCT

The first two parts of this book followed British debates over badgers and bTB as the two previously separate issues collided in the early 1970s, tracing the formation and development of three epistemic communities engaging with badger/bTB—animal health, disease ecology and animal protection.[1] It explored the historical backstories of each of these and documented how they engaged with the news of tuberculous badgers; created and contested new knowledge; and shaped new policies to deal with the problem. The last part of this book will bring these stories back together to help us understand what has happened since the 1990s to create the situation we see today: to ask once again, 'How did we get into this mess?'[2] From here on in, we will address the overall knowledge controversy around badger/bTB, to help us understand how and why this relatively obscure science-policy problem has transformed into the extensively reported, highly polarised and political public controversy we see today.[3] To this end I will adopt a metaphor of events in the 'backstage' and the 'frontstage' of the controversy as an aid to analysing this situation. Policy is usually constituted by interactions between: informal and internal communications; formal policy documents and technical information (open to public scrutiny, but engaged with by specialists); and material circulating around the wider public sphere, including mass media coverage, campaigning materials and political statements, aimed at and involving public audiences.[4] These sit on a spectrum of 'publicness', which is getting messier as new communications technologies make it possible for relatively closed communications (such as private emails and policy documents) to be brought into the wider public sphere.[5] While it is only possible to gain access to informal/internal interactions via first-hand observation (e.g. ethnography) or in hindsight using archives (as in the first two parts of this book), the increased accessibility of specialist policy documents makes today's 'backstage' much more visible than in the past.

Badger/bTB debates have always had an aspect of publicness which emerged from time to time—as seen in animal protection activist Ruth Murray's attempts to prosecute the Farming Minister (Chap. 2), or the controversy following the 1980 Zuckerman review. However, these were specific incidents, with most of the dialogue still taking place between people already deeply involved with the issue. Towards the end of the last decade this started to change, and since 2010 the controversy has become more consistently public, attracting widespread mainstream media coverage, involving larger and more diverse media audiences, and stepping firmly onto the 'frontstage' of British political life. In order to understand this shift into the broader public sphere, we must first gain a deeper understanding of the 'backstage' of badger/bTB by asking a number of questions: how have scientists, veterinarians, farmers, journalists, campaigners, policymakers and politicians negotiated what we know about badger/bTB; what that knowledge means and what to do about it? Who has been considered to be an 'expert', by whom, and how has this expertise been established? What have scientists and policymakers expected from each other, have these expectations been fulfilled, and what have been the consequences? How, when and why has policy learned from past mistakes, and if not, why not? This chapter will analyse the 'backstage' of bTB policy since the mid-1990s, demonstrating how past events and expectations of the future have contributed to decision-making in the present, creating a repeating cycle of science–policy interaction.[6] In the long term, this has created mutual disillusionment and mistrust on all sides: however, I will argue that it may also have enabled some success in advancing 'backstage' policy agendas both within and beyond badger/bTB.

6.1 Experts, Evidence and Policy

By the end of 2018, the problem of badgers and bTB in Britain will have been the responsibility of nine prime ministers, and twenty-one cabinet ministers—initially of the Ministry for Agriculture, Fisheries and Food (MAFF) and since 2001, the Department for Environment, Food and

Rural Affairs (Defra). Between them, these ministers have weathered eleven general elections, bringing them into and out of power. Over this time, badger/bTB has also provided scientists and veterinarians (as researchers in government and academia) with intellectual, funding and career opportunities, as well as applied roles in government, NGOs and private companies. Badger/bTB has also become a battleground for the increasingly tense relationships between science, policy and politics in the UK. Between 1980 and 2018, there have been nine expert-led reviews of the evidence and/or policy surrounding the issue, starting with the Zuckerman report discussed in Chap. 3. The most recent of these was chaired by population biologist and bTB policy veteran Professor Sir Charles Godfray and was published in October 2018.[7] Given the long-standing nature of the problem, on one level it is entirely unremarkable and indeed sensible that there have been so many of these reviews, especially given the centrality for policy of rapidly changing scientific knowledge about badger/bTB. These reviews take place in the context of wider traditions across British policymaking, whereby publics sceptical of government and ambitious politicians have required them to support and justify their decisions with expert knowledge. This expertise must in turn be recognised as legitimate—and in the UK this takes the form of a combination of technical qualifications, professional reputation and social standing (hence all the 'Sirs' and 'Lords' chairing bTB reviews).[8]

As we have explored through the earlier parts of this book, the first twenty years of badger/bTB was shaped and reshaped by a broader 'sea change' in interactions between science, policy, publics and wider society. Historian Jon Agar argues that this took the form of experts starting to disagree in public much more often, while publics (particularly via new social movements) have contested Establishment views on many fronts, including environmental and animal politics.[9] During the 1990s and early 2000s, the UK saw a further wave of changes in relationships between scientists, publics, politicians and policymakers, precipitated by a series of crises centring upon agriculture, food and animal health. These included failings in decision-making under uncertainty in the case of Bovine spongiform encephalopathy (BSE); mismatches between expert, policy and public understandings of 'risk' in the case of genetically modified foods; and disciplinary rivalries, policy–community disconnects and the traumatic loss of thousands of animals following an outbreak of foot and mouth disease (FMD).[10] As well as impacting on wider debates about science and society,[11] these crises exposed governance flaws which eventually led to the reorganisation of MAFF into Defra in 2001.[12] This period saw the widespread embedding of environmental concerns into UK national, European and international policy. This created new policy mechanisms to curb pollution and CO_2 emissions, protect biodiversity and encourage sustainable farming; while environmental NGOs further professionalised and embedded themselves in policy. The UK also saw a 'third wave' of renewed activism on environmental issues, this time driven by a plethora of ad hoc 'grassroots' campaigns, more willing than ever to take direct action on a wide range of issues.[13] Since 2010, long-standing government agendas for implementing policy via markets have combined with internal tensions in political parties to create further shifts in the politics of expertise, environment and agriculture.[14] In recent years we have seen the public dismissal of 'experts' by some politicians and campaigners, and widespread concerns that many countries, including the UK, are entering a 'post-truth era', in which science itself is becoming politically polarised.[15] Most famously, this has been in relation to the US Trump administration's hostility to science and environmental interests: of more relevance to badger/bTB would be the pro-Brexit politician (and current Secretary of State for Defra) Michael Gove's 2016 comment that 'people in this country have had enough of experts'.[16]

Given these changes—including several transitions back and forth between Conservative and Labour governments—the persistence of the 'authoritative expert' bTB review in the face of ongoing controversy requires explanation. Why have successive generations of politicians, policymakers and scientists continued to commission, conduct and cooperate with these reviews? Recalling the timeline presented in Chap. 1 (Fig. 1.1), it is noticeable that such reviews have often been commissioned at politically significant moments, such as transitions between government administrations (e.g. Major–Blair, or Blair–Brown). Whether and how they end up effecting policy change is—as we saw with the Zuckerman report—another matter. Policy scholars have not been optimistic about the bTB case: it has been characterised as following in the footsteps of BSE and FMD—yet another classic example of 'policy failure', one which may even be 'intractable'.[17] Since the 1990s badger/bTB has been further complicated by the devolution of agricultural policy powers to Scotland, Northern Ireland and Wales: resulting in an increasingly diverse patchwork of regional policies, sometimes at direct odds to those of national government in Westminster. As political administrations have changed, so bTB policies have swung back and forth, often justified by multiple interpretations of the same substantive evidence base.[18] This situation has led some to characterise bTB as a 'pathology of policy learning'—a situation 'where learning processes degenerated as the result of various weaknesses in government's management of its relationship with an epistemic community established to advise it.'[19]

This chapter will build on this research, explaining how today's situation has come about by tracing the development of the badger/bTB controversy since the mid-1990s, through the course of two Labour governments (Blair and Brown), the Coalition government of 2010–2015 and into Theresa May's Conservative administration. Over the longer history of badger/bTB, I see a pattern of repeatedly building and breaking the mutual *expectations* that have been built between science, policy and wider society. As in other cases where promises made in the present about what science and technology will do in the future (e.g. *there will be a cure for cancer in five years*) then go unfulfilled, I argue that this has created disillusionment and alienation between scientific, policy, political and campaign actors, and contributed to a long-term politicisation of the debate.[20] Expanding on the situation outlined in Chap. 1, I will also explore the complexities of 'the science' of bTB, drawing out the knowledge practices of the epistemic communities involved in badger/bTB, and demonstrating their strategic deployment to support multiple positions in the debate.

Before exploring the post-1990s history of badger/bTB in depth, a brief reminder about epistemic communities: these are groups of people who work together to produce reliable knowledge about a particular policy area. In the above quotation, the 'epistemic community' referred to was a group of scientists known as the Independent Scientific Group (ISG), appointed by government in 1998 to conduct a specific piece of research about badger/bTB. We will learn more about the ISG later in this chapter, but for now it is important to note that, as we have traced through this book, the ISG has not been the only epistemic community involved with badger/bTB. While much of the literature on epistemic communities regards them as conventional 'experts' by default, here I have drawn upon an expanded definition which includes the contributions of other actors with specialist knowledge, including farmers, naturalists and animal advocates.[21] I have applied this to the worlds and work of three overlapping but identifiable cultures of care arising from the epistemic communities around badger/bTB. We started with *animal health* (veterinary scientists and clinicians, farmers and agricultural policymakers) and the long-established policy of 'stamping out'—controlling contagion with animal slaughter and movement restriction. We then traced the development of a parallel epistemic community also concerned with animals and infectious disease: that of government pest control scientists and their colleagues in *disease ecology*, natural history and conservation. They were primarily concerned with understanding 'organisms in their environment', gaining support by applying their research to boosting agricultural productivity. MAFF scientists become involved in disease ecology when dealing with myxomatosis in rabbits during the 1950s and were drawn into the bTB issue because of their expertise in working with wildlife. Our third epistemic community is the most fuzzy—and has experienced rapid change—the complex alliances involved in campaigning for *badger protection*. While the British 'badger debate' has been ongoing for hundreds of years, it was reignited in the mid-1960s by canny and charismatic animal advocates. When tuberculous badgers were found in the early 1970s, campaigns for badger protection were already in full swing.

While initially the three cultures worked closely together to investigate the previously unknown connections between *M. bovis*, cattle and badgers, tensions rapidly manifested—initially between MAFF and animal advocates, then with conservationists and ecologists. The epistemic communities around animal health and pest control moved apart as their theories and methodologies diverged, creating new internal and external pressures on traditionally veterinary-dominated animal health policy. This came to a head during the early 1990s, when a new 'live' test for bTB in badgers turned out to be ineffective. When the expectations of politicians and policymakers (that new technologies would solve the bTB problem) were broken, disease ecology advocates renewed lobbying for a new approach to scientific investigation of the problem.[22] In the meantime bTB faded into the background, as the emergence of BSE fully occupied the attention of MAFF scientists, policymakers, ministers and wider publics. The policy and political failures associated with animal health, particularly the attempts of ministers to reassure the public that British beef was 'perfectly safe' during the BSE crisis, contributed to a disintegration of voters' trust in the Conservative party and their defeat in the 1997 General Election.[23]

6.2 'A Proper Experimental Assessment'

On 23 July 1996, the last Conservative Agriculture Minister of John Major's government had announced the third independent scientific review into policy on 'TB in cattle and badgers' since 1980: the report was delivered to Labour's new Minister, Dr Jack Cunningham, a year later.[24] The enquiry was chaired by a senior ecologist, Professor John Krebs, and included a highly distinguished team including three Fellows of the Royal Society, several ecologists, an epidemiologist, a microbiologist, immunologists and a statistician.[25] Krebs et al. concluded that while MAFF's existing research findings supported the idea that bTB in badgers was being passed to cattle, the evidence was 'indirect'.[26] The various culling policies that had been implemented involved different scales, geographical features, quantities, frequencies and timings of culls, making it impossible to coherently understand their effects. To counter this problem, the Krebs group recommended conducting a major field experiment testing the effects of badger culling on bTB in cattle—a study directly comparing several culling strategies with a 'control' (with no culling), where the application of each condition was randomly applied.[27] The scientists envisaged that such a study would take about five years, could provide better evidence about whether culling worked, and therefore would be able to directly shape policy:

> A proper experimental assessment is the only way to test rigorously the effectiveness (and cost-effectiveness) of different strategies and to provide a sound basis for future policy. Although this would have significant resource implications for Government, these must be considered in the context of the actual and potential costs of TB. An analogy might be the evidence required to recommend the widespread use of a new therapeutic drug.[28]

By drawing this analogy with biomedicine, Krebs et al. presented their proposed experiment as a randomised controlled trial (RCT), considered to be the 'gold standard' for research in evidence-based medicine, as well as in agricultural and ecological research.[29] They appealed to a core idea of the new Labour government—evidence-based policy—suggesting that the best way of resolving the bTB controversy would be to put politics to one side and let policy be determined by the evidence that their proposal would deliver.[30] Cunningham was convinced, and appointed a new Independent Scientific Group (ISG). The group was chaired by Prof. John Bourne (former director of the government Institute for Animal Health), and included former members of the Krebs group, plus the economist member of the 1986 Dunnet group and two further statisticians.[31] The new ISG was charged with designing and implementing the proposed experiment, which they named the Randomised Badger Culling Trial (or

RBCT, sometimes known as the 'Krebs trial'). The RBCT is probably the largest field trial yet conducted in the UK: it was carried out across over 3000 km² of the South West of England, took over nine years, culled approximately 10,000 badgers and cost just over £49 million.[32] By the end of the trial, the ISG had met 103 times, published six formal reports and at least twenty-eight peer reviewed journal articles.[33] Since then their findings have been cited, presented, interpreted, contested, analysed, *re*analysed and *re*interpreted by multiple actors in the bTB debate, who sometimes refer to it as 'the science' or the 'sound science' of badger culling. While much more research has been conducted since (including analyses of the long-term effects of culling after the RBCT, studies of badger–cattle interactions, sophisticated epidemiological models and comparisons with other countries), RBCT data still provide the core of most contemporary research about bTB in the UK.[34]

The ISG was charged with the design, implementation and monitoring of the RBCT experiment, but from the start the group claimed a wider remit: 'to recommend a combination of measures which, taken together, will provide information essential for the establishment of future policy.'[35] The ISG drew up a list of research questions, on topics including cross-species disease transmission, wildlife ecology, the genetics of bTB and alternative 'control strategies' beyond culling. The experiment was designed to compare three experimental conditions: culling badgers *reactively* on an ad hoc basis in response to bTB outbreaks in cattle herds; culling *proactively* across an entire area; and a *control* condition where information was gathered but nothing else was done. The ISG decided that these conditions would be implemented across ten 'triplet' areas in parts of the country where bTB was prevalent—adjacent circles of land, each with an approximate area of 100 km². In the process of implementing the design, some modifications were made. Rather than starting the experiment across all ten 'triplets' at the same time, it was implemented as and when land became available in different places. Krebs had emphasised the need to remove *all* badgers in areas assigned to the culling conditions, including repeating culls to prevent 'recolonisation'.[36] However, the ISG culls were undertaken on a more restricted basis than had been employed in MAFF's earlier culling trials such as at Thornbury. The ISG was at pains to ensure that its work was as 'humane' as possible, employing cage-trapping with care, closely monitoring trapped animals and only culling outside of the badger breeding season of 1 February to 30 April. This

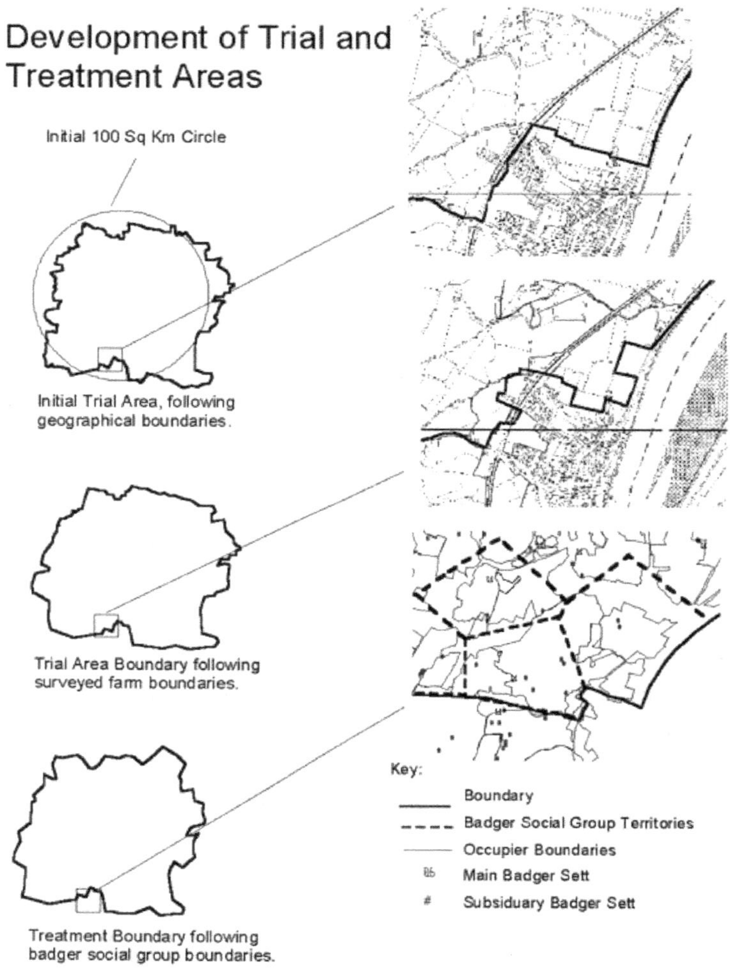

Fig. 6.1 Translating experimental design into lived landscape. Source: Bourne et al., 'Bovine TB: Second Report of the Independent Scientific Group on Cattle TB' (27).

continued the practices of conservation and animal welfare care which had been developed at the Pest Infestation Control Laboratories (PICL); responded to concerns of external animal advocates; and ensured that the trial complied with the UK's international legal commitments.[37]

The next job was to translate the planned 'triplet' design into the landscapes of the South West of England, resulting in a shift from idealised interlocking circles to messily bordered specific places, taking account of human and badger social boundaries (Fig. 6.1). A year in, the ISG reported a series of complications and delays—relating to surveying potential trial areas, gaining consent from landowners, recruiting staff to do the culling and other fieldwork, and localised 'interference' with staff and equipment.[39] 'Interference' was MAFF and the ISG's term for the actions of badger protection activists who opposed culling for various reasons. While some advocacy groups campaigned in more conventional ways, others acted directly against the RBCT. As had happened intermittently in the past, these activists destroyed cage-traps, released trapped badgers and damaged equipment: threats were also made against ISG members, MAFF officers and government ministers.[40] It was three years before the ISG had surveyed all ten of the proposed triplet areas, although it had started culling in seven of these. The experiment had only just gotten into full swing when the situation was further complicated by a major outbreak of FMD in February 2001. The outbreak brought much of the British countryside to a standstill and the RBCT experiment with it. The severity of FMD was such that all meat exports were stopped, as were animal and human movements in affected areas. Most of MAFF's animal health officers and scientists were seconded into the FMD control effort, suspending not only the RBCT experiment, but routine bTB controls.[41] By the end of the outbreak approximately 10 million animals had been slaughtered, with economic and social impacts on farming communities for years to come.[42] When bTB testing resumed in January 2002, it soon became clear that bTB incidence had risen sharply (see Chap. 1, Fig. 1.2), creating renewed pressure from farming and veterinary groups for policy action, rather than more research.[43] This had a further knock-on effect for the RBCT trial, which was dependent on routine cattle testing to proceed: there was now a year's backlog to catch up with.[44]

Once the experimental fieldwork finally resumed and the ISG was able to start analysing the preliminary data, an unexpected finding emerged, which the scientists advised ministers of immediately:

> … the incidence of herd breakdowns in reactively culled areas has been consistently greater than expected. This increase was estimated to be 27%, though it could be as small as 4.3% or as large as 53%. This increase was consistent in all nine triplets that had received reactive culls by the time of

> analysis (triplet J has not yet been reactively culled). While the larger adverse effects may be implausible on general grounds, even a 10% deterioration, if it persisted, would clearly be of major concern. (ISG advice to DEFRA, 29 October 2003)[45]

Not only was culling not reducing bTB in cattle, it looked like the 'reactive' condition was actually making things worse. The ISG recommended completing data collection for that season, then stopping the reactive condition as it was 'not a viable base for a future policy option'.[46] However, Labour ministers instead decided that the implications for farming were so severe that they stopped reactive culling immediately, leaving the dataset incomplete. As the decision was announced, the ISG published its preliminary analysis in the scientific journal *Nature*.[47] While these events received relatively little attention, the 2005 publication of the 5th ISG report, combined with a public consultation, did stoke controversy. Ex-MAFF veterinarian and bTB pioneer John Gallagher resigned from Defra's science advisory group, mustering 420 veterinary colleagues to sign a letter of no confidence in the Ministry; opposition MP Owen Paterson asked over 600 questions in Parliament about bTB; while National Farmers Union (NFU) spokesmen called for an immediate 'blitz cull' in the press.[48] In the meantime, Defra's public consultation had come back with responses that were overwhelmingly (over 90%) against badger culling: backstage, political pressures on the ministry were building.[49]

Perturbing Findings, Policy Recommendations

For the next few years, the ISG concentrated on publishing findings from the 'proactive' culling condition. These seemed contradictory: while bTB incidence had dropped by 19% inside areas where badgers had been culled, it went up by 29% in areas surrounding these cull zones.[50] It was not until the ISG published its Final Report on 18 June 2007 that the findings were seriously discussed in wider public contexts. This 289-page document, (published ten years after Krebs) laid out the ISG's data, analyses, findings, key conclusions and policy recommendations. From inception to final report, the ISG's research had taken over nine years to complete, over which time MAFF/Defra's policy on badger culling could best be summarised as 'wait for the science'. The report revealed that there had been further adjustments to the original research design: as well as cutting short reactive culling, it transpired that several of the 'triplets' (meant to provide comparable conditions) had migrated significant distances apart, in one case to the very different landscapes of North and South Devon.[51] We can surmise that this was due to the complications of conducting a controlled experiment across a living countryside instead of a laboratory: one populated by reluctant landowners, disillusioned farmers and angry animal rights protestors, all intervening in unanticipated and unwelcome ways.

The ISG summarised its overall findings: that *reactive* culling appeared to increase bTB in cattle, while *proactive* culling decreased it where badgers were culled, but seemed to make things worse in surrounding areas. The report also provided a coherent explanation for these apparently contradictory findings—the perturbation effect:

> The disruption of the social organisation or structure of badger populations, such as that which is caused where trapping/culling has taken place.[52]

Badgers in Britain tend to live in unusually large family groups defending well-defined territories over long periods of time. The ISG argued that badger culling, particularly when undertaken on an ad hoc, localised basis (as in the 'reactive' intervention), disrupts this social organisation. As Infestation Control Division (ICD) staff had known since at least the 1960s, an emptied territory was likely to be 'recolonised' by badgers from adjacent areas; just as Eunice Overend had predicted, this resulted in *M. bovis* spreading further. While the scientific term 'perturbation' is used throughout the sciences to indicate any kind of unusual interaction, ecologists use it to characterise and explain the consequences of human disturbance of ecosystems on populations and their movements.[53] By the mid-1990s, mammal and disease ecologists had already linked perturbation to the spread of rabies in foxes and were already speculating about its effects on the disease ecology of bTB.[54] While the ISG had anticipated that perturbation might play a role, devoting an entire subprogramme of the project to badger ecology, it had not anticipated the strength of the effect on the spread of bTB. It was not until 2007 that the ISG foregrounded the idea and term 'perturbation',[55] arguing that perturbation explained both the acute increases in cattle bTB following 'reactive' culling and the increases in neighbouring areas around 'proactive' culling.

Drawing on perturbation theory alongside their own economic analyses, the ISG made a series of policy recommendations. These not only pushed back against years of denial (from badger protection campaigners) that the animals harboured *M. bovis*, but also against agricultural interests' lobbying for a cull:

> First, while badgers are clearly a source of cattle TB, careful evaluation of our own and others' data indicates that badger culling can make no meaningful contribution to cattle TB control in Britain. Indeed, some policies under consideration are likely to make matters worse rather than better. Second, weaknesses in cattle testing regimes mean that cattle themselves contribute significantly to the persistence and spread of disease in all areas where TB occurs, and in some parts of Britain are likely to be the main source of infection.[56]

The ISG argued that badger culling was simply too expensive and risky to be economically or practically viable, and that tightening the existing regulatory framework of bTB testing and movement control was the most viable way forwards for policy. On the day the Final Report was published, four members of the ISG gave evidence to a parliamentary enquiry on bTB, while John Bourne gave a series of media interviews.[57] Unlike their earlier 'backstage' approach to working with policymakers, (private briefings and publicly available but technical reports), the scientists had decided to take the conversation about badger culling onto the 'frontstage': it was now critical that their ideas reached wider public audiences.

6.3 'Cutting the Cake' of Science and Policy: The Aftermath of the RBCT

As soon as the report was published, the ISG came under fire from representatives of the NFU, Conservative politicians and media, who renewed their calls for culling. Government responses to the report were lukewarm, stating only that ministers would 'consider carefully' the findings.[58] All went quiet until four months later, when the government's Chief Scientific Adviser, Sir David King, published a second report on 'Bovine Tuberculosis in Cattle and Badgers'.[59] King, a chemist known for his climate change advocacy, had convened an alternative expert panel (comprising a mammal ecologist, an immunologist and three veterinary scientists): their report was endorsed by the Chief Veterinary Officer (CVO). Directly rebutting the ISG, but drawing on RBCT data, King et al. concluded that culling in high-incidence areas was the 'best option available at the moment to reduce the reservoir of infection in wildlife'. How was this possible? From the start, the ISG had adopted a deliberately broad remit, integrating scientific questions with policy considerations, while King's group had framed the problem narrowly, only considering the effects of 'badger removal' on bTB without weighing it against other policy options. The report justified this move as addressing the 'scientific basis', enabling them to also disregard considerations of animal welfare, practicality and the economic implications, including the crucial cost–benefit analysis conducted by the ISG.[60] King's group only considered the RBCT data on proactive culling, including their estimates of how many animals needed to be killed and how large an area was necessary to make the strategy viable. They combined these figures with their own modelling, looking only at the impacts inside culling areas, projecting forwards over longer periods of time and exploring the possibility of using 'hard' geographical boundaries (such as rivers or major roads) to prevent perturbation. While the King group drew upon the same data as the ISG, the different boundaries drawn around 'science' and 'policy' enabled them to reach the opposite conclusion.[61]

The ISG immediately defended its claims, arguing that King's conclusions were unrealistic for policy practice. The ISG, King, politicians and others campaigning for and against badger culling then engaged in a heated debate, fought out in mass media as well as an enquiry conducted by the House of Commons Environment and Rural Affairs Committee:

> The scientists—Professor John Bourne, Christl Donnelly, Rosie Woodroffe and Sir David King—gave evidence before us. The atmosphere between them was interesting; it was probably more of an atmosphere than we sometimes have in here for Prime Minister's Question Time, such was their commitment to the work they had done.[62]

Further critiques of the ISG emerged, this time from ex-MAFF veterinary officers and scientists, focusing on the detailed design and implementation of the RBCT. These included the adjustments that the ISG had made to adapt to policy, welfare and practical requirements, the curtailment of the 'reactive' condition and the disruptive effects of badger protection activism. The vets argued that this meant *not enough* badgers had been culled in the trial areas, *increasing* the likelihood of disruption to their social groups. This resulted in a flawed experiment which could not support the ISG's claims; some argued that the RBCT was actually designed to induce perturbation and was not comparable to the culling regimes used in past trials such as Thornbury, which they believed had removed more badgers more effectively.[63]

As the still-ongoing Parliamentary enquiry continued, it unravelled the 'backstage' sequence of events contributing to the appearance of badger/bTB onto the 'frontstage' of rural politics.[64] As its work approached completion, the ISG sent Defra ministers a near-final draft of the report on 23 May, but received little or no feedback—while they had attempted to communicate directly with ministers when possible, as the ISG's findings about perturbation had emerged, the relationship between Defra and the ISG had deteriorated.[65] Until a few weeks prior to the publication of the ISG's final report, Defra was briefing that culling was about to be reintroduced, and correspondence published in 2015 confirms that Prime Minister Tony Blair had supported this position.[66] Once again, political expectations of scientists had not been met, as was forcefully explained by the Defra minister who had overseen much of the ISG, Jeff Rooker:

> I have gone back and looked at what we were told the trials would deliver 10 years ago—that we would find out the extent of TB in the badger population, how badgers transmit TB to cattle, that we might have a vaccine, and that we would have all the answers. Well, frankly we haven't, have we? The fact that they can't tell us how TB is spread from badgers to cattle, other than it's respiratory, is not a lot of bloody help to us.[67]

Shortly after reading the ISG's final report, the Secretary of State for Defra, David Milliband, contacted Sir David King and asked him to 'undertake a short objective assessment of the key scientific issues', which 'did not extend to economic or other practical issues'.[68] The King report was written and delivered to Defra within six weeks: however, it was not made public until October 2007, after which ministers finally met with the ISG to discuss its findings.

This was due to a critical political transition: on 27 June, only ten days after the ISG publication, Gordon Brown took over from Tony Blair as Prime Minister, and as part of this shift within Labour, a new Defra minister, Hilary Benn, was appointed. It was therefore Benn who took delivery of the King report, releasing it to the public in October and then meeting the ISG scientists. In July 2008, Benn announced that 'after a great deal of consideration', he had decided not to resume culling, primarily on the advice of the ISG scientists.[69] Instead, there would be major investment in vaccination as a long-term solution to bTB, including further clinical research and a new field trial testing badger vaccination. While the announcement was welcomed by badger advocates, it produced correspondingly negative responses from culling advocates, some of whom had nicknamed the Minister 'Veggie Benn', who interpreted this rapid policy reversal as politically motivated. While Krebs and the ISG's original intention that scientific research would directly inform bTB policymaking had been met, it was at a deep cost. The disease ecology epistemic community—of which the ISG was a part—were now regarded as allies by badger advocates, environmentalists and political interests on the left; and as opponents by farming advocates and right-wing political interests.[70] While these actors had not changed their positions on badger culling, some curious reversals had taken place in their rhetoric about science and evidence. In 1998, the Badger Trust had campaigned vociferously against the trial, critiquing the validity of the science and appealing to EU law to try and stop the research. However, by the time that the ISG delivered its final report they were effusive in their praise for the 'sound science' that demonstrated culling did not work.[71] Correspondingly, NFU representatives had initially welcomed the RBCT, anticipating that it would provide evidence to support culling. When the ISG instead reached the unexpected and unwelcome conclusion that culling could make things worse, the NFU also reversed their position, criticising the ISG and selectively citing David King's report to argue for immediate 'action'.[72] Since then, it has become increasing common for both pro- and anti-culling actors to argue that 'the science' of bTB supports their arguments, while selectively drawing on different experts or interpretations of research findings to do so.

From 'Evidence-Based Policy' to 'Veterinary Advice': The Post 2010 Return to Badger Culling

Benn's decision not to cull badgers had less than two years to embed into policy before being upended by the outcome of the next General Election in May 2010, when the Brown Labour government was ousted in favour of the first Coalition Britain had seen since the Second World War. David Cameron became prime minister of an administration formed between his own Conservative Party and the Liberal Democrats. While much of the rapidly formulated Coalition Agreement involved careful fudging of the two parties' rather different positions, one easy point of agreement was over badgers and bTB. The Conservatives had made a manifesto pledge to reintroduce badger culling: while the Liberal Democrats held a similar position.[73] Within months, the new Farming Minister, Jim Paice, announced their plans: the vaccination trials were cut back and replaced by a new 'science-led' policy, in which licences would be issued 'to enable farmers and landowners to cull badgers at their own expense'.[74] Departing from Defra's established best practice, this would be undertaken by a new technique referred to as 'free' or 'controlled' shooting. The idea was to adapt existing practices for shooting foxes and deer to 'free ranging' badgers, even though the risks of causing suffering were 'unknown'.[75] Extrapolating from the rather different practices of deer shooting, policymakers estimated that free shooting would cost half as much as the long-established procedure of cage-trapping followed by shooting badgers (used in the RBCT).[76]

Two new 'pilot culls' were announced, to be carried out in bTB 'hotspots' in Somerset and Gloucestershire—unlike the RBCT, but like the vaccination trials, these were not experimental tests of the effects on bTB but were instead intended to 'test' out the application of the new policy in the field. Ministers took care to flag their engagement with science, holding an open meeting at the Royal Society and drawing once more on the RBCT data and King et al. to set out the licencing conditions. These stipulated the size, geography and number of badgers that would need to be killed in a given area to achieve a 16% reduction of bTB in cattle.[77] They also appointed not one but two new expert groups—one to 'provide a succinct summary of the natural science evidence base underlying bovine tuberculosis policy in the UK'[78], and a new 'Independent Expert Panel' (IEP), asked to 'look at the effectiveness, humaneness and safety of controlled shooting as a culling method'.[79] While the plans were criticised by badger and animal welfare advocates, as well as Labour politicians in opposition, the idea that the government's strategy was 'science-led' seemed to hold.[80] However, there was a shift in emphasis—while the new policy was based upon 'the available scientific evidence', it was also critically supported by 'veterinary advice'. While scientists could only provide evidence for later interpretation by policymakers, veterinarians were visible again as publicly trusted experts on animal health, providing advice and directly shaping bTB policy.[81]

The Coalition's policy was beset with problems from the start. Following high-profile anti-culling campaigns, the first round of culling 'trials' was delayed. Badger/bTB was debated several times in Parliament, and a group of senior scientists (including Krebs, members of the ISG and other epidemiologists and ecologists) publicly criticised the culling policy, predicting it would not work and would be a 'costly distraction' from bTB control.[82] When the pilots finally started in the summer of 2013, they were further disrupted by anti-cull campaigners directly sabotaging attempts to kill badgers (as happened during the RBCT), as well as indirect 'badger patrols' who guarded setts or monitored culling operations in the field. Contractors were not killing enough animals to meet government targets, and chronic uncertainties over how big the badger population was in the first place meant that this figure was adjusted several times, changing the success rates of the pilot culls.[83] It was this uncertainty which led Defra minister Owen Paterson to famously state that 'the badgers are moving the goalposts'—a comment we will return to in Chap. 7.[84] Then in 2014 the IEP investigating badger shooting delivered its final report to the Minister. The IEP's report, like those of its predecessors, did not fulfil the expectations of policymakers and politicians to calm public controversy or provide legitimacy for bTB policy. Instead, the IEP's conclusions were deeply critical not only of 'free shooting' but of the implementation of the new policy in general. While the IEP had been charged with assessing free shooting only, they found that both pilots had also used cage-trapping, without recording exactly how much, confounding the study. The IEP concluded that while the trials had been *safe* (in terms of risks to the public), they had not been *effective* (had not killed enough badgers) or *humane* (too many animals had been shot that took longer than five minutes to die).[85]

Shortly after the IEP's report, Defra published their *Strategy for Achieving Officially Bovine Tuberculosis Free Status for England*, which set out their full policy plans, including the overall goal—to bring bTB incidence below a threshold set by EU law, lifting some trade restriction—confusingly, this was referred to as 'eradication'. The strategy document emphasised the need to use 'all available tools' up to and including badger culling: while it discussed the commissioning of the IEP, their disruptive conclusions were not discussed.[86] Instead, culling (by whatever method) was framed as an established policy approach, used successfully in the past in Britain and in the present in other countries, including Ireland and New Zealand. In an unprecedented shift, the new strategy moved away from a uniform policy to one using different approaches according to the level of bTB in the area—from 'low risk' in the North and East to 'high risk' in the

South and West, with an 'edge' zone between the two.[87] The bTB control 'tools' included tightening of testing and movement regimes for cattle, biosecurity practices, badger culling, but also its publicly abandoned counterpart, badger vaccination. The new strategy also brought in a stronger emphasis on 'partnership working' with industry, veterinary practitioners and other 'stakeholders'. This came hand in hand with an expectation that government would bear less of the costs of bTB control and that 'risk-based trading'—in which bTB risks factor into market valuations of cattle, meat and milk—would be introduced.[88] As we will explore in the next chapter, little of this complexity was made visible in the 'frontstage' of the bTB debate. Shortly after publishing their strategy document, Defra proceeded with a second year of culling, a move which was publicly criticised by IEP and ISG scientists.[89] This elision and then open conflict with scientific expertise contrast starkly with the early 1980s (see Chap. 3), when scientific recommendations that a culling method was ineffective and inhumane resulted in the swift and public withdrawal of Cymag 'gassing' from use.

The 2015 General Election saw the replacement of the Coalition government by a Conservative administration (led initially by David Cameron and then by Theresa May), opening the most recent phase of bTB policy. The intensity of public controversy has subsided somewhat, in part due to its displacement by debates leading up to and following the UK referendum on withdrawal from the EU on 23 June 2016. Meanwhile the 'backstage' negotiation of bTB policy has continued, with a curious mix of continuity and change. Further culling licences have been granted, for culls no longer characterised as 'pilots', while Defra have progressively adjusted licencing criteria away from the original conditions, which were shaped by the ISG, the King group and the IEP. The next Defra Secretary, Michael Gove, showed a subtler approach to science, environment and agriculture than expected, as he worked to persuade scientists, farmers and conservationists alike into backing his proposals to replace EU agricultural subsidies with 'public money for public goods'.[90] In March 2018, Gove commissioned the ninth expert review on badger/bTB to be conducted since 1980, to 'reflect on progress being made with implementation of the bTB Strategy'. Even though this third Godfray Review had not yet reported, Defra also announced the further rollout of culling across the country, citing drops in bTB incidence in the initial 'trial' areas in Gloucestershire and Somerset.[91] As we will explore in the next chapter, while media coverage of badger/

bTB has died down from a media 'storm' which peaked in 2013, the 'frontstage' of the controversy remains highly polarised. Locally based anti-cull activism continues, in the form of public protests, as well as direct 'sabbing' activities, disrupting culls out in the field: the ongoing conflict has become deeply divisive for many communities across the South West.[92]

Meanwhile, in the backstage of badger/bTB new complexities have emerged, alongside renewed signs of interest from all sides in finding alternative, more productive approaches to research, policy and practice. To start with, long-standing processes of reorganisation and privatisation in government research have continued. The Food and Environment Research Agency (or FERA, of MAFF's Agricultural Science Service) was privatised in 2014, while the scientists of Woodchester Park were placed alongside Defra's veterinarians in a newly merged Animal and Plant Health Agency. As we have seen, earlier reorganisations tended to move around the placement of research, policy and implementation functions within government, but maintained broad organisational distinctions between animal health and agricultural science (including ecological) expertise. The impacts of this organisational shift have yet to be documented, but the decision was justified in terms of 'One Health'—the need to address multisectoral problems like bTB in a more coordinated way. However, as is often the case with One Health, other agendas are at work—in this case the Conservative-led 'bonfire of the quangoes', in which many arm's-length government agencies and regulators have been closed, privatised or scaled back since 2010.[93] This broader political agenda has also knocked on to bTB policy via Natural England (NE), a descendent of the Nature Conservancy Committee (NCC), whose scientists had been so critical of animal health approaches to badger/bTB during the 1970s and 1980s. NE remains the regulatory body which monitors and grants licences for interventions in conserved landscapes and legally protected species, and is therefore also responsible for licencing the return to badger culling. Government 'austerity' agendas have hit Defra particularly hard, with NE's budget being cut in half, undermining its core expertise and ability to provide independent advice on conservation, or to fulfil its regulatory functions.[94] The devolution of agricultural policy to Scotland, Wales and Northern Ireland has also contributed to the 'backstage' diversification of complexity in bTB policy, fostering a range of attempts to target and tailor bTB control measures (including culling) geographically.[95]

While Defra's CVO regards the culls to be 'safe, effective and humane', since 2015 the British Veterinary Association (BVA) has opposed free shooting (but not culling with other methods) on animal welfare grounds—breaking a forty-year history of solidly pro-cull support from the veterinary profession.[96] Scientific research on the topic has expanded and diversified, involving a wider range of methodologies and disciplines than ever before, including an increasing emphasis on social research.[97] New testing technologies are being developed which may open up new possibilities for bTB policy—by differentiating between vaccinated and infected cattle (which the current regime cannot do); and by directly identifying the presence of mycobacteria in living animals and environments.[98] While debates continue about the applicability of these tests for regulatory frameworks, they are already being marketed for private use to farmers and veterinarians.[99] This diversity has been accompanied by a new willingness to engage in dialogue: a good example of this would be a shift in tactics from Brian May's 'Save Me' organisation (see Chap. 7) towards sponsoring scientific conferences, farm trials of new technologies and undertaking more direct policy engagement.[100] Behind the scenes at least, there appears to be more potential for exploring the possible 'diplomatic spaces' of mutual interest and even agreement around badger/bTB than at any time since the early 1970s.[101]

6.4 Epistemic Rivalries in bTB Policy

By tracing the developing 'backstage' story of how bTB policy has changed over time, we can gain further insights into the peculiarities of this case, as well as into broader changes and problems in science–policy relations in the UK. A central feature of British policymaking—the expert-led policy review—has been deployed with increasing frequency since the 1990s. However, it seems to have become less and less effective (for all concerned) as tensions between the epistemic communities of badger/bTB, as well as between scientists and politicians in general, have become dramatically visible. The first two parts of this book have charted the origins and development of the *animal health*, *disease ecology* and *badger protection* epistemic communities, their engagement with the new problem of badger/bTB, and the changing 'cultures of care' developed by these communities along the way.[102] Between 1971 and 1996, relations between the three changed from a collaborative effort directed at solving the new and urgent problem of tuberculous badgers, to open conflict between policy insiders and outsiders, and backstage tensions between government veterinarians and ecologists. The twists and turns of badger/bTB since the 1990s can therefore be understood as the outcome of intensifying epistemic rivalries, entrenched by the reorganisation of government research and policy following Krebs and the RBCT culling trial. The incoming Labour government's decision to accept Krebs's recommendations marked a major shift away from MAFF's traditional approach to bTB, characterised by 'stamping out' in infectious disease control and close working relationships with the animal health epistemic community. The long-standing 'Badgers and Bovine TB' research programme, led by animal health policymakers, and involving Ministry veterinary and ecological scientists, was closed. While MAFF's own bTB research continued, it was under the aegis of the new programme formulated by the ISG—scientists from outside the Ministry. As such, the commissioning of Krebs and then the ISG signified a loss of influence for the animal health epistemic community, which had already been the target of significant criticism for their roles in government mishandling of BSE. Around this time, the inclusive but powerless Badger Consultative Panel was shut down and replaced by the narrower TB Advisory Group (TBAG). While the former was designed to draw all parties into the policy process, including representatives from conservation, animal welfare, veterinary, landowner and farming bodies, the latter was focused on bTB control, and largely comprised veterinary and farming interests.[103] Research on the insider–outsider distinction suggests that due to their lack of access to policy processes, outsiders tend to focus their activities on the public sphere—in other words the 'frontstage': for this reason we will return to badger protection in the next chapter.[104]

As has already been emphasised, epistemic communities are not conventionally disciplinary entities—therefore it should be no surprise that the Krebs, King and ISG committees were all multidisciplinary, nor that the King group included a badger ecologist, while the ISG was chaired by a Professor of Animal Health. These review groups are better understood as entities connected to the various epistemic communities of badger/bTB, which in turn form a wider 'ecology of knowledge' subject to constant renegotiation and change over time.[105] The Krebs and ISG groups were both connected with *disease ecology* (explored in Chap. 4)—most obviously through Krebs himself, whose primary expertise is in behavioural ecology. This field combines the traditions of Elton's ecology with Tinbergen's ethology (animal behaviour): Krebs trained in these groups at Oxford University, and has close links with another influential grouping of

British ecologists engaged in interdisciplinary, policy-oriented research: the 'Silwood Circle' of Imperial College London.[106] Prior to chairing his bTB review, Krebs was the head of the UK Natural Environment Research Council and afterwards ran the Food Standards Agency for five years: he continues to command considerable influence through his appointment to the House of Lords.[107] The Silwood group also includes epidemiologist Roy Anderson, a pioneer in the mathematical modelling of disease—work which directly informed Defra's drastic FMD culling policy and further fuelled tensions with animal health and farming.[108] The Krebs and ISG groups both included other members of the Silwood and Oxford research networks. These connections are also visible in the research design of the RBCT, which drew upon classic ecological research methods, including randomised, controlled experiments, cost–benefit analysis and mathematical modelling—all intended to make field research more like the controlled space of the laboratory and the lab more like the field.[109]

The hostile reactions to the ISG's final report from farming representatives, the more specific criticisms from ex-MAFF veterinarians and the contradictory conclusions of the King report become much easier to understand as part of this process of epistemic rivalry. Contra to recent policy scholarship on bTB, these were not coming from a 'counter-epistemic community' formed in reaction to the ISG, but instead from core members of the much older *animal health* community explored in Chap. 3.[110] While animal health was still integral to Defra's policy implementation by 2007, it had been challenged by the BSE and FMD crises as well as by the reorganisation of a ministry devoted solely to agriculture and food (MAFF) to one also charged with protecting the environment (Defra). Veterinarians have a long history of engaging in disciplinary rivalries aimed at expanding or defending their own epistemic authority, and so the conflict with the ISG can be understood as a continuation of these traditions.[111] Krebs and the ISG had taken full advantage of biomedicine's 'rhetoric of control', gaining policy influence by positioning their approach to bTB as more 'scientific' than MAFF's earlier veterinary-led research.[112] In turn, the animal health critics of the ISG pointed out the contrasts between the ideal experiment pitched by Krebs and the multiple compromises that had to be made while implementing the RBCT in the field. The controversy has become subject to what historian Amanda Rees has described as the 'field experimenter's regress'—the ease with which scientific findings can be critiqued and unpicked by pointing out the contingencies, compromises and sheer messiness involved in doing field research.[113] Veterinarians and farmers have highlighted these limitations and the abstracted nature of ecologists' expertise, while effectively contrasting it with their own professional expertise and experiences of dealing with bTB in the 'real world'.[114]

The responses of Defra and their changing political masters to the ISG can also be better understood as an outcome of these epistemic rivalries. Krebs had persuaded the New Labour government that a new approach was needed, and gained the support of sceptical farmers and landowners with the promise of providing evidence to support policy. However, the envisaged experiment was not designed to test whether culling worked in the first place, but which form of culling worked best, building expectations that the RBCT would provide scientific legitimacy for badger culling. When the unexpected and unwelcome findings—that localised (reactive) culling might make bTB in cattle worse—started to emerge, the research left policymakers with few practical courses of action.[115] This explains the subsequent distancing between policymakers and the ISG, the pro-cull briefings coming out of Defra in 2007, and the commissioning of King (with the help of government veterinarians) to reinterpret RBCT data in a more useful direction. This 'cutting of the cake' of what counts as 'science' and what counts as 'policy' can also be interpreted as boundary-work: drawing rhetorical boundaries around the category of 'science' to further a specific aim.[116] Hilary Benn's reversal to a 'no-cull' decision (informed by the ISG) reflects political differences between the new Brown and old Blair administrations, but was also an attempt to redirect the institutional inertia of Defra away from the long-standing pro-culling stance of animal health.[117] However, there was not enough time for this decision to embed into policy before the next election, while the ISG's findings and post-publication dispute had further politicised the problem. The breaking of high expectations—this time that science could provide 'all the answers' to a notoriously thorny problem—has created widespread disillusionment between scientific, political, policy and campaign actors.

The Coalition and the following Conservative governments' decisions to return to badger culling can also be interpreted in this light. These politicians have returned to a trusted epistemic community who can offer them authoritative expert advice under ongoing uncertainty (the classic working conditions of the veterinarian). Animal health experts can also help the current government to deliver a policy that has been increasingly vocally demanded by key political supporters in right-leaning and rural constituencies. But how can we explain the 'backstage' situation? Recent years have seen a breakdown of the distinctions between animal health and disease ecology research, and a new willingness to engage in direct dialogue. Scientists working with and particularly inside Defra have worked hard to redraw the boundaries of science, policy and politics blurred by the ISG, arguing that they should lay out 'the science', but leave decisions to politicians.[118] Policy scholar Paul Cairney has written of the British government's 'imaginative use' of evidence to make policy—in a study of family policy, he demonstrates how policymakers work with, around and through developing evidence in order to achieve their own, longer-term policy goals.[119] A longer view of badger/bTB reveals another agenda at work beyond 'the science' of bTB control, which I argue has directed the overall direction of policymakers' work on bTB. In contrast to the expansions of the 1970s and 1980s, Defra's research budget has been cut repeatedly since the 1990s—a consistent trend across Labour and Conservative governments. Indeed the Krebs report notes the need to cut the costs of bTB control, and a wider 'cost-sharing' agenda for animal health was fully articulated by Defra under Labour.[120] However, cost-sharing requires the cooperation of industry, opening up badger culling as a potential quid pro quo and negotiating tool. In October 2007, the chair of Defra's TBAG wrote to the farming minister as follows:

> We were struck by the farming industry's willingness to consider additional cattle controls, but they made clear that going down this route without addressing the wildlife reservoir could only have a partial impact on levels of TB in cattle and, in their view, would not be acceptable given the need to control the disease. As we move further towards cost and responsibility sharing for animal health and welfare, including bovine TB, we were also encouraged to learn that the farming industries were exploring the costs and benefits of the ISG's recommendations for increased cattle measures and would welcome the opportunity to discuss these in more detail with Government.[121]

In other words, the chair of TBAG was saying that industry was willing to cooperate with government on tightening up cattle controls (as per the ISG's recommendation) as well as on cost-sharing only if government was willing to give them badger culling. As we have already seen, Hilary Benn's decision to not cull would have gone directly against this 'backstage' negotiation process, perhaps driving some of the intensity of farming reactions and the politicisation of scientific expertise we have seen. While the post-2010 reversal of Benn's decision and return to culling has further driven public polarisation of the debate, it is worth noting that behind the scenes Defra has since been more successful at implementing these cost-sharing and regulatory agendas. At present, bTB policy (including the tightening of cattle controls recommended by the ISG) is (albeit with reluctance) being supported (and paid for) by farmers, who in turn have been permitted to cull badgers for themselves.[122] In Chap. 8, we will revisit the long-term retreat of the state in animal health and disease control and explore the implications of this for the longer history of bTB beyond the culling controversy in Britain.

Notes

1. For epistemic communities, see Claire A. Dunlop, 'Knowledge, Epistemic Communities and Agenda-Setting', in *Handbook of Public Policy Agenda-Setting*, ed. N. Zahariadis (Cheltenham: Edward Elgar, 2016), 273–96; Meyer and Molyneux-Hodgson, 'Introduction: The Dynamics of Epistemic Communities'.
2. Reynolds, 'Case Study'.
3. As discussed in Chap. 1, a knowledge controversy is an academic and/or policy and/or public debate centred upon questions of scientific knowledge, expertise and evidence: Pinch and Bijker, 'The Social Construction of Facts and Artefacts'; Barry Barnes, David Bloor and John Henry, *Scientific Knowledge: A Sociological Analysis* (Chicago: University of Chicago Press, 1996); Whatmore, 'Mapping Knowledge Controversies'; Barry, 'Political Situations'.
4. Backstage–frontstage was originally developed by Goffman as an analysis of how people behave and think differently when 'in private' compared to 'in public': Erving Goffman, *The Presentation of Self in Everyday Life* (Garden City, NY: Doubleday, 1959). For this analysis, I draw upon research applying the idea to museums and 'public science': Sharon Macdonald, *Behind the Scenes at the Science Museum* (Oxford: Berg, 2002); Angela Cassidy, Simon J. Lock and Georgina Voss, 'Sexual Nature? (Re)Presenting Sexuality and Science in the Museum', *Science as Culture* 25(2) (2016): 214–38; science–policy relations: Stephen Hilgartner, *Science on Stage: Expert Advice as Public Drama* (Stanford, CA: Stanford University Press, 2000); Göran Sundqvist et al., 'One World or Two? Science–Policy Interactions in the Climate Field', *Critical Policy Studies* 12(4) (2018): 448–68; and policy–political negotiations: Raymond Alan Friedman, *Front Stage, Backstage: The Dramatic Structure of Labor*

Negotiations (Cambridge, MA: MIT Press, 1994); Ayres, Sandford and Coombes, 'Policy-Making "Front" and "Back" Stage'.

5. For an accessible discussion of 'publicness', see Nick Mahony, Janet Newman and Clive Barnett, *Rethinking the Public: Innovations in Research, Theory and Politics* (Bristol: Policy Press, 2010); for the complicating effects of social media and online communications, see Nancy K. Baym and danah boyd, 'Socially Mediated Publicness: An Introduction', *Journal of Broadcasting & Electronic Media* 56(3) (1 July 2012): 320–29.
6. To clarify, I use the term 'science' in the inclusive sense of the German term *Wissenschaft* (any field of systematic research); i.e. this would encompass natural sciences such as ecology and epidemiology; medical fields such as veterinary science; engineering and mathematics; and the social sciences, arts and humanities. See Angela Cassidy, 'Communicating the Social Sciences: A Specific Challenge?' in *Handbook of Public Communication of Science and Technology*, 2nd ed., ed. Massimiano Bucchi and Brian Trench (New York: Routledge, 2014), 186–98.
7. In date order, the reviews have been: Zuckerman, 'Badgers, Cattle and Tuberculosis'; Dunnet, Jones and McInerney, 'Badgers and Bovine Tuberculosis'; Krebs et al., 'Bovine Tuberculosis in Cattle and Badgers'; Godfray et al., 'Independent Scientific Review of the Randomised Badger Culling Trial and Associated Epidemiological Research'; Bourne et al., 'Bovine TB'; King et al., 'Bovine Tuberculosis in Cattle and Badgers'; Godfray et al., 'A Restatement of the Natural Science Evidence Base Relevant to the Control of Bovine Tuberculosis in Great Britain'; Munro et al., 'Pilot Badger Culls in Somerset and Gloucestershire Report by the Independent Expert Panel'; Godfray et al., 'A Strategy for Achieving Bovine Tuberculosis Free Status for England'.
8. Regarding social status and badger/bTB, we should note that while several highly eminent women have participated in bTB expert review committees, all have been chaired by senior white men. For a detailed analysis of the contrasting 'civic epistemologies' of science-policy in the USA, Germany and Britain, see Sheila Jasanoff, *Designs on Nature: Science and Democracy in Europe and the United States* (Princeton: Princeton University Press, 2005). For relationships between experts, the state, NGOs and publics in Britain, see Hilton et al., *The Politics of Expertise.*
9. Agar, 'Transition'.
10. For BSE see, Miller, 'Risk, Science and Policy'; Patrick Van Zwanenberg and Erik Millstone, 'BSE: A Paradigm of Policy Failure', *The Political Quarterly* 74(1) (January 2003): 27–37. For GM foods, see Brian Wynne, 'Creating Public Alienation: Expert Cultures of Risk and Ethics on GMOs', *Science as Culture* 10(4) (2001): 445–81; Renata Motta, 'Social

Disputes over GMOs : An Overview', *Sociology Compass* 8(12) (2014): 1360–76. For FMD in 2001, see Bickerstaff and Simmons, 'The Right Tool for the Job?'; B. Nerlich, 'War on Foot and Mouth Disease in the UK, 2001: Towards a Cultural Understanding of Agriculture', *Agriculture and Human Values* 21(1) (2004): 15–25; Convery et al., 'Death in the Wrong Place?'

11. G. Blue, 'Food, Publics, Science', *Public Understanding of Science* 19(2) (April 2009): 147–54; Melanie Smallman, 'Science to the Rescue or Contingent Progress? Comparing 10 Years of Public, Expert and Policy Discourses on New and Emerging Science and Technology in the United Kingdom', *Public Understanding of Science* 27(6) (1 August 2018): 655–73.
12. Neil Ward, 'Rethinking Rural Policy under New Labour', in *New Labour's Countryside Rural Policy in Britain since 1997*, ed. M. Woods (Bristol: The Policy Press, 2008), 29–43.
13. Griggs and Howarth, 'Protest Movements, Environmental Activism and Environmentalism in the United Kingdom'; Hilton et al., *The Politics of Expertise.*
14. Neil Carter and Ben Clements, 'From "Greenest Government Ever" to "Get Rid of All the Green Crap": David Cameron, the Conservatives and the Environment', *British Politics* 10(2) (1 June 2015): 204–25.
15. Chloe Lucas and Russell Warman, 'Disrupting Polarized Discourses: Can We Get out of the Ruts of Environmental Conflicts?' *Environment and Planning C: Politics and Space* 36(6) (16 May 2018): 987–1005; Matthew Motta, 'The Polarizing Effect of the March for Science on Attitudes toward Scientists', *PS: Political Science & Politics* (July 2018): 1–6.
16. This is something of a misquote as Gove was cut short, but his comments were widely reported in this form, suggesting deep resonances during the UK's EU membership referendum campaign: Henry Mance, 'Britain Has Had Enough of Experts, Says Gove', *Financial Times*, 3 June 2016.
17. Grant, 'Intractable Policy Failure'.
18. Spencer, 'One Body of Evidence, Three Different Policies'; Dunlop, 'Contestation and Contingency in Advisory Governance'.
19. Claire A. Dunlop, 'Policy Learning and Policy Failure: Definitions, Dimensions and Intersections', *Policy & Politics* 45(1) (17 January 2017): 3–18; Claire A. Dunlop, 'Pathologies of Policy Learning: What Are They and How Do They Contribute to Policy Failure?' *Policy & Politics* 45(1) (17 January 2017): 19–37.
20. On building and breaking expectations around science and technology, see Nik Brown and Mike Michael, 'A Sociology of Expectations: Retrospecting Prospects and Prospecting Retrospects', *Technology*

Analysis & Strategic Management 15(1) (March 2003): 3–18; Nik Brown and Siân M. Beynon-Jones, '"Reflex Regulation": An Anatomy of Promissory Science Governance', *Health, Risk & Society* 14(3) (2012): 223–40. On science as *political* but *politicisation* as a process that science can still be drawn into, see Brown, 'Politicizing Science'.

21. Meyer and Molyneux-Hodgson, 'Introduction'.
22. Stephen McGinness, 'Bovine Tuberculosis', *House of Commons Library Research Paper* 63 (1998): 29.
23. Miller, 'Risk, Science and Policy'.
24. HC Deb 23 July 1996 vol. 282 c262W.
25. The full Krebs review group were: Prof. John Krebs, Prof. Roy Anderson, Prof. Tim Clutton Brock, Prof. Ivan Morrison, Prof. Douglas Young and Dr Christl Donelly, assisted by Dr Simon Frost and Dr Rosie Woodfroffe. See Krebs et al., 'Bovine Tuberculosis in Cattle and Badgers'.
26. Krebs et al., 'Bovine Tuberculosis in Cattle and Badgers', 6.
27. Ibid., 6–7.
28. Ibid., 128.
29. For evidence-based medicine in animal health see Jean-Michel Vandeweerd et al., 'Is Evidence-Based Medicine so Evident in Veterinary Research and Practice? History, Obstacles and Perspectives', *The Veterinary Journal* 191(1) (January 2012): 28–34. For RCTs in agricultural and ecological research, see Berry, 'The Resisted Rise of Randomisation in Experimental Design'.
30. The Agriculture Minister, Jack Cunningham, trained as a scientist and was also a key architect of Labour's reform and evidence-based policy agendas: Cabinet Office, 'Modernising Government' (London: HMSO, 1999). Cunningham received the first report of the ISG and initiated the post-BSE reform of MAFF, which led to the creation of Defra.
31. John Bourne et al., 'Bovine TB: Towards a Sustainable Policy to Control TB in Cattle', Independent Scientific Group on Cattle TB (London: Defra, July 1998).
32. Bourne et al., 'Bovine TB: The Scientific Evidence, Final Report of the Independent Scientific Group on Cattle TB'; Defra, 'A Strategy for Achieving Officially Bovine Tuberculosis Free Status for England'.
33. The full ISG group were: Prof. John Bourne, Prof. Christl Donnelly, Sir David Cox, Prof. George Gettinby, Prof. John McInerney, Prof. John McInerney, Prof. Ivan Morrison and Prof. Rosie Woodroffe. The full documents of the ISG are held in the UK Government Web Archives at: http://webarchive.nationalarchives.gov.uk/20081107202002/http://www.defra.gov.uk/animalh/tb/isg/index.htm.
34. For recent reviews, see Godfray et al., 'A Restatement of the Natural Science Evidence Base Relevant to the Control of Bovine Tuberculosis in Great Britain'; McDonald, 'Animal Health'.

35. Bourne et al., 'Bovine TB: Towards a Sustainable Policy to Control TB in Cattle', 3.
36. Krebs et al., 'Bovine Tuberculosis in Cattle and Badgers', 128.
37. John Bourne et al., 'Bovine TB: Second Report of the Independent Scientific Group on Cattle TB', Independent Scientific Group on Cattle TB (London: Defra, December 1999).
38. Bourne et al., 'Bovine TB: Second Report of the Independent Scientific Group on Cattle TB', 27.
39. Bourne et al., 'Bovine TB: Second Report of the Independent Scientific Group on Cattle TB'.
40. CBAG, 'A History Lesson of Direct Action & Badger Culls. | Badger Killers', Badger Killers—Coalition of Badger Action Groups, 14 April 2014.
41. Environment, Food and Rural Affairs Committee, Bovine TB, 2 April 2003, HC 432 2002–3, EV 32–3.
42. Convery et al., 'Death in the Wrong Place?'
43. Environment, Food and Rural Affairs Committee, Bovine TB, 13 July 2004, HC 638 2003–4, 6.
44. John Bourne et al., 'An Epidemiological Investigation into Bovine Tuberculosis: Towards a Science Based Control Strategy', Independent Scientific Group on Cattle TB (London: Defra, December 2004), 23.
45. Ibid., 120.
46. Ibid., 121.
47. Christl A. Donnelly et al., 'Impact of Localized Badger Culling on Tuberculosis Incidence in British Cattle', *Nature* 426(6968) (December 2003): 834–37.
48. C. Booker, 'Paterson finally prods Defra into action on bovine TB', *Sunday Telegraph* 18 December 2005, 35; S. Mitchell, 'TB OR NOT TB? Badgers are on trial, accused of spreading tuberculosis', *Daily Telegraph Weekend*, 4 March 2006, 1.
49. Defra, 'Public Consultation on Controlling the Spread of Bovine Tuberculosis in Cattle in High Incidence Areas in England: Badger Culling Summary of Responses' (London: Defra, July 2006).
50. John Bourne et al., 'Independent Scientific Group on Cattle TB: Report of the Work of the Group & Its Published Findings in 2005', Independent Scientific Group on Cattle TB (London: Defra, 2005).
51. Bourne et al., 'Bovine TB: The Scientific Evidence, Final Report of the Independent Scientific Group on Cattle TB', 46. For a visual illustration of this point, see Cassidy, '"Big Science" in the Field', 313.
52. Bourne et al., 'Bovine TB: The Scientific Evidence, Final Report of the Independent Scientific Group on Cattle TB', 288.
53. Y. Loya, 'Recolonisation of Red Sea Corals Affected by Natural Catastrophes and Man-Made Perturbations', *Ecology* 57(2) (1976): 278–89.

54. Krebs et al., 'Bovine Tuberculosis in Cattle and Badgers'; J. Swinton et al., 'A Comparison of Fertility Control and Lethal Control of Bovine Tuberculosis in Badgers: The Impact of Perturbation Induced Transmission', *Philosophical Transactions of the Royal Society of London. Series B, Biological Sciences* 352(1353) (May 1997): 619–31; F. A. M. Tuyttens, D. W. Macdonald and B. Long, 'Spatial Perturbation Caused by a Badger (Meles Meles) Culling Operation: Implications for the Function of Territoriality and the Control of Bovine Tuberculosis (Mycobacterium Bovis)', *Journal of Animal Ecology* 69 (2000): 815–28.
55. Bourne et al., 'Bovine TB: The Scientific Evidence, Final Report of the Independent Scientific Group on Cattle TB', 85.
56. Ibid., 5.
57. Environment, Food and Rural Affairs Committee, 'Badgers and Cattle TB: The Final Report of the Independent Scientific Group', vol. I, 3 February 2008, HC 130-I 2007–8, EV 63.
58. C. Clover, 'TB crisis "needs funds, not badger cull"', *Daily Telegraph*, 19 June 2007, 10.
59. King et al., 'Bovine Tuberculosis in Cattle and Badgers'.
60. Ibid., 3–4.
61. Dunlop, 'Contestation and Contingency in Advisory Governance'.
62. HC Deb 25 Oct. 2012, vol. 551, col. 1148. Prime Minister's Questions is a weekly session in Parliament where the PM is directly questioned by other MPs. It is a notoriously oppositional and rowdy event.
63. Environment, Food and Rural Affairs Committee, 'Badgers and Cattle TB: The Final Report of the Independent Scientific Group', vol. II, Oral and written evidence, 3 February 2008, HC 130-II 2007–8, EV 29, EV 164, EV 172; Godfray et al., 'Independent Scientific Review of the Randomised Badger Culling Trial and Associated Epidemiological Research'; R. M. Q. Sainsbury and J. Gallagher, 'TB Controls', *Veterinary Record* 161(4) (28 July 2007): 143; Simon J. More, 'What Is Needed to Eradicate Bovine Tuberculosis Successfully: An Ireland Perspective', *Vet J* 180(3) (June 2009): 275–78.
64. Environment, Food and Rural Affairs Committee, 'Badgers and Cattle TB', vol. I, EV 21–25.
65. Dunlop, 'Pathologies of Policy Learning', 17 January 2017, 26.
66. E. Woolf, 'Cull of badgers is given the go-ahead by Blair', *Independent*, December 11 2005, 9. Blair's views emerged when the 'black spider' correspondence of culling advocate HRH Prince Charles was published: Cabinet Office, 'Prince of Wales Correspondence with the Prime Minister', GOV.UK, 13 May 2015.
67. EFRAC, 'Badgers and Cattle TB', vol. I, EV 23.
68. EFRAC, Badgers and Cattle TB', vol. II, EV 82.

69. BBC, 'Benn Confirms TB Cull Rejection', *BBC News Online*, 7 July 2008.
70. R. Page, 'Dairy drop is udderly disgraceful', *Daily Telegraph* Weekend, 14.
71. B. Mouland, 'Animal rights against human livelihoods in battle of the badgers', *Daily Mail*, 5 December 1998, 19; compared with James Meikle, 'English Badgers Earn a Reprieve, as Government Rejects Mass Cull', *The Guardian*, 4 July 2008, sec. UK news.
72. G. Gibbs, 'Friends and foes threaten the badger cull', *Guardian*, 14 July 2000, 7; compared with C. Clover, 'Chief Scientist urges badger cull', *Daily Telegraph*, 23 October 2007.
73. Johann Tasker, 'In the Hot Seat: Tim Farron of the Lib Dems', *Farmers Weekly*, 14 September 2009; Cabinet Office, 'The Coalition: Our Programme for Government' (London: HMSO, 2010).
74. Jim Paice, 'New Measures to Control Bovine TB in Badgers', GOV.UK, 15 September 2010.
75. Defra, 'The Government's Policy on Bovine TB and Badger Control in England' (London: HMSO, 2011), 34.
76. Ibid., 21, annex F.
77. Ibid.
78. Godfray et al., 'A Restatement of the Natural Science Evidence Base Relevant to the Control of Bovine Tuberculosis in Great Britain'.
79. Defra, 'Badger Culling Pilots: Independent Expert Panel', GOV.UK, 2013.
80. *The Times*, 'Editorial: A Necessary Cull: Controlling the badger population is good science to prevent the spread of disease', 29 August 2013, 20.
81. Defra, 'The Government's Policy on Bovine TB and Badger Control in England', 20.
82. Damian Carrington and Jamie Doward, 'Badger Cull "Mindless", Say Scientists', *The Observer*, 13 October 2012, sec. Environment.
83. T. Bawden, 'Badgershambles', *Independent*, 12 October 2013, 16; see also Phoenix, 'Local Understandings of Bovine Tuberculosis (Working Title)'.
84. BBC, 'Badgers "moved Goalposts" in Cull', *BBC News*, 9 October 2013, sec. England.
85. Munro et al., 'Pilot Badger Culls in Somerset and Gloucestershire Report by the Independent Expert Panel'.
86. Defra, 'A Strategy for Achieving Officially Bovine Tuberculosis Free Status for England'; Dafydd Saunders-Jones, 'Bovine TB Eradication Programmes in Europe', Nuffield Farming Scholarships Trust Report, August 2016.
87. Defra, 'A Strategy for Achieving Officially Bovine Tuberculosis Free Status for England', 33–34. For an up-to-date picture of how govern-

ment is allocating bTB risks across the UK, see http://www.tbhub.co.uk/risk-map/.

88. Defra, 'A Strategy for Achieving Officially Bovine Tuberculosis Free Status for England', 33–34. For further analysis and farmers' reactions to this new system, see also G. Enticott, 'Market Instruments, Biosecurity and Place-Based Understandings of Animal Disease', *Journal of Rural Studies* 45 (2016): 312–19; Damian Maye, 'Geography Matters: Farmer Perceptions of a Voluntary TB Risk-Based Trading System', *The Veterinary Record* 180(6) (February 2017): 146–47.
89. M. Bagot, 'Badger Bodgers: Officials "give up on the scientific basis of cull but still carry on killing"', *Daily Mirror*, 24 June 2014, 22.
90. Defra, 'Press Release: Landmark Agriculture Bill to Deliver a Green Brexit', GOV.UK, 12 September 2018; Eustace, 'Bovine TB'.
91. Defra, 'Bovine Tuberculosis (BTB) Strategy Review 2018: Terms of Reference', GOV.UK, 15 March 2018.
92. A. Coles, 'Taunton's MP and Michael Eavis resign as vice presidents of Wildlife Trust amid badger cull row', *Somerset County Gazette*, 22 June 2018.
93. For organisational agendas and One Health, see Angela Cassidy, 'One Health? Building an Interdisciplinary Bandwagon at the Interfaces of Animal Health, Human Health and the Environment', in *Investigating Interdisciplinary Collaboration: Theory and Practice across Disciplines*, ed. Scott Frickel, Mathieu Albert and Barbara Prainsack (New Brunswick, NJ: Rutgers University Press, 2016). For APHA and One Health, see Veterinary Record, 'Combining Plant and Animal Health', *Veterinary Record* 175(8) (August 2014): 182.
94. Prospect, 'The State of Natural England 2018–2019' (London: Prospect: the trade union for professionals, 2018).
95. Spencer, 'One Body of Evidence, Three Different Policies'; G. Enticott, Alex Franklin and Steven Van Winden, 'Biosecurity and Food Security: Spatial Strategies for Combating Bovine Tuberculosis in the UK', *The Geographical Journal* 178(4) (December 2012): 327–37.
96. Giesler and Ares, 'Badger Culling in England'.
97. For an accessible overview to developments in natural science see Robertson, 'TB Knowledge Exchange'; for social aspects see e.g. J. M. Broughan et al., 'Farm Characteristics and Farmer Perceptions Associated with Bovine Tuberculosis Incidents in Areas of Emerging Endemic Spread', *Preventive Veterinary Medicine* 129 (1 July 2016): 88–98; Damian Maye, G. Enticott and Rhiannon Naylor, 'Using Scenario-Based Influence Mapping to Examine Farmers' Biosecurity Behaviour', *Land Use Policy* 66 (October 2016): 265–77; Stephan Price et al., 'From Contradiction to Contrast in a Countryside Conflict: Using Q

Methodology to Reveal a Diplomatic Space for Doing TB Differently', *Environment and Planning A* 49(11) (23 August 2017): 2578–94.

98. Benjamin M. C. Swift, Thomas W. Convery and Catherine E. D. Rees, 'Evidence of Mycobacterium Tuberculosis Complex Bacteraemia in Intradermal Skin Test Positive Cattle Detected Using Phage-RPA', *Virulence* 7(7) (2 October 2016): 779–88; L. McCallan et al., 'Assessment of Serological Tests for Diagnosis of Bovine Tuberculosis', *Veterinary Record* 181(4) (22 July 2017): 90.
99. E.g. Saved and Safe Ltd, 'BeatbTB', 2014; PBD Biotech, 'APHA Grants Access to New Actiphage Technology for Chronic TB Breakdowns | PBD Biotech', 21 May 2018.
100. Save Me Trust, 'Bovine TB Symposium 2017—Save Me Trust', Dr Brian May's Save Me Trust: Giving Animals a Voice, 28 March 2017.
101. Price et al., 'From Contradiction to Contrast in a Countryside Conflict'.
102. Davies et al., 'Science, Culture, and Care in Laboratory Animal Research'.
103. For further analysis of this transition, see Grant, 'Intractable Policy Failure: The Case of Bovine TB and Badgers'. The current version of this group is the TB Eradication Advisory Group (TBEAG), https://www.gov.uk/government/groups/bovine-tb-eradication-advisory-group-for-england.
104. Marsh David et al., 'Policy Networks and the Distinction between Insider and Outsider Groups: The Case of the Countryside Alliance', *Public Administration* 87(3) (27 July 2009): 621–38.
105. Charles Rosenberg, 'Chapter 15—Toward an Ecology of Knowledge: On Discipline, Context, and History', in *Rise of the Knowledge Worker*, ed. James W. Cortada (Boston: Butterworth-Heinemann, 1998), 221–32; Cassidy, 'Evolutionary Psychology as Public Science and Boundary Work'.
106. Gay, *The Silwood Circle*.
107. Who's Who, 'Krebs, Baron, (John Richard Krebs) (Born 11 April 1945)', in *WHO'S WHO & WHO WAS WHO* (Oxford: Oxford University Press, 2018).
108. Bickerstaff and Simmons, 'The Right Tool for the Job?'; Gay, *The Silwood Circle*, 282.
109. Burkhardt, 'Ethology, Natural History, the Life Sciences, and the Problem of Place'; Beale, 'Tinbergian Practice, Themes and Variations'; Berry, 'The Resisted Rise of Randomisation in Experimental Design'; Cassidy, '"Big Science" in the Field'.
110. Dunlop, 'Policy Learning and Policy Failure', 32.
111. Worboys, 'Germ Theories of Disease and British Veterinary Medicine, 1860–1890'; Keir Waddington, 'The Science of Cows: Tuberculosis, Research and the State in the United Kingdom, 1890–1914', *History of*

Science 39(3) (September 2001): 355–81; Abigail Woods, 'The Farm as Clinic: Veterinary Expertise and the Transformation of Dairy Farming, 1930–1950', *Studies in History and Philosophy of Biological and Biomedical Sciences* 38(2) (June 2007): 462–87; Woods, 'From Practical Men to Scientific Experts'.

112. Martin Edwards, *Control and the Therapeutic Trial: Rhetoric and Experimentation in Britain, 1918–1948* (Leiden: Brill, 2007).
113. Rees, *The Infanticide Controversy.*
114. For the 'fieldworker's regress', see Rees, *The Infanticide Controversy*; for the reinterpretation and contestation of the RBCT, see Dunlop, 'Contestation and Contingency in Advisory Governance'; Dunlop, 'Pathologies of Policy Learning', 17 January 2017; Rhiannon Naylor et al., 'The Framing of Public Knowledge Controversies in the Media: A Comparative Analysis of the Portrayal of Badger Vaccination in the English National, Regional and Farming Press', *Sociologia Ruralis* 57(1) (2017): 3–22; Cassidy, '"Big Science" in the Field'.
115. Dunlop, 'Pathologies of Policy Learning', 17 January 2017.
116. T. F. Gieryn, 'Boundaries of Science', in *The Handbook of Science and Technology Studies*, ed. S. Jasanoff (Thousand Oaks, CA: SAGE, 1995), 393–456; Cassidy, 'Evolutionary Psychology as Public Science and Boundary Work'; Cassidy, '"Big Science" in the Field'.
117. Andre Sorensen, 'Taking Path Dependence Seriously: An Historical Institutionalist Research Agenda in Planning History', *Planning Perspectives* 30(1) (2 January 2015): 17–38.
118. I. Boyd, 'Making Science Count in Government', *ELife* 2 (July 2013): e01061–e01061.
119. Cairney, 'The UK Government's Imaginative Use of Evidence to Make Policy'.
120. Krebs et al., 'Bovine Tuberculosis in Cattle and Badgers', 8; Caroline Stocks, 'DEFRA faces angry silence from producers', *Farmer's Weekly*, 18 July 2008.
121. Defra TB Advisory Group, 'TB Advisory Group Letter to Jeff Rooker', 16 October 2007.
122. Enticott, 'Relational Distance, Neoliberalism and the Regulation of Animal Health'; Enticott, 'Market Instruments, Biosecurity and Place-Based Understandings of Animal Disease'.

7

Interactions between Media, Politicians and Pressure Groups

In the last chapter, we explored the interactions between the three epistemic communities of badger/bTB (*animal health*, *disease ecology* and *badger protection*), policymakers and politicians taking place 'backstage'—specialist interactions open to, but rarely scrutinised by, the wider public sphere.[1] It demonstrated how the backstage manoeuvrings of experts, campaigning interests, policymakers and politicians have been constituted in relation to the 'frontstage' of debates taking place in the wider public sphere. For example, it was after the breakdown of working relationships with policymakers that the Independent Scientific Group (ISG) ensured that their Final Report received wider public attention by giving media interviews, and crafting a clear, quotable message: 'culling cannot meaningfully contribute to the future control of cattle TB in Britain'.[2] As we saw through the first half of the book, such interactions between policy and public spheres have punctuated the history of badger/bTB. Examples would include Ruth Murray's attempt to prosecute the Farming Minister using his own badger protection legislation; the controversy following the publication of the Zuckerman review in 1980; and the argument between the ISG and David King. At various points in time, the arguments and decisions made in the relatively restricted spaces of scientific and policy fora have been mutually shaped by both mass media coverage and that poorly understood and unpredictable creature, public opinion. This has changed in recent years: as Britain saw the return of badger culling, badger/bTB moved dramatically from the margins to the mainstream of politics. However, this appears to have been a temporary shift. Following a brief 'storm' of media interest peaking in 2013, coverage levels have dropped off and have been occluded by bigger political issues, most obviously the highly divisive debate over whether, when and how the UK will 'Brexit'—leave the EU.

This chapter will investigate the interactions of media, politicians, pressure groups, journalists and audiences, who between them have made badger/bTB into a hotly contested issue which receives widespread media attention. In the process, it also addresses a wider question for the sociology and history of science: what makes a knowledge controversy become a public knowledge controversy, and how do controversies affect policy-making?[3] In today's professionalised sciences, disagreements and controversies are mostly fought out by qualified academics in the relatively constrained fora of journal articles, conferences and personal correspondence. While public controversies between and questioning of experts have become more common over the past fifty years, compared to everyday routines of scientific communication, they are still unusual.[4] When science does become controversial in public, it is often the implications of new scientific ideas or technologies which are contested, for example as seen in 1990s debates over genetically modified foods.[5] Less commonly, scientists make and contest knowledge claims in the public sphere instead of or alongside their usual fora of academic journals. This makes scientific uncertainties, changing knowledge and questioning of established ideas publicly visible, with significant implications for policy. A good example would be public controversies over Bovine spongiform encephalopathy (BSE) in the UK during the late 1980s and early 1990s. At this time, policy decisions about BSE and food safety had to be made in the face of deep 'unknown unknowns'—when the properties and existence of the transmitting agent, a molecule called a *prion*, were utterly unanticipated, and scientific understandings of the disease had to be developed under intense public and political scrutiny.[6] Public knowledge controversies therefore demonstrate that scientific communication and 'popularisation' are not always one-way processes of communicating established science to wider publics; they are also multidirectional and can contribute to the process of building scientific knowledge. They tend to be driven by a combination of internal factors pushing them out of specialist fora (e.g. rapidly changing situations; communications blocks; disciplinary rivalries); and external factors pulling them into mass media (e.g. the power of a good story; direct risks to people; political implications).[7] As seen in the BSE case, the uncertainties and complexities of 'science in the making' exposed during public controversies[8] raise critical questions about how 'experts', politicians and policymakers can best work together to make sustainable policy decisions that can work in the long term.

This chapter will examine key contours of British press coverage of badgers and bTB and how it has changed since the middle of the last century, as well as how badger/bTB has come to be framed in mass media. It will then return to the sequence of events recounted in Chap. 6 to explore how badger/bTB has been debated in the frontstage of British policy and mass media. We will explore how the long-standing public concerns of the British badger debate and of bTB have repeatedly been brought together and drawn apart over the past fifty years, as well as how in recent years the two have become tightly linked. There has been a series of key changes in badger protection campaigning, wider political debates and mass media working practices since 2010. I argue that these have all contributed to the mainstreaming, polarisation and politicisation of badger/bTB and its movement from the 'backstage' to the 'frontstage' of British animal health policy.[9] Finally, we will explore how and why this has happened and speculate on the consequences for the underlying problems which have made badger/bTB into such a notorious policy failure.[10]

7.1 UK Newspaper Coverage: Some Key Indicators

The digitisation of newspaper archives has made it easier than ever to use press coverage as a blunt indicator of where and when media pay attention to a given issue, providing insights into changes in the public profile of a topic over time. It has also made it possible to collect a large sample of national press coverage of badger/bTB, which has been analysed alongside the archival material, policy documents and interviews used as sources throughout this research. To this end, three sets of keywords were used to search the digital archives of the *Guardian/Observer*, *Independent*, *Times*, *Telegraph*, *Mail* and *Mirror* (plus their Sunday editions) from 1950 to 2000. They were also used to search the Nexis UK database of modern print media (narrowed to these titles) from 1995 to 2017. The first ('badger' AND 'animal') was designed to capture overall coverage of badgers while excluding the unrelated usage of 'badger' as a verb and as a name. The second ('bovine tuberculosis' OR 'bovine TB') was designed to find coverage of bTB itself; while the third ('badger' AND ['TB' OR 'tuberculosis']) found articles discussing badgers and bTB together. The articles brought up by these searches were downloaded and added to two databases (alongside interview transcripts, scans of archival sources and images), before and after the publication of the Krebs report in 1997. This search process also yielded quantitative data about how the British press has covered the issue, which will briefly be presented here.[11] This quantitative data offers some useful insights into how media coverage of badgers, bTB and the controversy about their connection has changed over the past half century.

The broad trends shown in Fig. 7.1 reflect and confirm the stories surrounding badgers and bTB over the second half of the twentieth century. Early press coverage about bTB focused on the success of the Ministry for Agriculture, Fisheries and Food's (MAFF) Area Eradication Scheme, and the 1960 announcement that the whole country had been 'attested'.[13] Following this, bTB ceased to be of interest until 1975, when MAFF announced its new research and policy programme addressing the new problem of tuberculous badgers. From then on, most articles mentioning bTB also mentioned badgers, but not necessarily the other way around, as can be seen by the close correspondence between 'bovine TB' and 'badger + TB'. By contrast, 'badger + animal' brought up a broad range of material, including natural history columns,

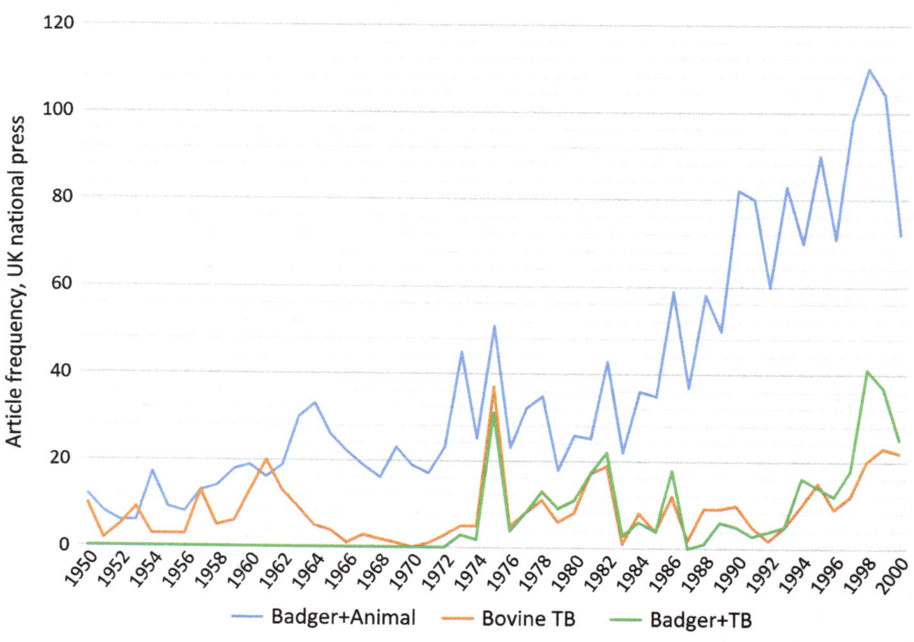

Fig 7.1 UK national newspaper coverage about badgers and bTB, 1950–2000[12]

articles about toys, holidays and the latest adaptation of *Wind in the Willows*, as well as news coverage relating to bTB. The growing popularity of badgers in the public sphere can be traced from a handful of nature columns in the 1950s, to around eighty articles a year by the 1990s. Peaks in this coverage can be linked to key events in wildlife politics: from the 1955 Scott Henderson report, through the initiation of badger protection campaigns in 1964, to the passing of the Badgers Act in 1973.[14] Between 1975 and 1986, coverage of badgers and of bTB was linked together, as suggested by the shared spikes in coverage in 1975 (the start of state-led culling) and again in 1982 (when badger gassing ended).[15] Through the rest of the 1980s and into the 1990s, bTB once again faded from media attention, but badgers received more coverage than ever before. Animal and environmental politics underwent a radical turn at this time, with protests targeted at road expansion, animal experimentation and fox hunting all hitting the headlines.[16] While substantive policy change on these issues was limited, animal advocates made significant gains on the issue of badger protection, whereby the 1973 Badgers Act was strengthened in 1992 and 1993.[17] Campaigning leading up to and following this success recreated badgers as a media story in their own right, decoupled from bTB.

As we moved into the twenty-first century, while badgers continued to be covered more than bTB, the two stories started to align once again. Peaks in coverage can be linked to key events in the culling controversy, such as the start of the Randomised Badger Culling Trial (RBCT) trial and the ISG/King controversy in 2007. As the Brown Labour government became weaker and General Election campaigning started, coverage of badger/bTB dropped away as news agendas turned towards mainstream political events. This pattern—of highly episodic coverage, linked to key policy or political events—has been present since the early 1970s in badger/bTB and is highly characteristic of environmental news coverage in general.[19] Since Labour lost power in 2010 and subsequent administrations have started returning to culling, the media debate has changed. As can be seen in Fig. 7.2, press coverage of badger/bTB started climbing as soon as the incoming Coalition announced its intention to return to culling in 2011, peaking in 2013 but then returning to mid-2000s levels by the end of 2017. In the process, media coverage of badgers and of bTB have become more closely linked than ever before. While of course we don't know what will happen next, this post-2010 pattern seems different. Not only was the 2013 peak three

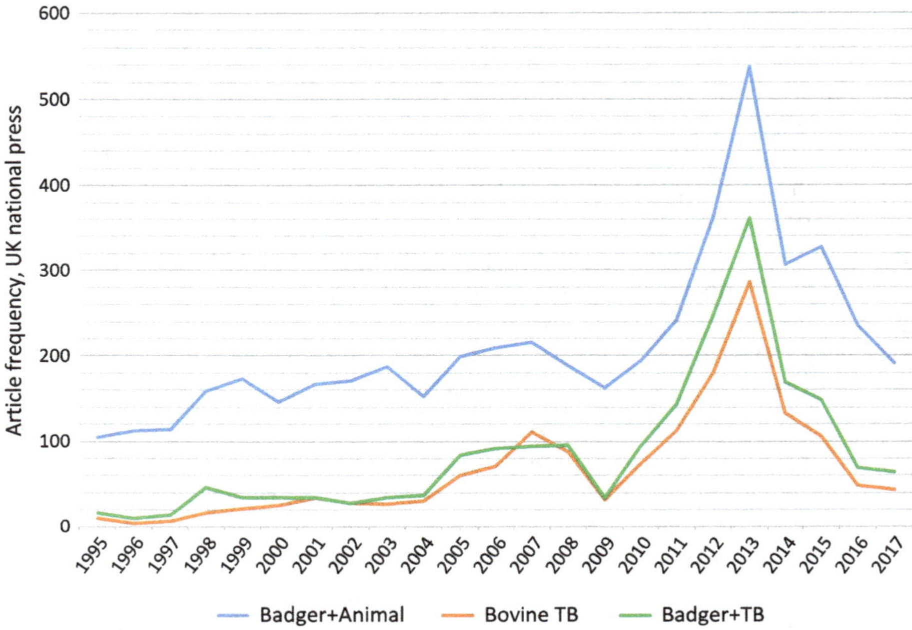

Fig. 7.2 UK national newspaper coverage about badgers and bTB, 1995–2017[18]

times higher than ever before, it cannot be easily attributed to any single event—we will explore the implications of this shift in Sect. 7.4.

British national newspapers operate an overtly politically 'partisan' system, whereby each title has a distinctive and widely understood political orientation, manifesting (for example) as endorsements of political parties during General Elections. As well as differing in their political orientations, newspapers can be further characterised as 'broadsheet', 'mid-market' and 'tabloid' titles, and while the physical differences between newspapers have blurred, it is clear from their content and design that these distinctions are still meaningful (see Table 7.1). These titles cater to significantly different demographics in their readership, particularly in terms of social class, income and political opinions (broadly congruent with those expressed in the newspaper they buy).[20]

Figure 7.3 shows the distribution and amount of coverage of badger/bTB across the sampled titles, as well as how this has changed over the decades. We can see that, on the whole, badger/bTB has been covered more by right-wing titles than left-wing, reflecting these newspapers'

Table 7.1 UK national newspapers by format and political orientation

	'Tabloid'	*'Mid-market'*	*'Broadsheet'*
'Left'	*Mirror* *Morning Star*		*Guardian/Observer* *Independent/'i'*
'Centre' / no clear orientation	*Star* *Sunday People* *Metro* (freesheet)		*Financial Times*
'Right'	*Sun / Sun on Sunday / News of the World*	*Mail* *Express*	*Times* *Telegraph*

alliances with rural interests. It has been covered far more by broadsheets than tabloids, in a pattern consistent with much scientific and environmental news.[21] Of more significance is the increasing levels of coverage from the mid-market *Mail* and tabloid *Mirror*, particularly since 2010. This is consistent with overall increases in coverage, but also marks a shift in the visibility of badger/bTB to new audiences—and given the higher circulation of these titles, many more people than ever before.

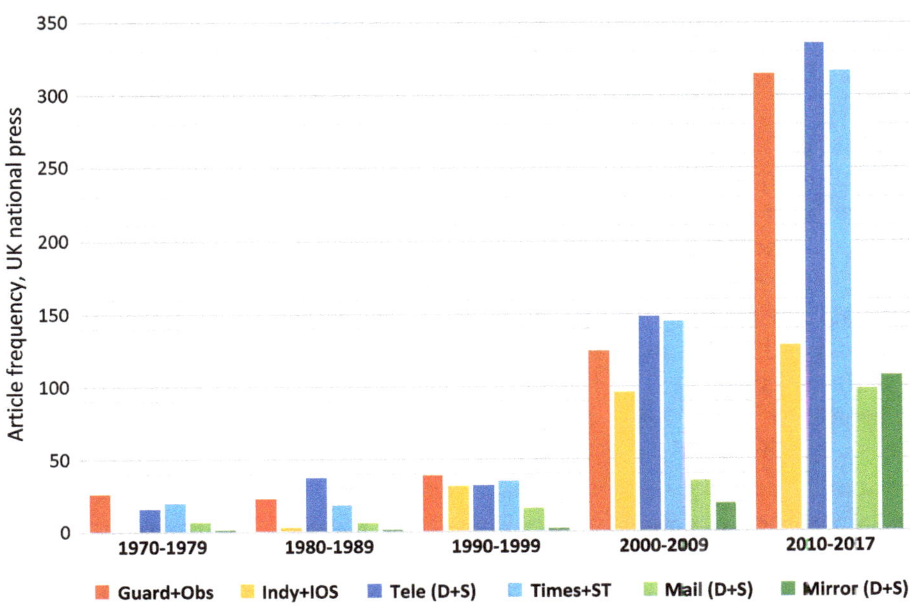

Fig. 7.3 UK national newspaper coverage of badger/bTB, by newspaper title and decade

7.2 Agricultural Malaise or Environmental Risk? Media Framings of Badger/bTB

These bare figures can be fleshed out into a richer picture by looking at the content of newspaper stories about badger/bTB, and particularly at how the issue has been 'framed'. Like historians of medicine, scholars of mass media use framing to analyse how and why particular issues come to the attention of journalists. Their focus tends to be more specific, documenting what gets included in a story and what doesn't, as well as the other issues any given topic is linked to. Media framings are not independently created: instead they are a product of the interactions of advocates' attempts to 'set the agenda'; the judgements of journalists and their editors about what makes a 'good story'; and the preferences of audiences, expressed through sales and increasingly via social media.[22] Since the 1990s, press coverage of badger/bTB can be characterised as framed in one of two ways: either bTB as an agricultural problem; or badger culling (one of several policies for controlling bTB) as an environmental risk. From the late nineteenth century up to the 1960s, bTB was primarily framed as a (human) public health problem: today risks to human health are only sporadically and strategically discussed. Even so, these framings of badger/bTB are broadly consistent with contemporary 'social representations' of infectious disease, also visible in discussions of diseases like HIV/AIDS and influenza. Each has clearly identified 'victims, villains and heroes': although who (or what) gets to play each of these roles is different in each framing.[23]

Framing One: An Agricultural Malaise. The first way of writing media stories about badger/bTB should be familiar from the ***animal health*** cultures of care explored in Chap. 3. The agricultural frame positions the disease as a resurgent problem severely affecting rural communities and the national economy. Farmers are portrayed as the primary victims (via the loss of their cattle), but also as key professional experts—curiously, they appear much more frequently and prominently than veterinarians. The seriousness of the bTB problem is emphasised by highlighting the zoonotic nature of the disease, and cases of bTB in other livestock (such as llamas), pets and particularly in humans receive a great deal of attention. Despite this, sick cows do not feature, primarily because Britain now rarely sees such cases. The collective slaughter of cattle testing positive for *M. bovis* is emphasised through large numbers: individual cows rarely appear, except (for example) during the 2007 conflict in Wales over the sacred bull

Shambo.[24] In line with animal health, the primary symptom of bTB is depicted as its economic impact—upon government, industry and individual farmers. The heroic stories of such farmers—struggling financially but also emotionally with bTB—provide personal depth to this reporting. They also place the disease into an ongoing narrative about the failures of animal health policy in Britain by connecting current problems to earlier disasters, including the 2001 outbreak of foot and mouth disease (FMD), and further back to BSE.[25] This links bTB into broader discourses of 'marginalised rurality'—the idea that rural perspectives are sidelined in British society—which have become increasingly politicised in recent years:

> A beef and sheep producer with arable interests, [incoming NFU President] Ms Batters says farmers are the best custodians of the countryside. But she warns that they are coming under increasing fire from animal rights activists, environmentalists and militant vegans. With consumers more interested in where their food comes from, growers and livestock producers 'cannot afford to be silent', or this void will be 'filled by others', she adds.
>
> Under attack: 'We have seen it with veganism, the badger cull and crop protection. We have been an industry under attack, but reacting to the noise is the worst thing farmers can do', she tells *Farmers Weekly*. 'Actually, farmers should be really proud of what we do and we need to get those messages across. It's about being more positive, less reactive.'[26]

Farmers are recognised as having immediate 'experiential expertise', and their first-hand testimony is used in a similar way to that of patients in health reporting.[27] Yet they are also portrayed as helpless victims, unable to do anything in the face of an unstoppable plague, while 'urban elites' are imagined as indifferent or hostile to the agricultural sector. While veterinarians do feature as legitimate experts dealing with the problem, policymakers and government are deeply distrusted.[28] When scientists appear they tend to be those supportive of culling, such as Sir David King, and the 'sound science' of such experts is also invoked. Finally, the history of the controversy features, in discussions of the 'Thornbury experiment' of the 1970s, or of earlier culling policies such as gassing.[29] This demonstrates the strategic role of memory in public controversies: while these past policies are recalled, the compelling reasons for their abandonment are not.

A second victim of bTB, curiously only visible in the agricultural frame, is the sick and suffering badger. The effects of tuberculosis on badgers themselves are discussed in some detail, and concerns may be expressed for their suffering. In this framing, killing sick or 'dirty' badgers can be understood as 'taking care'—of sick wildlife, of livestock populations, and of agricultural communities and businesses.[30] Again in line with animal health and farming cultures of care, the proper role of people in relation to animals and environments should be to restore a 'natural balance' and take on stewardship of the countryside. This natural balance is seen as currently disrupted by overly strict protective legislation, leading to badger populations growing 'out of control'.[31] More often, the diseased badger is not sympathetic but a 'guilty victim', to be feared, stigmatised and excluded just as we do with human disease victims who lack power.[32] Badgers were constructed as the chief agents or causes of the bTB epidemic, therefore positioning culling as the most obvious solution to the problem. Today's agricultural framings of bTB have continued to highlight other negative traits of badgers unrelated to the disease, such as violence, predation on other charismatic wildlife such as hedgehogs, disruptive digging and crop destruction. This is emphasised by the frequent reuse of stock images of badgers and cows together: a situation so rare in life that some biologists think that these photographs were staged.[33] The Bad Badger, present in British culture for centuries, persists and has been transformed by its connection with bTB into more of a villain than ever before.

Framing Two: An Environmental Risk. The second way of talking about badger/bTB in mass media eclipses and elides infectious disease almost entirely, focusing instead on the favoured 'agricultural frame' solution to bTB: culling wild badgers. This framing tends to downplay disease problems and risks, acknowledging the existence of bTB, but treating it as largely absent—by inference (like its human equivalent), a solved problem of the past.[34] Sick cattle are never seen, badgers do not become ill and human health risks are not discussed. Up until the ISG's findings were made public, the idea that badgers could carry tuberculosis at all was disputed by many badger advocates.[35] While the connection between cows, badgers and *M. bovis* is now generally acknowledged, the significance and direction of badger–cattle transmission (compared to cattle–cattle transmission) and the extent to which badgers show clinical symptoms are still heavily contested. Instead, farming practices—including cattle trading, stress, poor hygiene and intensive breeding—are highlighted as the main causes of the resurgence of bTB. These causes are also rooted in accounts of the recent past: in this case the intensification of farming and its consequences, for livestock, wildlife and environments. The possibility of avoiding culling in the first place through vaccination has been widely advocated as an alternative, implicitly drawing upon audiences' familiarity with human medical care.[36]

Instead, the focus shifts to badger culling as an environmental risk. The consequences of culling for animals, ecosystems, public order and the popularity of politicians are highlighted. The political and economic risks of culling policies are emphasised, with widespread citation of high policing costs (due to protests) and cost–benefit analyses suggesting culling is not economically viable. Casting government in general or particular politicians as the villains, this framing assumes that 'the public' is strongly opposed to badger culling.[37] As in the agricultural framing, experiential experts—in the form of animal rescue volunteers and activists—loom large, providing first-hand accounts of badger persecution, as well as heroic stories from the 'front line' of confrontations with those undertaking the Conservatives' new 'trial culls'.[38] Campaigners are attributed the role of experiential and moral experts, not only bearing witness, but also arguing that humans bear the responsibility for preventing and alleviating non-human suffering. Scientists and conservationists are prominently depicted as the professional experts who know most about badger/bTB. When the Badger Trust opposed the RBCT trial in the 1990s, it drew heavily upon the scientific credentials of their then spokesperson, Dr Elaine King, and her PhD in badger ecology.[39] More recently, the ecologists and scientists associated with the ISG—particularly Krebs, Bourne and Woodroffe—have been most prominent, as have famous 'telenaturalists' such as Chris Packham. While specific scientific issues are discussed (such as the perturbation effect, or the consequences of culling for rural ecosystems), science also features as a generalised source of authoritative knowledge. The trope of 'sound science' is fully mobilised by anti-cull campaigners; these tactics are also deployed by scientists themselves when criticising the current culling policy:[40]

> The government's chief vet, Christine Middlemiss, said the first cull areas, in Gloucestershire and Somerset, were starting to see drops in TB in cattle, and a full analysis of the data was under way. [ISG scientist Rosie] Woodroffe said: 'Claims that the culls are reducing cattle TB is based on cherry-picking data from a report produced by government scientists. It states explicitly that "these data alone cannot demonstrate whether the badger control policy is effective in reducing bovine TB in cattle".' Middlemiss did not mention

> another cull area, Dorset, where TB rates appear to be rising. Dominic Dyer, the chief executive of the Badger Trust, said: 'This is the largest destruction of a protected species in living memory. By the end of 2018, the government will have spent over £50m of public funds killing over 67,000 badgers (since 2013), which could push the species to the verge of local extinction in areas of England where it has lived since the ice age. The badger cull is a cruel, costly and ineffective policy and its continuation is a national disgrace.'[41]

While disease victims are absent, the central victim—not of bTB but of human capriciousness—is instead the Good Badger, constructed as a charismatic wildlife species and symbol of idealised British 'nature'. Culling is the human intervention disturbing the 'balance of nature', which in this framing is best achieved by the withdrawal of humans altogether. Badgers are further described as a 'scapegoat' for the bTB problem, enabling farmers, rural interests, policymakers or politicians to avoid addressing a problem implicitly caused by their own actions.[42] The actual or potential suffering of wild badgers has provided a focus for highly emotive coverage, whether the culling method is free shooting or the more well-established cage-trapping technique.[43] While gassing has been long abandoned, the rhetoric that badgers are victims of a human inflicted 'holocaust' persists (at times to the dismay of British Jews), emphasising the large numbers killed. Unsurprisingly, these deaths were linked with illegal practices of badger persecution and killing (thought by campaigners to be on the rise), the politics of fox hunting and representations of pro-cull actors as psychologically unbalanced.[44] In the agricultural framing, British wildlife politics is presented as an aspect of 'urban–rural conflict'. By contrast, in environmental framings opposition to culling is presented as an aspect of a broader ethical outlook, part and parcel of a pro-environmental worldview and identity. Visual images also reinforce the Good Badger—by using wildlife photography these framings immediately recall the long, affectionate history of badgers' appearances on natural history television in Britain.[45] Cute and literally fluffy animals feature prominently (particularly cubs in animal rescue settings), alongside shocking images of dead and/or suffering badgers: both these tropes draw upon long-standing traditions of animal campaigning.[46]

Not only do these mutually exclusive framings talk about badger/bTB differently, but which media they appear in, and the cast of characters who are interviewed, cited and discussed are very different. The agricultural frame appears most often in right-wing national, farming and South West local press and tends to be written by journalists specialising in agriculture, the countryside or by conservative columnists. Key institutional actors include Defra, the NFU, the Farmers' Union of Wales and the National Beef Association. Given their centrality to animal health policy, veterinary associations rarely appear, but practising veterinarians do feature in this coverage. Farmers were the most frequently interviewed source: other individual sources include Conservative Party politicians, celebrities and various members of the British royal family. Stories using the environmental frame tend to appear in left-wing national newspapers and conservation magazines, and are mostly written by environmental and science journalists, or left-wing commentators. Barring Defra, an entirely different set of institutional actors appear, the most prominent of which is the Badger Trust. Considering its small size and tiny budget compared to many NGOs, the Trust's public prominence evidences a continuing tradition of highly skilled media relations. Other actors include the much larger RSPCA and more recently a coalition of animal welfare groups under the banner of 'Team Badger'. Instead of farmers and vets, we see animal rescue volunteers, protesters on marches, and activists directly disrupting culling. Since founding his Save Me Trust, the rock star Brian May has become a key source, and a wave of other celebrities have appeared in the environmental frame. While most coverage has used one of these two framings, some articles have sought to take a more traditionally journalistic, neutral stance, in which both were deployed, using the flip from one to the other as a narrative device. While publics' knowledge and views of badger/bTB are less well studied, similar framings can be discerned in social media and other online fora focused on the topic.[47]

7.3 Constituting and Contesting Badgers, bTB and Culling

Throughout this book, I have used 'badger/bTB' as a shorthand for the central question under debate in this public knowledge controversy—Do wild badgers carry and pass bTB to domestic cattle, and if so, what should be done about it? As we have seen, over the past fifty years, it has taken a lot of work to bring the previously separated issues of badgers and bTB together into the single issue we see today. Research on environmental and public communication has shown how journalists, audiences, campaigners, politicians and experts of various sorts work together to constitute an issue into something that is paid attention to in the public sphere. This involves making and contesting knowledge claims; writing (and convincing editors to publish) pieces in media; and taking on board (or ignoring) coverage about the topic at hand.[48] In turn, media debates can set, shape, build and break political and policy agendas, perhaps increasingly so in an era where policy actors use coverage as a proxy for wider public opinion, and campaigners put huge resources into gaining it.[49] Dramatic events, claims, counter-claims and appealing stories attract coverage and draw audience attention not only to the topic but to the various actors' framings of the issue—as demonstrated above. Others with differing views respond with their own counter-claims, which may or may not be persuasive. In the longer term, this is how political, social, scientific and environmental issues become constituted, reconstituted and dissolved in the 'public arenas' of mass media.[50] Having explored the general characteristics of contemporary UK media coverage of badger/bTB, the rest of this chapter will trace the public constitution and development of badger/bTB in the long term. It will return to the sequence of events recounted in Chap. 6; but will shift the focus to the 'frontstage' of policy debates as they have played out in mass media. As we will see, while the key events are the same, the details and dynamics of the debate have been very different: subtle rivalries and detailed interpretations of evidence are replaced by dramatically performed protests and emotive rhetorical flourishes.

As suggested by the data in Fig. 7.1, up until the 1990s, the distinct issues of badger protection and of bTB control came together and moved apart several times in the 'frontstage' of the debate.[51] When it was considered at all, bTB provided a classic narrative of the triumph of modern (veterinary) public health programmes over disease—until it was connected to badgers. By contrast, the public story of the badger was one of increasing visibility, initially through popular natural history across multiple media forms, and then through the energetic media work of badger protection campaigners, drawing in a diverse coalition of actors, including amateur naturalists, professional field biologists, animal welfare campaigners, the Women's Institute (WI) and politicians across party lines. They successfully reframed the older British 'badger debate' in relation to public concerns over environmental damage and the politics of wildlife welfare. This meant that by the time the news of tuberculous badgers broke, it was reported in terms of concern for wildlife rather than cattle: the initial news triggers were the passing of protective legislation and Ruth Murray's attempt at prosecuting the Farming Minister.[52] Coverage of bTB as animal health was largely confined to specialist contexts—agricultural correspondents and local and farming press.[53] From this point onwards, bTB was mostly reported in terms of badger protection, while badger protection continued to be covered in addition to bTB.

Given that media were foregrounding farmers' illegal 'gassing' of badgers, and that naturalists had already established themselves as accessible, articulate and authoritative experts on the matter, it was relatively easy for them to set the public agenda on bTB.[54] MAFF tried to argue that their research was 'aimed at settling once and for all the old argument over whether badgers infect cattle with bovine tuberculosis', but this was rarely reported.[55] Backstage, MAFF had managed to form a broad consensus that culling using Cymag ('gassing') was the most humane way of dealing with the problem. However, media responses to the new policy were very different, with naturalists directly challenging the causal links drawn between badgers, *M. bovis* and cattle, while illegal gassing by farmers was presented as continuous with illegitimate gassing by Ministry officials. Rhetorics of the 'mass extermination' of badgers by authorities would have been particularly resonant for the post-war generations making up public audiences of the time.[56] This coverage—present in newspapers across the political spectrum—continued into the pre- and post-publication controversy around the Zuckerman review and MAFF's abandonment of gassing in 1982. It was congruent with the broader convergence of the 'cultures of care' of conservation, environmentalism and animal rights discussed in Chap. 5. Moving into the 1980s and 1990s, bTB receded as a public issue, while wildlife politics (including badger persecution and fox hunting) became even more prominent. Further badger protection campaigning, including the adoption of media-friendly public spectacle (see Chap. 5, Fig. 5.4) was highly successful, culminating in the passing of the Badgers Act (1991), the Protection of Badgers Act (1992)—making it illegal to interfere with a sett without a government licence—and the further scaling back of culling for bTB control.[57]

The adeptness of badger advocates at setting media agendas continued in the early coverage of the RBCT experiment, sometimes referred to as the 'Krebs trial'. The National Federation of Badger Groups (NFBG, now Badger Trust) acquired a new media team: Dr Elaine King, a scientist who had trained at Woodchester Park, and PR specialist Trevor Lawson.[58] Together, they mobilised King's own expertise to critique the new government plans, arguing it was based on 'weak science': 'The experiment is fundamentally flawed. In some of the target areas farmers are already killing badgers illegally and this will affect the outcome … In other places landowners are denying access to land. And the traps cannot be guaranteed to catch all the badgers in an area.'[59] Backstage, the RBCT had been supported by the RSPCA, National Trust, British Veterinary Association (BVA) and NFU because they were persuaded that 'better evidence' was needed.[60] Frontstage, farmers were more equivocal: 'Something has to be done. I don't know if it's badgers. You say thousands of badgers have been killed. Well, 31,000 cows have been killed as well. I just know this experiment is the best thing we've been offered. I'm imploring it all to go forward. It's affecting us all.'[61] Public debates were laying bare the growing differences between the epistemic communities of badger/bTB. While farmers cared for their cattle and their livelihoods, badger protection advocates were primarily concerned with the prospect of 'their' species being killed. Both found themselves at odds with policy-facing actors, whose cultures of care operated at a broader scale, concerned with (for example) the economic welfare of agricultural industries, preservation of landscape or minimising animal suffering.

When the emerging RBCT data suggested that badger culling might make bTB worse, the response from ministers was to shut down part of the experiment, while policymakers distanced themselves from the ISG. While the news was made public, it did not receive much attention, and MAFF continued planning for re-implementing culling, briefing to the press that this would happen.[62] When the ISG eventually went public with their conclusions about culling and perturbation in 2007, the response from the NFU was one of shock and surprise: 'Sir John's [Bourne] report is a counsel of despair. We are not prepared to accept it.'[63] Conservative commentators echoed these sentiments, describing the ISG's work as a 'bombshell' and citing bTB as another issue in which an increasingly beleaguered countryside was ignored by the 'metropolitan' interests allegedly dominating the Labour government. This narrative, also fostered by the burgeoning Countryside Alliance, placed bTB alongside the outlawing of hunting with hounds, animal health problems such as BSE and FMD, and environmental reforms of the EU's Common Agricultural Policy.[64] These responses of shock, surprise and rejection of the ISG's research intensified when the following year Defra Secretary Hilary Benn reversed bTB policy, taking the scientists' advice, and decided not to cull: 'a move welcomed by environmentalists but condemned as a disaster by farmers'—widely interpreted as politically motivated.[65] Even the Badger Trust appeared to be surprised by the ISG's findings.[66] Given that MAFF specialists had been aware of 'badger movement' and 'recolonisation' since the 1970s, that ecologists had been researching perturbation and infectious disease since the mid-1990s, and that the ISG had been flagging the possibility for some years, the degree of surprise evidenced in media reporting suggests implies an widening gap between the 'backstage' and 'frontstage' of the policy debate.

The Return of Culling: Public Polarisation of bTB. In recent years, media debates over badgers and bTB seem to have undergone a significant—if possibly temporary—shift in visibility. During the pre-election year of 2009, levels of press coverage dipped as news agendas became occupied with mainstream politics. Since the incoming Coalition government announced their intention to return to badger culling (a policy agenda which has been progressively implemented ever since), these coverage patterns have changed. Rather than the long-standing pattern of episodic spikes, after 2010 press rose steeply to over 350 articles in 2013, before returning to similar levels to the mid-2000s. While the knowledge controversy over badger/bTB has always had a public aspect to it, over the past ten years it has become significantly more public. So what happened? Why did this relatively obscure, chronic and complex policy problem suddenly become so much more newsworthy? In other words, why did we see 'peak badger' during 2013? Furthermore, what are the implications—for badger/bTB, for science-policy and for wider political debates—of wider media interest in the issue having faded almost as quickly as it appeared?

The post-2010 story of the return to badger culling has been one of progressive policy expansion, punctuated by deep uncertainties, persistent contestation of 'the science', many public protests and some spectacularly ridiculous news stories. While it was important to government that their policies were seen to be 'science-led' (albeit reliant on careful interpretations of the RBCT), we have seen increasingly strident criticisms of badger culling from scientists. These criticisms initially came from Lord Krebs and members of the ISG, but are now voiced across much wider scientific and policy networks. These public tensions were magnified when one of two expert panels appointed by Coalition ministers reached the conclusion that culling using 'free shooting' was neither humane nor effective, government ignored this advice, and members of the panel joined in scientific criticisms of government policy (see Sects. 6.3–6.4). As had happened after the Zuckerman report in 1980, the Krebs report in 1997 and the ISG report in 2007, once again an expert report had had the effect of opening up public debates, drawing media attention to the problem and creating further controversy. While these tensions have become much more public, they are continuous with the post-ISG situation of the mid-2000s, itself the outcome of a history of rivalries between the epistemic communities clustered around *animal health* and *disease ecology* policy.

As with most public knowledge controversies, a combination of 'push' and 'pull' factors has been responsible for moving the topic further into the public sphere.[67] Epistemic rivalries acted as a strong 'push' for scientists connected with *disease ecology* to turn to public channels to make their case, particularly since 2007. In response, government *animal health* experts have changed their communications strategy, with the Chief Veterinary Officer (CVO) and Chief Scientific Adviser (CSA) taking on a new role:

> … to provide information to those having to make decisions, including the public, and to ensure that the uncertainties around that information are made clear. When scientists start to stray into providing views about whether decisions based upon the evidence are right or wrong they risk being politicised.[68]

In contrast with the ISG's broad ambitions to make recommendations that would directly establish bTB policy, this position neatly re-circumscribes the boundaries of science and politics, putting the responsibility for decision-making firmly on the shoulders of politicians. However, this move may risk further politicising the problem.[69]

These 'backstage' drivers have been accompanied by a series of more visible 'frontstage' shifts, particularly relating to NGO campaigning, the alignment of the issue with partisan divides in British politics and media working practices. While badger protection groups have been active since the 1970s, it was not until 1996 that the NFBG registered as a charity, renaming itself Badger Trust in 2006.[70] In 2014, the Trust acquired a new 'CEO', professional lobbyist Dominic Dyer, already involved in badger/bTB in his previous position with the animal advocacy group Care for the Wild.[71] In line with wider trends in the NGO sector, the Trust has professionalised significantly since 2010, moving away from its roots in popular natural history and becoming more involved with fundraising and lobbying activities.[72] A wider range of conservation and animal campaign groups have become involved with the badger/bTB debate, including the Save Me Trust, a wildlife charity founded and funded by the rock star Brian

May. May has acted as the focus for a campaigning coalition known as Team Badger, which coordinates formal organisations with broader public activities, including protest marches and 'Wounded Badger Patrols' monitoring local culls.[73] There has also been widespread illegal and semi-legal direct action conducted against the cull trials including protest camps, 'sabbing' of traps and equipment, and targeting of individuals.[74] Since 2010 campaigners have also brought a series of court cases against the British and Welsh governments over culling policies: while these have been unsuccessful so far, they have enabled further public scrutiny of the scientific basis used to support policy.[75]

Despite its long-term entanglement with British conservation, environmental and animal politics, until quite recently badger/BTB has not been aligned clearly with the left–right partisan divides of British party politics. Early badger protection campaigners built broad alliances of support for legal changes and against culling which included both Conservative and Labour politicians. Similarly, while changes in bTB policy have been associated with transitions in governments, they have been equally symptomatic of rivalries and shifts *within* political parties as *between* them. This changed in 2008, when Labour minister Hilary Benn ruled out a culling policy. While his decision seems to have been driven by an openness to advice from a broad range of scientists and a reaction against the previous Blair government's pro-culling agenda, it was interpreted (by commentators on both left and right) in the context of increasingly politicised debates over agriculture, rurality, class and the environment. The 2010 election campaign saw Conservatives adopt a manifesto pledge to return to badger culling, and since 2011, Labour in opposition has actively campaigned against culling, working closely with NGO campaigners.[76] Labour have now folded their opposition to badger culling into broader commitments to strengthening animal welfare policy.[77] Conservative internal politics around badger/bTB have been equally complicated. By 2010, liberal modernisers (led by David Cameron) had adopted a pro-environmental stance, symbolised by his election promise to deliver the 'greenest government ever'. However, this was resisted by more traditional factions in the party, who—allied with right-wing press commentators and landowning/agricultural interests—took an increasingly partisan position on environmental issues including climate change and regarded a return to badger culling as a key goal.[78] During the Coalition government, both factions were needed to maintain party unity, making badger culling a relatively easy way of doing this (alongside commitments to a referendum on membership of the EU). As such the 2012 replacement of Caroline Spelman (a moderniser) in the role of Defra Secretary by Owen Paterson (a traditionalist) was an early signal of the shifting balance of power. This was particularly because Paterson was known to have long campaigned for badger culling, as well as being a climate- and Eurosceptic.[79] While Paterson lost his job in 2014, the culling policy stayed and was further rolled out following the election of a Conservative government in 2015. In the 'front-stage' of bTB policy, the controversy has now settled into a politically partisan, binary debate for and against badger culling, in line with wider trends towards the public polarisation of environmental issues in the USA and UK.[80]

Making News. Together, these changes created many more stories appealing to 'news values' (factors which journalists and editors believe will appeal to audiences).[81] After so many years of scientific research, arguments over interpretations of 'the evidence', briefing and counter-briefing, *something was happening*. Not only had politicians said culling was going to happen, but then it actually did, with two 'pilot' culls implemented in 2013 and more rolled out year on year. The increase in anti-cull campaigning activity and adoption of social media by all sides, carnivalesque protest marches (Fig. 7.4) and dramatic stories of intrepid animal activists and badger shooters chasing each other around the Gloucestershire countryside all drew journalistic attention, while the story was further sustained by a series of legal challenges. Controversy is itself a powerful news value, in which 'every action triggers a countermove by an opponent, with a series of sub-conflicts that become news again'—once a controversy like this becomes active in the media, nearly every story will generate another one.[82] Finally, the badger/bTB story was increasingly populated by celebrities, whose actions and opinions are newsworthy in and of themselves. This was most obvious with Brian May, who wrote opinion pieces, attended protest marches and generally used his fame to bring the issue to public attention, up to and including his performance at the 2012 Olympic opening ceremony. He joined an increasingly long list of eminent but disgruntled scientists; 'telenaturalists' (including Bill Oddie, Chris Packham and David Attenborough); and other celebrities, all of whom drew print, broadcast and online media coverage far beyond the national press. This was not limited to anti-cull campaigning: celebrity chef Clarissa Dickson-Wright helpfully suggested that one solution to the badger

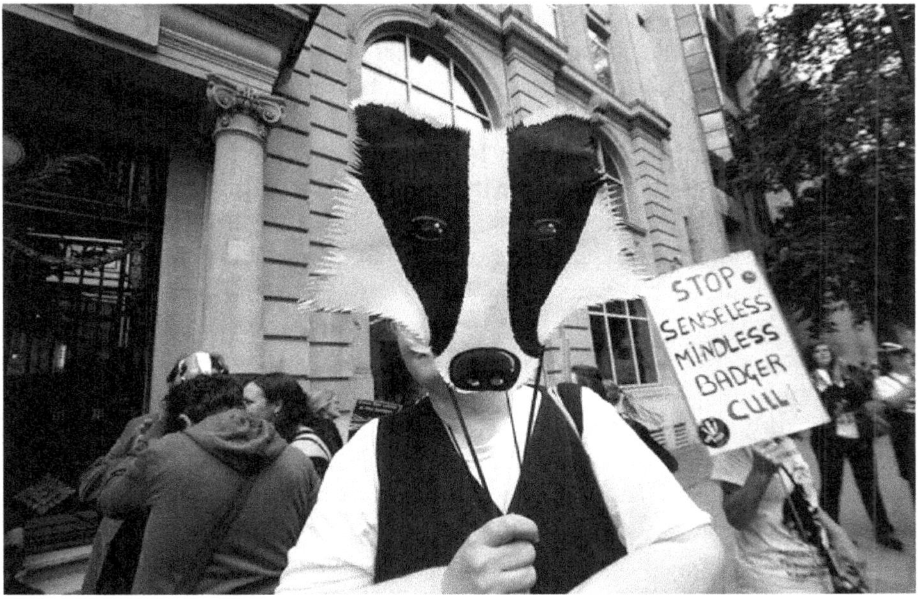

Fig. 7.4 Anti-cull demonstration, London, 1 June 2013. Credit: amer ghazzal/ Alamy Live News. Reproduced by permission of Alamy Stock Photos

problem could be to return to older practices of eating the animals, creating further outrage-cum entertainment from the story.[83]

The regular movement of politicians in and out of the role of Defra Secretary was always covered, but Owen Paterson's term of office (2012–2014) provided a particularly rich seam of material for journalists. Paterson was a colourful figure, outspoken on environmental and agricultural politics, with entertaining biographical details: '[he] kept two orphaned badgers named Bessy and Baz as pets while growing up'.[84] Paterson oversaw a series of disasters at Defra, including a scandal in which horsemeat was found to be (illegitimately) present in UK food supplies, and disastrous flooding events.[85] Notoriously, while being questioned about whether government was manipulating evidence relating to the pilot culls in 2013, Paterson stated, 'No, that's not right at all. The *badgers* have moved the goalposts. You're dealing with a wild animal! It's a *wild animal*, subject to the vagaries of the weather, and diseases and breeding patterns.'[86] From the perspective of someone familiar with badger/bTB (or wildlife in general) this statement makes sense, of a sort—

Paterson seems to have been trying to express the deep unpredictability of working with wildlife, particularly badgers who, as we have seen, have repeatedly thwarted human 'management' by refusing to stay where they are put. However, this was lost on wider audiences, for whom the idea that badgers 'move the goalposts' (but politicians don't) was inherently ridiculous. The story hit social media with a bang, inspiring a series of satirical responses (including an online game: 'Owen Paterson's Badger Penalty Shootout') and reviving an '#omnivoreshambles' social media hashtag invented specifically for Paterson.[87]

This episode highlights how the sudden explosion of badger/bTB into mainstream media was not just a consequence of the topic generating more stories than before, but also of transformations in mass media industries, working practices and what counts as 'news' as we have moved into the twenty-first century. These changes include the appearance and mass uptake of social and Internet-based media; the convergence and movement of 'traditional' formats (such as newspapers, television and radio) online; and an ongoing search for stable income models for commercial media.[88] Communications scholars argue that these pressures have changed journalistic working practices, particularly in terms of the time and resources available to develop complex stories, and a tendency for coverage to become self-referential, more subject to 'hype', 'storms' and external manipulation than ever before.[89] As discussed in the previous chapter, the movement of communications online has made the 'backstage' of policy and academic science more open and visible to the wider public sphere, while social media has facilitated direct interactions between journalists, news values and audiences, albeit with the specific groups of people using these platforms.[90] In turn, this appears to have changed the news values of British media, increasing the importance of factors such as 'conflict', 'shareability' (on social media) and 'arresting audio-visuals'.[91] Badger/bTB created a stream of striking visual stories (including badger masks, costumes, logos and a proliferation of political cartoons), lots of conflict, outrage and a good dose of ridiculousness. These stories, combined with a wider atmosphere of public polarisation around rural and environmental politics, made the issue perfect for a twenty-first-century media storm.[92] However, like any storm, this one seemed to blow itself out nearly as quickly as it had arrived.

7.4 A Passing Storm?

In this chapter, we have explored the increasingly dramatic dynamics of the 'frontstage' of the badger/bTB controversy, over the period of the RBCT culling trial, as well as the return of badger culling since 2010. We explored some basic contours of UK national newspaper coverage of the issue, which demonstrated how badger advocates have repeatedly been adept at setting media agendas, before and after the news of tuberculous badgers became public. This data also suggests that badger protection and bTB have become tightly linked together, and that together they were the subject of extremely high levels of media coverage between 2012 and 2014. Since the 1990s the issue has increasingly been framed in one of two mutually exclusive ways: bTB as an agricultural problem, or badger culling as an environmental risk. Within these framings, the centuries old British 'badger debate' continues, taking on new characteristics relating to infectious disease. As discussed in Chap. 1, these discourses are congruent not only with much older representations of the Good and Bad Badger, but with broader patterns in how people tend to talk and think about animals designated as 'pests'.[93] Since 2010 the public controversy seems to have changed, with badger/bTB increasingly present in mid-market and tabloid newspapers and an extraordinary rise in overall coverage levels, which peaked in 2013 and then receded once more. While experts and evidence have always played a central role in these debates, 'science' is now routinely invoked in a simplistic way to support arguments both for and against badger culling, while some scientists have started actively campaigning, particularly against culling. While badger/bTB has always been political (with a small 'p') and fiercely contested by those involved, it was still a relatively obscure topic, covered intermittently. Since 2010 it has shifted to become a consistent topic of wider media interest. Until 2008, questions of badger persecution and/or what to do about bTB were topics of division and debate within political parties, with policy change as often precipitated by internal power shifts as the passing of government from one party to another. However, since Hilary Benn's decision to take the advice of the ISG and not cull, the issue has increasingly become politically partisan, with right-wing agendas lobbying for badger culling and left-wingers against. While the terms 'politicisation' and 'polarisation' might imply the sullying of a previously 'pure' scientific debate with a political mess, they can be better understood as the widening of differences between positions in the debate, the increasing identification of those positions with those of political parties and increasing levels of hostility expressed between opponents. The badger/bTB debate can perhaps be best understood as a British version of the highly polarised climate debates seen in the USA. As such, it forms part of wider trends toward the public polarisation and politicisation of environmental issues in the twenty-first century.[94]

But what happened next? The wave of media coverage of badger/bTB that crested in 2013 rapidly receded, returning to similar levels to those of the late 2000s. While it is likely that media attention will return to the topic in future—if, for example, a left-wing government enters power and turns bTB policy on its head yet again—this extraordinary peaking and fading still requires explanation. In part, the answer is obvious: it is the nature of media storms to abate, more so in today's fast-moving online world, driven by momentary social media clicks and 'likes'.[95] There is also an underlying tendency for news coverage of environmental issues to focus upon dramatic events and move on to something else before the complexities of the underlying problems can be explored.[96] Novelty is yet another critical news value: when the pilot culls were expanded the same stories returned year after year, leading the ongoing 'YES!/NO!' narrative of the story to get stale. There has been a series of further changes since 2015, potentially contributing to an abatement in the public controversy. The culling policy has hardened, transforming from 'pilots' to a 'rollout', with licences planned even in areas with little or no bTB; while at the same time the 'backstage' of bTB policy and scientific research has diversified and depolarised a little, as explored in the previous chapter. In the latest turn of the long story of the RSPCA's engagement with wildlife politics (see Chap. 5), the UK's oldest animal welfare charity has recently pulled back from an assertive anti-cull campaign running from 2011. While the RSPCA is still opposed to culling, the charity has undergone both internal and external criticism that it had become too 'political', resulting in changes in leadership and campaigning around wildlife politics.[97] However, the major factor contributing to the receding of media interest in badger/bTB is most likely to be the appearance of another, much bigger polarised political controversy, which continues to dominate news agendas at the time of writing: Brexit.

On one level, the 2016 UK referendum decision of Britain to withdraw from the EU has little to do with badger/bTB: it is entirely plausible that the former displaced the latter in media agendas simply through the sheer volume of Brexit news. The causes and consequences of Brexit are still being played out: it is already the subject of a plethora of academic and non-academic opinion and analysis. While central drivers of the Brexit debate (such as the politics of immigration) do not seem to map directly onto badger/bTB (although I note the significance of the badger as a British 'native' species), some shared factors drive both controversies. Most obviously, this can be seen in broader rural and environmental politics, and the rhetoric of 'marginalised rurality', ignored by urban elites and bureaucracies (whether located in London or Brussels). These have gathered strength over the past twenty years, driven by a cluster of environmental/agricultural problems including BSE, FMD, environmental reforms of the Common Agricultural Policy, fox hunting, supply chain dominance by retailers, regulation of pesticides, rural poverty and lack of infrastructure—and badger/bTB.[98] The referendum outcome made visible wider urban–rural differences in Leave–Remain support, while a majority of farmers voted to Leave, despite the NFU supporting the Remain campaign and the potential devastation of their livelihood by the loss of EU subsidies.[99] Key policy decisions were outcomes of tensions within political parties, particularly the attempts of moderniser David Cameron to maintain the support of right-wing Conservatives; but also tensions within Labour. Finally, both issues have become notoriously polarised, creating deep social divisions over specific points of contention, which appear to symbolise a broader constellation of political differences—including crucially the social roles of *science, knowledge and expertise*. At the time of writing, evidence is emerging suggesting that social media debates (about Brexit in Britain among others) have been subject to manipulation, creating public divisiveness and fostering mistrust in political systems.[100] To purely speculate: was the 2012–2014 badger/bTB media storm a rehearsal or prefiguring of the Brexit debate yet to come?

Having explored the parallel development of the 'backstage' and 'frontstage' controversies over badger/bTB since the 1990s, several things are clear. In the earlier stages of the debate, explored in the first two parts of this book, the initially separate issues of badger protection and bTB have come together and moved apart several times, according to changes in the activities of animal advocates as well as shifts in bTB policy. Since the late 1990s, and particularly since the return to badger culling policies since 2010, the two issues have become increasingly tightly linked. While badgers still draw media coverage by themselves, it is less so than in the past, while bTB is almost never discussed without mentioning badgers. Even though the 'backstage' of policymaking is far more visible to the 'frontstage' of the public sphere than ever before, in the case of badger/bTB, it seems that policy and public debates have become increasingly disconnected. During the 1970s, MAFF sought to head off public controversy by enrolling as wide a range of interests as possible in bTB policy processes. This was implemented explicitly by the creation of the Badger Consultative Panel, which, even if it had limited power, created a forum where key actors could engage directly with each other; and implicitly via the involvement of naturalists in MAFF's research and wider publics in a long-term project measuring bTB in badgers found dead on the roads.[101] From the inception of the RBCT, these and other features of MAFF's previous policy approach were gradually abandoned, largely for reasons of cost, meaning that structures for direct engagement have been eroded, particularly for 'wildlife interests'. Increasingly the only forum available for all actors in badger/bTB to interact with each other has been via mass media: as we know from other cases of environmental controversy and policy formation, this removes opportunities for more subtle forms of negotiation and communication.[102] This may also help to explain the increasingly tight focus of mass media on a highly dichotomised debate: to cull or not to cull, largely ignoring the complexities of how or when or the broader underlying causes of the problem. We have seen politicians on all sides benefiting from this process, as have campaigners claiming to speak on behalf of animals, environments and farmers. While much is still unclear about changing relationships between frontstage/backstage policymaking in the twenty-first century, policy scholars agree that imbalances or divergences between the two can contribute to policy failure and political problems.[103] We will examine the implications of this disjunct—and what could possibly be done to bring the public and private aspects of badger/bTB policy back together—in the final chapter.

Notes

1. Ayres, Sandford and Coombes, 'Policy-Making "Front" and "Back" Stage'; Dunlop, 'Knowledge, Epistemic Communities and Agenda-Setting'.
2. Bourne et al., 'Bovine TB: The Scientific Evidence, Final Report of the Independent Scientific Group on Cattle TB', 14.
3. Whatmore, 'Mapping Knowledge Controversies'; Naylor et al., 'The Framing of Public Knowledge Controversies in the Media'; Amelia Sharman and Richard Perkins, 'Post-Decisional Logics of Inaction: The Influence of Knowledge Controversy in Climate Policy Decision-Making',

Environment and Planning A: Economy and Space 49(10) (1 October 2017): 2281–99.

4. Agar, 'Transition'.
5. Motta, 'Social Disputes over GMOs'.
6. Kim, *The Social Construction of Disease.*
7. Lewenstein, 'From Fax to Facts'; Bucchi, *Science and the Media*; Cassidy, 'Evolutionary Psychology as Public Science and Boundary Work'.
8. Bruno Latour, *Science in Action: How to Follow Scientists and Engineers through Society* (Cambridge, MA: Harvard University Press, 1987).
9. Ayres, Sandford and Coombes, 'Policy-Making "Front" and "Back" Stage'; Hilgartner, *Science on Stage.*
10. Grant, 'Intractable Policy Failure'.
11. Because these newspaper digital archives are organised differently to the Nexis database the results are not directly comparable. Therefore, the results of these searches are depicted separately in Figs. 7.1 and 7.2.
12. Sources: *Daily Mail* Historical Archive (1896–2004); *Daily Mirror* Archive (1903–present); *Guardian* and *Observer* Archive (1791–2003); *Independent* Digital Archive (1986–2016); *Telegraph* Historical Archive (1855–2000); *Times* Digital Archive (1785–2011), excluding advertisements, crosswords, TV and racing listings.
13. See Sect. 3.1.
14. See Sect. 5.2.
15. See Sects. 3.3 and 5.3.
16. Griggs and Howarth, 'Protest Movements, Environmental Activism and Environmentalism in the United Kingdom'.
17. Sect. 5.3.
18. Source: Nexis-UK print media database: *Daily Mail/Mail on Sunday*, *Daily/Sunday Mirror*; *Guardian/Observer*; *Independent/Independent on Sunday*; *Daily/Sunday Telegraph*; *Times/Sunday Times.*
19. M. Djerf-Pierre, 'When Attention Drives Attention: Issue Dynamics in Environmental News Reporting over Five Decades', *European Journal of Communication* 27(3) (September 2012): 291–304.
20. Raymond Kuhn, *Politics and the Media in Britain* (Basingstoke: Palgrave Macmillan, 2007), 213–25.
21. Mike S. Schäfer, 'Taking Stock: A Meta-Analysis of Studies on the Media's Coverage of Science', *Public Understanding of Science* 21(6) (December 2012): 650–63.
22. M. C. Nisbet, 'Framing Science: A New Paradigm in Public Engagement', in *Understanding Science: New Agendas in Science*, ed. LeeAnn Kahlor and Patricia A. Stout (New York: Routledge, 2009), 40–67.
23. P. Wagner-Egger et al., 'Lay Perceptions of Collectives at the Outbreak of the H1N1 Epidemic: Heroes, Villains and Victims', *Public Understanding of Science* 20(4) (March 2011): 461–76.

24. Maya Warrier, 'The Temple Bull Controversy at Skanda Vale and the Construction of Hindu Identity in Britain', *International Journal of Hindu Studies* 13(3) (2009): 261–78.
25. Van Zwanenberg and Millstone, 'BSE'; Mort et al., 'The Health and Social Consequences of the 2001 Foot & Mouth Disease Epidemic in North Cumbria'; Döring and Nerlich, *The Social and Cultural Impact of Foot and Mouth Disease in the UK in 2001.*
26. S. Roberts, 'New NFU president issues rallying cry for "Team Agriculture"', *Farmers Weekly*, 23 February 2018.
27. Collins and Evans, 'The Third Wave of Science Studies'; Chloe Silverman, *Understanding Autism: Parents, Doctors, and the History of a Disorder* (Princeton: Princeton University Press, 2012).
28. Pile, 'A Load of Bloody Idiots'.
29. In an interview on the BBC's *Countryfile* in 2014, Princess Anne called for a return to gassing on animal welfare grounds; David Lowe, 'Princess Anne: Gas Is Much Nicer Way of Culling Badgers', *Countryfile* (BBC Television, 8 April 2014).
30. Anon., 'A diary of the badger cull—a marksmen tells his story', *Western Morning News*, 15 Oct. 2016, 20–21; see also Enticott, 'Techniques of Neutralising Wildlife Crime in Rural England and Wales'; G. Enticott, 'Public Attitudes to Badger Culling to Control Bovine Tuberculosis in Rural Wales', *European Journal of Wildlife Research* 61 (2015): 387; Naylor et al., 'The Framing of Public Knowledge Controversies in the Media'.
31. Robin Page, 'Country diary: Badgers are out of control', *Daily Telegraph*, 15 June 2013, 17. Farming claims of rising populations have recently been confirmed by new research; however, there seems to be a complicated, counter-intuitive relationship between population density and the epidemiology of bTB. See Judge et al., 'Abundance of Badgers (Meles Meles) in England and Wales'.
32. Wagner-Egger et al., 'Lay Perceptions of Collectives at the Outbreak of the H1N1 Epidemic'.
33. Daniel Cressey, 'Scientists Track Badger–Cow Encounters to Understand Cattle TB', *Nature News*, 5 August 2016. One of these images is definitely staged (on closer inspection the animal is stuffed)—see the second picture in Brian May, 'This Cruel Badger Cull Is Pointless—and I Can Prove It, Says Queen Guitarist Brian May', *Mail Online*, 20 October 2012.
34. Counter to prevailing narratives, beyond the well-off and well-regulated Global North, neither TB nor bTB are 'solved' or a 'problem of the past'; for the history of (human) TB and public health, see McMillen, *Discovering Tuberculosis.*

35. See Sect. 5.3.
36. Naylor et al., 'The Framing of Public Knowledge Controversies in the Media'.
37. Research on public attitudes to culling is still quite sparse. However, we do know that views are much less polarised and more subtle than is generally assumed; see Enticott, 'Public Attitudes to Badger Culling to Control Bovine Tuberculosis in Rural Wales'; Price et al., 'From Contradiction to Contrast in a Countryside Conflict'; OPM Group, 'Defra Bovine TB Citizen Dialogue. Cross-Cutting Summary' (London: Defra, April 2015).
38. Price, *Thinking through Badgers*; Phoenix, 'Local Understandings of Bovine Tuberculosis (Working Title)'.
39. M. Engel, 'Killing Zones: Ethnic cleansing is to be attempted in the English counties', *The Guardian*, 24 October 1998, 23.
40. Patrick Bateson, 'Culling Badgers Could Increase the Problem of TB in Cattle|Letters', *The Observer*, 14 October 2012, sec. Global.
41. Damian Carrington, 'Record 32,000 badgers shot in annual cull; Scientists accuse officials of cherry-picking data to defend disease-control scheme', *The Guardian*, Environment section, 18 December 2018.
42. S. Cowell, 'Call off the Cull', *Daily Mirror*, 1 September 2016, 12.
43. H. Weathers, 'Mother badgers are snared in rusty cages, parted from their screaming cubs and shot in the head', *Daily Mail*, 3 June 2000, 11; BBC, 'Anger after Badger Found Shot in Gut', *BBC News Online*, 23 September 2014, sec. Somerset.
44. L. Gray, 'Jews angered by star's claim that badger cull is genocide', *Daily Telegraph*, 11 September 2013, 15; Zoe Williams, 'Chris Packham: It has a psychopathic element, taking pleasure from killing', *Guardian*, 11 September 2015.
45. See also the BBC Trust's recent review of their rural coverage: Helen Hancock, 'BBC Trust Impartiality Review: BBC Coverage of Rural Areas in the UK', A BBC Trust report, June 2014.
46. Cronin, *Art for Animals*.
47. Rebecca Sandover, Samuel Kinsley and Stephen Hinchliffe, 'A Very Public Cull—The Anatomy of an Online Issue Public', *Geoforum* 97 (1 December 2018): 106–18; Clare Saunders and Caroline Keenan, 'Conflict Framing in the Control of Bovine Tuberculosis' (journal article, in prep.); Mehmet Mehmet and Peter Simmons, 'Kangaroo Court? An Analysis of Social Media Justifications for Attitudes to Culling', *Environmental Communication* 12(3) (September 2016): 370–86; Price et al., 'From Contradiction to Contrast in a Countryside Conflict'.
48. For accessible overviews of science, environment and media research, see Anders Hansen, 'Communication, Media and the Social Construction of the Environment', in *The Routledge Handbook of Environment and*

Communication, ed. Anders Hansen and Robert Cox (New York: Routledge, 2015), 26–38; A. Anderson, *Media, Environment and the Network Society* (Cham, Switzerland: Springer, 2014).

49. I. Petersen, H. Heinrichs and H. P. Peters, 'Mass-Mediated Expertise as Informal Policy Advice', *Science, Technology & Human Values* 35(6) (August 2010): 865–87; A. M. Scheu et al., 'Medialization of Research Policy: Anticipation of and Adaptation to Journalistic Logic', *Science Communication* 36(6) (September 2014): 706–34; Dunlop, 'Knowledge, Epistemic Communities and Agenda-Setting'.
50. Stephen Hilgartner and C. L. Bosk, 'The Rise and Fall of Social-Problems—A Public Arenas Model', *American Journal of Sociology* 94(1) (1988): 53–78.
51. See Chaps. 3, 4 and 5 for full accounts of the controversy between the 1960s and 1990s.
52. Anon., 'Ministry Seeks Powers to Gas Ailing Badgers', *Times*, 6 February 1975; 'Peart Cleared of Badger Cruelty Charge', *Daily Telegraph*, 29 January 1975, 3.
53. G. Brown, 'Gassing of Badgers Paying Off—Agriculture Correspondent', *Daily Telegraph*, 10 January 1978, 6.
54. Alongside Murray's ongoing media appearances, natural history books reinforced earlier accounts of badger persecution. The animal star of one of these fell victim to gassing just before MAFF announced their culling policy—anon., 'Death in a Sussex Gas Chamber', *Sunday Telegraph*, 13 July 1975, 13; Malins, *Bully & the Badger*.
55. G. Lakeman, 'Ministry Plans Mass Gassing of Badgers', *Daily Telegraph*, 28 July 1975, 3.
56. Anon., 'Ministry Gets Rap for "Blitz" on Badgers', *Daily Mail*, 23 Dec. 1980, 9. While Cymag was a different compound to that used during the Holocaust (Zyklon B), both work by releasing deadly hydrogen cyanide gas.
57. R. J. Delahay et al., 'Managing Conflict between Humans and Wildlife: Trends in Licensed Operations to Resolve Problems with Badgers Meles Meles in England', *Mammal Review* 39(1) (January 2009): 53–66.
58. Dr King is now Director of Wildlife Link, the coalition group of NGOs cited by Peter Melchett as instrumental in aligning conservation and animal advocacy during the early 1980s; Melchett and Brodie, *Peter Melchett Interviewed by Louise Brodie*; Elaine King, 'Elaine King|LinkedIn', 2018.
59. N. Fielding, 'Why Are They Slaughtering Our Badgers?' *Mail on Sunday*, 2 May 1999, 28.
60. Interviews with RSPCA scientific officer, 28/01/10; ISG member, 17/03/10.

61. M. Engel, 'Killing Zones: Ethnic Cleansing Is to be Attempted in the English Counties', *Guardian*, 24 October 1998.
62. See Sect. 6.3.
63. Charles Clover, 'Badger Cull "Off" as Study Concludes It Would Make TB Worse', *Daily Telegraph*, 16 June 2007, 14.
64. Clive Aslet, 'It's Up to You Now, Gordon', *Daily Telegraph*, 1 Aug. 2007, 21; see also work on discourses of 'marginalised rurality' during the 2001 FMD outbreak by K. Bickerstaff, P. Simmons and N. Pidgeon, 'Situating Local Experience of Risk: Peripherality, Marginality and Place Identity in the UK Foot and Mouth Disease Crisis', *Geoforum* 37(5) (2006): 844–58. On the 'prohibition' of hunting by New Labour, see Marvin, 'English Foxhunting'. On Euroscepticism, environmental issues and rural politics in the UK, see Michael M. Bell, Sarah E. Lloyd and Christine Vatovec, 'Activating the Countryside: Rural Power, the Power of the Rural and the Making of Rural Politics', *Sociologia Ruralis* 50(3) (June 2010): 205–24; Matthew Reed, '"This Loopy Idea": An Analysis of UKIP's Social Media Discourse in Relation to Rurality and Climate Change', *Space and Polity* 20(2) (May 2016): 1–16.
65. D. Derbyshire, 'Farmers' Fury as Badger Cull to Fight Cattle TB Is Called Off', *Daily Mail*, 5 July 2008.
66. Fiona MacRae, 'Cull Badgers to Protect Cattle from TB Threat', *Daily Mail*, 23 Oct. 2007, 4.
67. Bucchi, *Science and the Media*; Cassidy, 'Evolutionary Psychology as Public Science and Boundary Work'.
68. Boyd, 'Making Science Count in Government', 1. It was around this time that Defra started using social media for public communication, including enrolling their Chief Scientist and CVO to make the case for badger culling.
69. The recent Godfray review makes similar recommendations re science and policy: Godfray et al., 'A Strategy for Achieving Bovine Tuberculosis Free Status for England'. However, for the potential pitfalls of this move see also Daniel Sarewitz, 'How Science Makes Environmental Controversies Worse', *Environmental Science & Policy* 7(5) (October 2004): 385–403.
70. Charity Commission, 'Charity Details: National Federation of Badger Groups', Registered Charities in England and Wales, 2006; Charity Commission, 'Charity Details: Badger Trust', Registered Charities in England and Wales, 2016.
71. L. Gray, 'Strip Badger Cull Farmers of Organic Status', *Daily Telegraph*, 21 September 2012; Lancashire Badger Group, 'Badger Trust's New CEO Is Leading Anti-Cull Spokesman', *Lancashire Badger Group* (blog), 24 February 2014.

72. Hilton et al., *The Politics of Expertise*.
73. See also www.save-me.org.uk and http://news1.teambadger.org, alongside Charity Commission, 'Charity Details: The Save Me Trust', 2017.
74. See http://badgeractionnetwork.org.uk/; Price, *Thinking through Badgers*; Phoenix, 'Local Understandings of Bovine Tuberculosis (Working Title)'.
75. Patrick Bishop, 'Badgers and Bovine Tuberculosis: The Relationship between Law, Policy and ScienceBadger Trust v Welsh Ministers [2010] EWCA Civ 807', *Journal of Environmental Law* 24(1) (1 March 2012): 145–54; Martin Lodge and Kira Matus, 'Science, Badgers, Politics: Advocacy Coalitions and Policy Change in Bovine Tuberculosis Policy in Britain', *Policy Studies Journal* 42(3) (August 2014): 367–90; Enticott, 'Public Attitudes to Badger Culling to Control Bovine Tuberculosis in Rural Wales'; Steven P. McCulloch and Michael J. Reiss, 'Bovine Tuberculosis and Badger Control in Britain: Science, Policy and Politics', *Journal of Agricultural and Environmental Ethics* 30(4) (1 August 2017): 469–84.
76. Damian Carrington, 'Pilot Badger Culls Get Go-ahead in England', *Guardian*, 15 December 2011, 19; Brian May, 'Vegetarian Rock Stars Don't Vote Tory. I Did. But I'll Never Vote for Cameron after His Bloody Badger Cull', *Mail Online*, 25 August 2012.
77. See https://labour.org.uk/issues/animal-welfare-plan/.
78. Carter and Clements, 'From "Greenest Government Ever" to "Get Rid of All the Green Crap"'.
79. C. Brooker, 'Paterson Finally Prods Defra into Action on bovine TB', *Sunday Telegraph*, 18 Dec. 2005; B. Brogan, and R. Winnett, 'We Want Our Country Back from Europe: Interview', *Daily Telegraph*, 8 Dec. 2012, 16.
80. Lucas and Warman, 'Disrupting Polarized Discourses'.
81. Tony Harcup and Deirdre O'Neill, 'What Is News? News Values Revisited (Again)', *Journalism Studies* 18(12) (2 December 2017): 1470–88.
82. Peter Vasterman, 'Introduction', in *From Media Hype to Twitter Storm*, News Explosions and Their Impact on Issues, Crises, and Public Opinion (Amsterdam: Amsterdam University Press, 2018), 18. See also Djerf-Pierre, 'When Attention Drives Attention: Issue Dynamics in Environmental News Reporting over Five Decades'.
83. B. Reade, 'NOW CLARISSA'S BADGER BASTING', *Daily Mirror*, 27 September 2012, 25.
84. J. Shute, 'Between the badger and the barrel of a gun', *Daily Telegraph*, 31 August 2013, 25; also Barkham, *Badgerlands*, chap. 15.
85. For 'horsemeatgate' see Yasmin Ibrahim and Anita Howarth, 'Contamination, Deception and "Othering": The Media Framing of the Horsemeat Scandal', *Social Identities* 23(2) (March 2017): 212–31.

86. BBC, 'Badgers "moved Goalposts" in Cull'.
87. Barkham, *Badgerlands*, 317–42; Price, *Thinking through Badgers*, 213–23; Political Scrapbook, 'Best of the Badger: The 5 Funniest Responses to Paterson's Own Goal', *Political Scrapbook*, 10 October 2013.
88. Vasterman, ed., *From Media Hype to Twitter Storm*; Anderson, *Media, Environment and the Network Society*.
89. H. Riesch, 'Changing News: Re-Adjusting Science Studies to Online Newspapers', *Public Understanding of Science* 20(6) (August 2010): 771–77; John Wihbey, 'Journalists' Use of Knowledge in an Online World', *Journalism Practice* 11(10) (November 2016): 1267–82; Joshua A. Tucker et al., 'Social Media, Political Polarization, and Political Disinformation: A Review of the Scientific Literature', SSRN Scholarly Paper (Rochester, NY: Social Science Research Network, 19 March 2018); Vasterman, ed., *From Media Hype to Twitter Storm*.
90. Aeron Davis, 'New Media and Fat Democracy: The Paradox of Online Participation', *New Media & Society* 12(5) (November 2009): 745–61; Baym and boyd, 'Socially Mediated Publicness'; Jonathan Mellon and Christopher Prosser, 'Twitter and Facebook Are Not Representative of the General Population: Political Attitudes and Demographics of British Social Media Users', *Research & Politics* 4(3) (1 July 2017).
91. J. H. Lee, 'News Values, Media Coverage, and Audience Attention: An Analysis of Direct and Mediated Causal Relationships', *Journalism & Mass Communication Quarterly* 86(1) (March 2009): 175–90; Harcup and O'Neill, 'What Is News?'
92. Cassidy, 'Badger–Human Conflict'. For the formation of 'issue publics' around badger/bTb in social media see Sandover, Kinsley and Hinchliffe, 'A Very Public Cull'.
93. Knight, 'Introduction'; Cassidy, 'Badger–Human Conflict'.
94. Dan M. Kahan et al., 'The Polarizing Impact of Science Literacy and Numeracy on Perceived Climate Change Risks', *Nature Climate Change* 2 (May 2012): 732–35; Lucas and Warman, 'Disrupting Polarized Discourses'.
95. Vasterman, ed., *From Media Hype to Twitter Storm*.
96. Djerf-Pierre, 'When Attention Drives Attention'.
97. J. Starkey, 'RSPCA backtracks on plan to shame farmers who take part in badger cull', *The Times*, 18 October 2017, 4.
98. Reed, 'This Loopy Idea'; Bickerstaff, Simmons and Pidgeon, 'Situating Local Experience of Risk'.
99. BBC, 'Farmers' Union Backs Staying in EU', *BBC News Online*, 18 April 2016, sec. UK; Philip Clarke, 'Farmer Support for Brexit as Strong as Ever, FW Poll Reveals', *Farmers Weekly*, 22 December 2017.

100. Tucker et al., 'Social Media, Political Polarization, and Political Disinformation'; Damian Maye et al., '"Present Realities" and the Need for a "Lived Experience" Perspective in Brexit Agri-Food Governance', *Space and Polity* 22(2) (4 May 2018): 270–86; Will Jennings and Martin Lodge, 'Brexit, the Tides and Canute: The Fracturing Politics of the British State', *Journal of European Public Policy* 26(5) (31 May 2018): 1–18.
101. Grant, 'Intractable Policy Failure'; Overy and Tansey, *A History of Bovine TB c.1965–c. 2000.*
102. Cassidy, 'Evolutionary Psychology as Public Science and Boundary Work'; Libby Lester and Brett Hutchins, 'The Power of the Unseen: Environmental Conflict, the Media and Invisibility', *Media Culture and Society* 34(7) (October 2012): 847–63.
103. Ayres, Sandford and Coombes, 'Policy-Making "Front" and "Back" Stage'.

Summary and Reflections

In this final chapter, I will draw together the threads of the various stories traced throughout this book to provide some answers to how the UK got into the tangled mess that is the badger/bTB controversy, and make suggestions on how we might go about getting out again. I will discuss the changing nature of our knowledge about wild badgers in Britain; about the microbe *M. bovis*; about farming and animal health; about the disease we call tuberculosis; and about the complex social and ecological relationships between them. In Chap. 1 (Sect. 1.1), I provided a summary of 'the science' of badger/bTB, in terms of how our knowledge has changed since the early 1970s, as well as areas of scientific consensus and contestation in contemporary research on the topic. However, as we have seen throughout this book, the idea that science and/or technologies are fixed, authoritative resources that we can expect to simply provide 'all the answers' has repeatedly turned out to be a canard. To be crystal clear, this problem *needs experts* and what they know, about a world we (humans) live in, which—as we are seeing with accelerating environmental change—pushes back when we do things to it.[1] However, it also needs all involved to adjust their understandings of what 'science' is and how it can relate to policy—to understand that 'experts' come from multiple backgrounds and often disagree; that science is a process, not a thing; and that knowledge is often provisional, uncertain and subject to change. As the cynical comments of Lord Rooker (quoted in Chap. 7) suggest, inflated expectations can simply store up trouble for later when research provides some answers (although not necessarily the expected ones), while also uncovering a plethora of new uncertainties and new questions.[2] As we have seen, they also open a space for misrepresenting 'the science' to support lobbying for multiple agendas, and for exploiting uncertainty to delay or avoid responsibility for policy decisions. My conclusions fall under four key themes: relating to the longer history of TB in humans and other animals; the history of wildlife conflicts in Britain; the changing 'cultures of care' of badger/bTB; and expectations of and around science, policy and society. Following these, I will outline some further questions that this work raises for researchers, and some suggestions for policymakers, politicians and others embroiled in this deeply sticky—but in my view, not insurmountable—problem.

8.1 TB in Humans, Other Animals and Environments

At the beginning of this book I discussed a core idea from the history of medicine which can help us understand the history of tuberculosis (a disease which has been with us for thousands of years)—that of disease 'framing'. Historians understand diseases as specific constellations of physical symptoms, organised and explained according to changing conceptual models of the body, health and illness, which come into existence when people collectively agree upon and label them as such.[3] The diseases 'phthisis', 'scrofula', 'consumption' and 'tuberculosis' have been built, rebuilt and in some cases abandoned over the last few hundred years, while mutually shaping changing social, political, technological and scientific contexts in the process. TB as we understand it today gradually took shape, from a generalised wasting illness indistinguishable from cancer, to several lung diseases caused by specific microbes. Similarly, the history of bTB—a disease contested back and forth as like, yet unlike human tuberculosis—can be understood as part of a broader reconfiguration of the domains of human and animal health since the late nineteenth century.[4] Eventually, the argument was settled by framing bTB (caused by *M. bovis*) as an animal disease, of importance because it was zoonotic (also infects humans); while TB (caused by *M. tuberculosis*) was recognised as solely human. This enabled scientists and medical professionals to assign the two diseases, respectively, to the separating domains of veterinary and human medicine—in science, clinical practice and policy. By the mid-twentieth century, bTB had been configured primarily as a cattle disease, and by the 1960s as one which had been successfully controlled by state-led animal health practices of 'stamping out' disease.[5]

Since the discovery of tuberculous badgers in the early 1970s, I think we have seen a further process of reconfiguring tuberculosis, this time towards an 'environmental' disease. Finding *M. bovis* in wild animals—primarily (although not exclusively) badgers in the UK, and a range of other mammals worldwide—disrupted the previous framing of bTB. It also brought new actors into the well-established domain of British animal health policy: professional ecologists (in government and academia), as well as naturalists and animal advocates, already involved with changing the social role of the badger. While they were new to bTB, these ecologists had their own understandings of microbes and infection from working with other wildlife diseases. Rather than infectious agents to be isolated and 'stamped out', disease ecology instead saw microbes as active elements of dynamically changing ecological systems.[6] This reconfiguration of bTB was aided by the development of new technologies for knowing wild animals in the field and their application by Ministry for Agriculture, Fisheries and Food (MAFF) researchers to following badgers and their traces. As we learned in Chaps. 2 and 4, once MAFF started looking for tuberculous badgers, they found more and more of them, changing their understanding of the scale and urgency of the problem—and in turn precipitating rapid policy action.

Recent years have seen rapid developments in biomedical technologies for rapidly detecting and diagnosing the presence of pathogenic microbes, including the notoriously difficult to detect mycobacteria, which are being tested and promoted by alliances of academics, NGOs, clinicians and private companies.[7] While these developments should be welcomed and I would agree that new tests are desperately needed, it would be deeply unwise to expect them to act as a panacea. There are two sets of reasons for this. First, earlier iterations of the badger/bTB debate involved similarly shared expectations that newly testing technologies could create a 'live' test for bTB in badgers, enabling MAFF to trace and eliminate the disease more accurately. When subsequent field trials indicated that the new test was not sensitive or accurate enough, MAFF's policy strategy collapsed.[8] The second set of reasons is subtler, but also more fundamental. Existing regulatory structures for controlling bTB are based around the tuberculin test. This diagnostic practice involves the skilled measurement of a body's inflammatory response to the injection of an extract of dead mycobacteria—the size of the lump that appears.[9] In other words, for all its problems, the tuberculin test provides a measure of *disease*—the bodily interaction between a pathogen and the immune response of the body it infects.[10] By contrast, many of the new rapid diagnostic tests work through means such as detecting 'biomarkers', the presence of 'bacteriophages' (species-specific viruses which infect bacteria, including *M. bovis*), and polymerase chain reaction (PCR) techniques for detecting DNA.[11] Just as new technologies (such as radio-tracking, infrared sensors and camera traps) have made it possible for scientists to follow, see and know about the lives of wild animals in completely new ways, these testing technologies are changing how we perceive and know *M. bovis*. Scientists are looking for—and finding—the microbe in places where they had thought it was absent: in the bodies of cows cleared by tuberculin testing, in soil and slurry, and even within the bodies of single-celled amoebae.[12]

Scientists and public health bodies—most significantly the World Health Organization (WHO)—have started renaming bTB from 'bovine TB' to 'zoonotic TB', flagging the capacity of *M. bovis* to pass beyond livestock into many other mammals, including humans and wildlife.[13] Because these new testing technologies often measure the *presence of microbes* rather than the *presence of disease*, their findings are likely to further disintegrate the twentieth-century livestock disease of bTB, recognising the complexities of an infection that passes across and between humans, other animals and wider environmental systems. Since it was first recognised in the late nineteenth century, bTB has been framed and reframed—initially as a disease shared between humans and other animals; then into an animal disease; then into a zoonosis; and perhaps now into an environmental disease. Just as scientists and veterinarians increasingly advocate a 'One Health' approach, I believe there is great value in thinking more broadly across humans, animals and environments about tuberculosis—there are important lessons to be learned when the histories of bTB and TB are brought together. This has potential not just for biomedical topics such as diagnostics and vaccination, but for public health problems such as surveillance, regulation and co-infection; and for the social, cultural and political aspects of TB such as inequality, stress, nutrition, stigma and economic factors.[14]

8.2 Wildlife Conflict and the Great British Badger Debate

My research has uncovered evidence of a long-standing 'wildlife conflict' (conflict between humans and animals as well as between humans about animals) involving badgers in Britain, at least a century before they were connected with bTB in cattle. Between the late nineteenth and mid-twentieth centuries, the social roles of these animals gradually shifted—from a 'vermin' animal (reviled, hunted and made to fight with dogs)—towards that of an iconic, British, charismatic wildlife species (to be valued and cared for).[15] In the 1960s the professional ecologists of MAFF's Infestation Control Division (ICD)—charged with deciding whether animals were officially regarded as 'pests' by government—found themselves caught between the supporters of the Good and Bad Badger. ICD eventually brokered a policy compromise based on the idea of the 'rogue badger'—aberrant individuals, to be eliminated, while the majority should be left alone.[16] This compromise was short-lived, as the Good and Bad Badger were strategically remobilised by badger advocates as they gathered a broad base of support for new protective legislation. Initially these campaigns gained little traction within government—until the discovery of tuberculous badgers made it necessary to create a legal framework that not only made the animals 'killable' for MAFF officers and government licensees, but also prevented their less ordered killing by others.[17] As the culling controversy continued into the 1980s and 1990s (intensifying since 2010) the Good and Bad Badger have survived, and are still alive and kicking in today's mass media, where they have been further transformed through mutually exclusive framings of the bTB controversy. Alongside the older roles of 'pest/vermin' and 'charismatic wildlife', association with *M. bovis* has created new social roles for the badger as a disease vector. These include more specific roles as infected 'guilty victims' (to be excluded or destroyed); and for others as targets of 'genocide' via government culling policies.[18]

These arguments demonstrate the strong continuities between how people argued about badgers in the past and how they are arguing about badgers and bTB in the present. In particular, we see aspects of contemporary debates which have little or nothing to do with bTB, such as badgers' habits of digging in awkward places, eating the wrong things and damaging crops. These continuities suggest that an underlying 'wildlife conflict' (comprising conflicts between humans and badgers and—more importantly—conflicts between humans *about* badgers) precedes and drives today's badger/bTB controversy.[19] The entanglement of disease narratives with this underlying wildlife conflict is likely to have further polarised and politicised people's relations with the animals themselves—as attested to by contemporary research into wildlife crime and animal advocacy in relation to badgers.[20] It follows that bTB policy—and perhaps animal health more widely—would benefit from sustained engagement with research and practice on managing wildlife conflicts. While scientists are already investigating badger–human interactions in relation to 'biosecurity'—that is how to block or break the transmission routes between cattle and badgers—these should be understood as only one aspect of a wider wildlife conflict with deep historical roots.[21]

8.3 Care as a Driver of Controversy

As we have explored the worlds and work of the three epistemic communities that have formed around badger/bTB (*animal health*, *disease ecology* and *badger protection*), we have seen how the knowledge practices (how they investigated the problem) of each of these were mutually shaped by 'cultures of care' developed in the processes of working together.[22] This analysis has drawn out the differences between these cultures of care, with respect to *whom* or *what* these groupings care about; whether care has been focused at the scale of individuals or populations; and what 'care' itself entails in practice. It has also drawn out the changing nature of these cultures of care as they have constantly reshaped themselves and each other, while also mutually influencing broader historical shifts in science–society relations and environmental, agricultural and animal politics.[23] This book has traced how ways of knowing and of caring about badger/bTB have changed since they were first connected in the early 1970s. For example, when MAFF's veterinarians and ecologists started working with naturalists to investigate the new problem of badger/bTB, they used similar methods of investigation—following organisms and their traces, and mapping their geographical distribution. Over time the methods and ideas of the two groups diverged, with veterinarians following a medical logic of case-based intervention; ecologists following one of randomised controlled experiments; and naturalists continuing to follow badgers, with an increasing emphasis on directly observing, interacting and empathising with wildlife. Since the late 1980s badger/bTB research has also drawn upon and contributed to the application of mathematical modelling in epidemiology and disease ecology, a methodology which has particularly come to the fore since the (expensive) completion of the Randomised Badger Culling Trial (RBCT) field trial provided more empirical data for refining these (cheaper) models.[24]

The contingent and changing nature of these cultures of care has also become clear as we traced the shifting alliances between and within these three epistemic communities over policies of bTB control. From the breakdown of an early consensus over the use of Cymag to 'gas' badgers in their setts, through disagreements between badger advocates about the ethics of killing badgers during the RBCT, to today's deep polarisation over culling, points of fracture have manifested over what it means *to care* in the first place. Participants in these debates have agreed—and disagreed—that technologies and practices of killing, catching, restraining and documenting animals could be 'humane' or not, marshalling evidence drawn from the knowledge practices of their own epistemic community. For some, working 'humanely' meant that minimising suffering always comes before preserving life, making killing (animals) a central act of care; for others the opposite is true, making killing the ultimate cruelty. Similar points of fracture/alliance have emerged, dissolved and been rearranged around the relative importance of individuals against populations, societies or wider environments; of economic constraints and who bears the costs of disease control; and of building reliable knowledge—'good science'—as a goal in and of itself.[25] As we have followed the story of badger/bTB over the past half-century, we have seen that these shifts have often directly determined policy outcomes, particularly relating to changing definitions of 'humaneness'—and whether these are considered to be important—in and outside of policy. The contrast between 1980s decisions (to rapidly withdraw badger gassing using Cymag following new scientific findings suggesting it was cruel and ineffective) and 2010s decisions (to elide and avoid similar findings about 'controlled shooting') is particularly stark.

Following the election of the Coalition government in 2010 and its decision to reinstate badger culling as a bTB control policy, badger/bTB has shifted into a pattern of partisan alignment of for/against culling with party-political positions of right and left. While the reasons for the public polarisation of the controversy have been explored in depth in Chap. 7, a key driver appears to have been widening differences in the politics of care, and particularly the public performance of this care, via mass media coverage and other 'public' statements. As we have seen, the longer history of badger/bTB has seen an overall change in policy strategy, from an inclusive mode which sought to involve all interests and keep important conversations 'backstage'; to one which has pushed many actors out towards the 'frontstage' of the wider public sphere.[26] This appears to have happened through a combination of design (e.g. going from an inclusive Consultative Panel to an exclusive Advisory Group) and accident (e.g. scrapping a long-term, citizen-led 'Badger Survey' on cost grounds): the outcome has been an erosion of opportunities for the full range of actors most involved in the problem to talk directly with each other about it.[27] This highlights the importance of care—in domains as diverse as science, medicine, farming, animal health, conservation, policy, politics, animal welfare and animal rights—not only for bringing people, animals and environments together, but also for driving conflict. The literature on care in science and medicine has demonstrated how care and caring practices enable shared work, new knowledge, collaborations, alliances and entanglements.[28] Similarly, scholarship on violent or enforced practices of care (including hunting, culling, euthanasia, surgery and quarantine) has tended to focus on processes of shared meaning-making and mutual support.[29] The badger/bTB case highlights how the creation of intense shared 'cultures of care' *within* social groupings can drive a corresponding intensity of opposition *between* them. If people think of themselves as heroes (who really care), does it become easier to think of those who oppose them as villains (who really don't)? Thinking through care as an aspect of conflict has great potential for helping us understand the drivers, propagators and eventual closure of knowledge controversies, and may also offer important insights into wider processes of political polarisation.[30]

8.4 Expectations

Since tuberculous badgers were first found by government veterinarians in the early 1970s, the exemplary 'policy failure' of badgers and bTB has now been the responsibility of nine prime ministers, fifteen government administrations and twenty-one cabinet ministers.[31] The 2018 bTB Strategy Review is the ninth government-commissioned, expert-led report on bTB in the UK since Lord Solly Zuckerman's in 1980.[32] Many of these reviews have been commissioned by politicians on the *expectation* that the views of authoritative experts and/or new scientific evidence will act to resolve the political controversies around bTB control. However, often the opposite has happened, whereby reviews have been criticised as a biased 'whitewash' (Zuckerman); or a 'betrayal' in which 'the science' invested in by government turned out to produce unexpected, uncertain and unwelcome findings (Krebs/ISG). In the meantime, further scientific research has revealed the deep complexity of the badger/bTB problem, finding new questions as much as it has provided answers. Often the outcome has been to drive media coverage of the problem, opening the issue up to wider public debate but also inflaming controversy. In the longer term, the repeated building and breaking of expectations between scientists, policymakers, politicians, campaigners and publics has contributed to an atmosphere of mistrust and the politicisation of 'evidence' both in and beyond the badger/bTB debate.[33] While this is in part symptomatic of wider problems in British policymaking, relating to expectation building/breaking, high turnover of civil servants and a wider lack of institutional memory, policy learning in badger/bTB has been further limited by rivalries within government between the animal health and disease ecology epistemic communities.[34]

As well as the mutual expectations that science can provide 'all the answers' and that politicians and policymakers will listen to what scientists say, this book has documented several other, equally corrosive expectation cycles in badger/bTB. We have seen repeated rounds of built and broken expectations about organisms, animals and environments—that they will be passive and amenable to policy decisions. Instead, the badger/bTB case has demonstrated how non-human actors play active roles in shaping history, policy and politics. This can be seen in in the long-term consequences of the 2001 foot and mouth disease (FMD) outbreak for the spread of bTB, for the science of the RBCT and for relationships between farmers and government. The most dramatic example of this is the idea of badger 'perturbation'—the awkward refusal of these animals to stay out of places we try and exclude them from. Even though specialists have known about the problem of 'badger movement' or 'recolonisation' since long before bTB entered the picture, whenever badgers exert their agency in this way, such events are greeted with surprise, shock and a continued refusal to anticipate that it will happen again. The badgers have indeed, repeatedly, moved the goalposts.[35] There have been similarly shared assumptions that people are not part of the badger/bTB problem—that this is entirely a phenomenon of the natural world. When research assumes that the densely lived-in landscapes of the South West of England can be controlled as easily as a laboratory, or policy assumes that culling livestock or wildlife has no implications for the people living alongside these animals, it then struggles to adapt when this turns out not to be so. Finally, there have been some peculiarly contradictory assumptions about publics—those directly concerned with badger/bTB, as well as wider audiences and voters.[36] On the one hand, 'lay' actors such as farmers, naturalists and badger advocates (also instrumental members of epistemic communities) have been assumed to passively accept policy decisions, and that they have no useful knowledge to contribute. When landowners have refused access, farmers insisted on 'taking care' of sick badgers themselves, naturalists have reported problems with gassing, and badger advocates have sabotaged culls in the field, policy has reacted with surprise and hostility, describing such actions as 'interference'. At the same time, and sometimes in the same documents, 'the public' has been widely assumed to be universally anti-cull, by actors on all sides of the controversy.

Even now, we still don't know that much about the opinions of the British population about badger/bTB: research conducted to date suggests that public attitudes vary according to demographic factors such as gender and regional location, and are highly contingent on culling having a more dramatic effect on bTB than it appears to.[37] We do know that when people are given the time, space and opportunity to engage with the complexities of bTB policy, their views tend to be more nuanced and productive than the YES!/NO! media debate over culling.[38] In line with other research on science and its publics, I think it is rhetorically useful for many involved in the badger/bTB debate to instead focus upon an 'imagined public', who can be strategically deployed to support arguments for or against culling, as well as to invoke a sense of marginalisation against which countervailing views can be justified.[39] These tactics feed into a wider tendency towards what I would describe as the politics of distraction—so culling is used to distract from the wider problems underlying badger/bTB, such as scientific complexity and uncertainty, the problems of testing, government cost-sharing agendas and the difficulties of living alongside awkward animals like badgers. In turn, bTB has provided a useful distraction away from a plethora of other political problems, as exemplified in Fig. 8.1. In 2011, these were a scandal over media 'hacking' of private citizens, the European debt crisis (and perhaps looming Russian influence?); in 2013 it may have been the internal tensions of the Coalition and Conservative Party; in 2019 we are constantly distracted by the political theatre of Trump, the Brexiteers and their political opponents. In all these cases, such tactics pull public and media attention towards heated, unproductive controversies and away from 'backstage' negotiation, engagement, compromise and building substantive, sustainable policy and political solutions for the long term.[40]

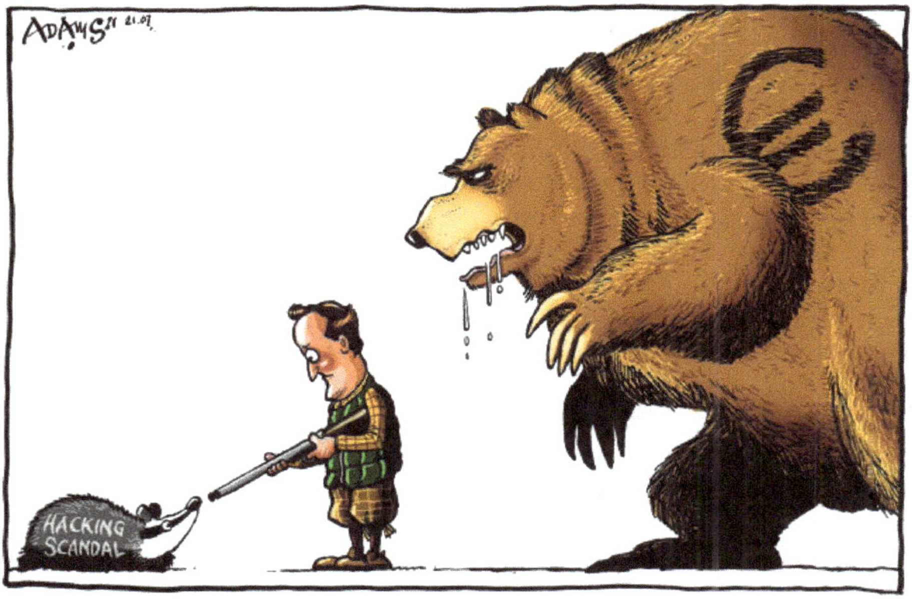

Fig. 8.1 David Cameron and the politics of distraction (Cartoon by Christian Adams, *Daily Telegraph*, 21 July 2011, 20.

8.5 Some Questions and Suggestions

At the beginning of this book, I said that this work has only scratched the surface of what we need to know about the history of badger/bTB in Britain. I stand by that view—like all research, this work has uncovered many more questions which bear further investigation. To start with, what would the history of badger/bTB look like viewed from outside the central perspectives of government archives and national media? Social, natural and historical research on bTB is increasingly highlighting stark differences in experiences of badger/bTB across the various countries and regions of the UK, as well as the need to think at multiple scales about the problem.[41] Therefore a key priority would be to use local, community and oral history approaches to investigate how the controversy since the 1970s was experienced by farmers, naturalists, activists and other publics living in places affected (and unaffected) by badger/bTB. While the unique history of the badger/bTB situation in Northern Ireland has been investigated, the critical experiences of people in the South West of England have yet to be documented.[42] Given that social research on bTB also points towards disjuncts in communication, engagement, responsibility, power and trust between central government and local actors as a key problem for bTB policy, the need to understand such histories is even more urgent. My work has also uncovered a further gap in the historiography of bTB—while late nineteenth- and early twentieth-century debates have been extensively investigated, and this volume traces the situation since the mid-1960s, we still have a rather sketchy understanding of how the disease was (mostly) brought under control in the post-war period. Other potentially fruitful areas of investigation include a comprehensive exploration of the shared histories of human and animal TB; more extensive research asking what wider publics in multiple places think about culling, animal health and the politics of wildlife in contemporary Britain; and the importance of care as a driver of knowledge controversies. I will end with some suggestions for policymakers, politicians, campaigners and anyone else involved with this messy and exhausting knowledge controversy. I build upon thoughts submitted to the 2018 Godfray Review on what I think the history of badger/bTB can tell us about where we might go next.[43] However, these cannot become properly useful or use-able policy recommendations without the input of those involved, and therefore I invite their thoughts.

Looking, Seeing, Knowing and Acting on TB in Humans and Other Animals. As outlined above, if bTB is being reframed as an environmental disease, this has deep epistemic implications—if what we know about badgers, cattle and *M. bovis* has been shaped by the technologies we use, where we decide to look, the presence of other microbes and environmental changes, and what we do with infected bodies, then both research and policy need to take account of this. Such insights can create more productive ways of understanding contradictory interpretations of 'the science' of bTB in relation to culling. For example, the Thornbury and other clearance trials of the 1970s are often held up as evidence that culling 'works', while the RBCT is used to support arguments that it doesn't. However, in my view both these approaches—as well as the early experiences of ICD officers trying to get rid of troublesome badgers—may in fact be telling us similar things. It looks like badgers can be culled, and if this is done thoroughly enough, for long enough, over a wide enough area, there appear to be positive effects on bTB incidence in cattle. However, that's a very big 'if'—as this history has shown, it takes a great deal of time, money, effort and systematic organisation to get rid of badgers and keep them away. Because *M. bovis* seems to pass between badgers–cattle, and between cattle–cattle, and (if newer research findings hold up) between these species and their environments, short-term, reactive, small-scale and ad hoc culling will risk disturbing local ecosystems and spreading the microbe further.[44] So the questions to ask of any bTB control measure would be: will this be this systematic enough? How do we determine this? How much effort and cost would be required to do the job properly? How big an effect can we expect, and once we know this, *is it really worth it*—ecologically, financially, politically and ethically? For many years, underlying policy agendas have advanced cost-sharing, decentralisation and reducing government oversight (particularly of culling), raising questions about the ability of government to systematically implement disease control. Given that historical research on how bTB risks were successfully managed in the first place points towards the importance of the state in coordinating and enforcing control measures, movement in the opposite direction does not bode well.[45] Thinking of bTB as an environmental disease also has wider implications for animal and human health policy. For example, if *M. bovis* and other mycobacteria can survive for longer outside the body, can *M. tuberculosis*? What would be the implications for global health? This cuts the other way: given that TB in humans has long been thought of as the 'social disease', then the social aspects of bTB should be taken much more seriously—not only as a political problem, but as a fundamental aspect of the disease.

Wildlife Conflicts and Care. Given that we can trace the British badger debate back to the Victorian era at least, and potentially as far as the Anglo-Saxons, the deep historical roots of this wildlife conflict also need to be taken seriously. Badger–human conflict (and human conflict about badgers) is deeply entangled with the bTB problem in this country. Therefore any sustainable bTB policy must also address those factors which make it difficult for badgers and people to co-exist, including their tendency to exercise their own agency, and the feelings this creates in people when for example their crops or other property gets damaged.[46] Practical frameworks for addressing these kinds of problems already exist, but have mostly been directed towards charismatic and rare species such as elephants, great apes and big cats, often in the Global South.[47] If we in Britain expect people elsewhere to live with (and care for) much more difficult and dangerous charismatic species, should we not learn to cope with one mildly cantankerous mustelid? Other historically awkward animals, including beavers, wild boar and polecats, are now returning to the British countryside: for them to flourish we need to find modes of co-existence which can take account of animal agency and benefit all publics, not just those who already care deeply for wildlife.[48] I noted at the end of Chap. 6 that there seems to be some 'backstage' potential for moving past the unproductive and bruising confrontations of today's public controversy. For this to happen, wider recognition is needed that all those involved do care a great deal—but what they care about and for may be different. We already know that, given time, space, in-depth information and opportunities for personal connection, people can engage with the deep complexities—and conflicting values—of this problem. Ultimately it is in the interests of those most involved and affected to work together and explore the 'diplomatic spaces' where there is potential for common ground. However, such processes need proper financial, institutional and practical support.[49]

Science, Policy and Expectations. The repetitive and unproductive cycle of building and breaking expectations seen over the past forty years or so suggests that some serious rethinking of UK science–policy relations—in and beyond animal health—is long overdue. Many people involved in the problem are already trying to do this, but my contributions follow. First, I would suggest that rather than calling for reviews at politically strategic moments, government should instead review this kind of complex and changing evidence base on a regular basis, with clearly established routes for research and policy activity to feed into one another, and for practical outcomes. What counts as 'evidence' needs to be broadened to include work from multiple STEM disciplines; quantitative and qualitative social science; humanities scholarship; the experiential expertise of professionals and volunteers closely involved with the situation; and should transparently take account of the contrasting and conflicting views of multiple publics. This could help politicians and policymakers to take a broader view of the situation and have a clearer understanding of the strategic redefinition and elision of evidence by campaigners on all sides—as well as what we *do not* know and perhaps *cannot* do.[50] As outlined above, there is strong potential for new technological developments—particularly in testing and possibly in vaccination—to create new possibilities for bTB policy. I believe that such potential should absolutely be explored, whilst also *anticipating* that they may not succeed, or if they do, will bring about new uncertainties and regulatory challenges. Technological solutions are indeed possible: the trap is to believe that the quick, easy, just-about-to-happen in five years technological fix means that nothing else needs to be done.[51] While I agree that the role of 'ministerial judgement' is essential and should be transparently acknowledged in badger/bTB, to cede all policy influence to elected politicians strikes me as a potential recipe for further manipulation of expertise and public polarisation.[52]

Instead, I suggest that properly supported mechanisms for regular, in-person interaction between the various interests concerned with bTB policy be reinstituted, at national and local level. While this seems be happening sometimes, behind the scenes, the creation of policy 'insiders' and 'outsiders' has contributed to the political polarisation of bTB.[53] As I argued in Chaps. 6 and 7, since the 1990s this has been exacerbated by increasing disconnects between the backstage of bTB policy and the front-stage of public debates. To move forwards, government may need to return to older, more inclusive styles of policymaking, no matter which political party is in charge. Experiments with dialogue and participatory governance suggest that, paradoxically, explicitly setting aside the goal of consensus can help opponents understand each other's points of view better and find ways of working together.[54] Finally, in line with the recommendations of other historians studying and working with policymakers, efforts to build more coherent institutional and public memories should be supported.[55] This would make it less likely that we keep revisiting past failures in bTB itself (such as gassing), but also more likely to draw wider lessons for applied research (such as the value of lab–field partnerships and independent regional expertise) and for science–policy relations (such as the dangers of unrealistic expectations). I believe that a more concerted effort to 'do TB differently'[56] and properly re-examine the situation from all those involved would greatly benefit the back-, front- and centre-stage of British animal health, agricultural and environmental policies.

Notes

1. For accessible primers on the natural science of bTB (from several angles), I refer readers to (1) TB Knowledge Exchange, run by my Exeter colleague Dr Robertson, 'TB Knowledge Exchange'; (2) the multi-agency-funded TB Hub: http://www.tbhub.co.uk/ and TB Advisory Service: http://www.tbas.org.uk/; (3) the badger/bTB briefing pages of the British Veterinary Association: https://www.bva.co.uk/News-campaigns-and-policy/Policy/Farm-animals/Bovine-tuberculosis/; (4) a recent briefing from the Zoological Society of London ZSL, 'Eradicating TB from Cattle and Badgers—A Review of Evidence'; and (5) the 2018 Godfray review of

government bTB policy, Godfray et al., 'A Strategy for Achieving Bovine Tuberculosis Free Status for England'.

2. See also Brown and Michael, 'A Sociology of Expectations'; V. C. Broto, 'Environmental Conflicts, Research Projects and the Generation of Collective Expectations: A Case Study of a Land Regeneration Project in Tuzla, Bosnia and Herzegovina', *Public Understanding of Science* 21(4) (November 2010): 432–46; Michaela Maier et al., 'Communicating Scientific Evidence: Scientists', Journalists' and Audiences' Expectations and Evaluations Regarding the Representation of Scientific Uncertainty', *Communications* 41(3) (2016): 239–64; Brown and Beynon-Jones, 'Reflex Regulation'.
3. See Sect. 1.3; also Rosenberg and Golden, *Framing Disease.*
4. Woods et al., *Animals and the Shaping of Modern Medicine*, 1–26.
5. See Sect. 3.1.
6. See Sect. 4.2.
7. See Sect. 6.4.
8. See Sect. 3.4.
9. Enticott, 'The Local Universality of Veterinary Expertise and the Geography of Animal Disease'.
10. As does a supplementary blood test known as interferon-gamma.
11. Sara H. Downs et al., 'Methodology and Preliminary Results of a Systematic Literature Review of Ante-Mortem and Post-Mortem Diagnostic Tests for Bovine Tuberculosis', *Preventive Veterinary Medicine* 153 (1 May 2018): 117–26.
12. Andrea Sanchez-Hidalgo et al., '*Mycobacterium Bovis* Hosted by Free-Living-Amoebae Permits Their Long-Term Persistence Survival Outside of Host Mammalian Cells and Remain Capable of Transmitting Disease to Mice', *Environmental Microbiology* 19(10) (October 2017): 4010–21; J. A. Barasona et al., 'Environmental Presence of Mycobacterium Tuberculosis Complex in Aggregation Points at the Wildlife/Livestock Interface', *Transboundary and Emerging Diseases* 64(4) (2 July 2017): 1148–58.
13. WHO, 'WHO|Roadmap for Zoonotic Tuberculosis'.
14. Bynum, *Spitting Blood*; Lukas Engelmann and Janina Kehr, 'Double Trouble: Towards an Epistemology of Co-Infection', *Medicine Anthropology Theory* 2(1) (2015): 1–31; McMillen, *Discovering Tuberculosis.*
15. See Sect. 1.4.
16. See Sect. 4.3.
17. See Sect. 5.3; for making animals 'killable' see Haraway, *When Species Meet*, 77–82.
18. See Sects. 7.2–7.4. For charismatic species see e.g. J. Lorimer, 'Nonhuman Charisma', *Environment and Planning D: Society and Space* 25 (2007): 911–32.

19. See Sect. 1.4, also e.g. Cassidy, 'Badger–Human Conflict'; Delahay et al., 'Managing Conflict between Humans and Wildlife'.
20. Enticott, 'Techniques of Neutralising Wildlife Crime in Rural England and Wales'; Phoenix, 'Local Understandings of Bovine Tuberculosis (Working Title)'.
21. E.g. Delahay et al., 'Managing Conflict between Humans and Wildlife'; Johanna Judge et al., 'Effectiveness of Biosecurity Measures in Preventing Badger Visits to Farm Buildings', ed. Justin David Brown, *PLoS ONE* 6(12) (December 2011): e28941–e28941.
22. See Sect. 1.2, also on epistemic communities, Meyer and Molyneux-Hodgson, 'Introduction'; Dunlop, 'Epistemic Communities'. For knowledge and cultures of care, see Davies et al., 'Science, Culture, and Care in Laboratory Animal Research'.
23. See Sects. 3.3, 4.4, and 5.4. For a broader perspective see also Agar, 'Transition'.
24. Conlan et al., 'The Intractable Challenge of Evaluating Cattle Vaccination as a Control for Bovine Tuberculosis'.
25. See Sects. 5.3–5.4; also e.g. Morris, 'Introduction'; Davies et al., 'Science, Culture, and Care in Laboratory Animal Research'; Druglitrø, '"Skilled Care" and the Making of Good Science'.
26. See Chs. 5 and 6 for these themes, also Ayres, Sandford and Coombes, 'Policy-Making "Front" and "Back" Stage'; Hilgartner, *Science on Stage*.
27. Grant, 'Intractable Policy Failure: The Case of Bovine TB and Badgers'.
28. Davies et al., 'Science, Culture, and Care in Laboratory Animal Research'; Richard Gorman, 'Therapeutic Landscapes and Non-Human Animals: The Roles and Contested Positions of Animals within Care Farming Assemblages', *Social & Cultural Geography* 18(3) (May 2016): 315–35; A. Martin, N. Myers and A. Viseu, 'The Politics of Care in Technoscience', *Social Studies of Science* 45(5) (October 2015): 625–41.
29. Van Dooren, 'A Day with Crows'; Haraway, *When Species Meet*; Morris, 'Introduction'; Marvin and McHugh, 'In It Together'.
30. On the public polarisation of science and environmental issues, see Kahan et al., 'The Polarizing Impact of Science Literacy and Numeracy on Perceived Climate Change Risks'; M. C. Nisbet and E. M. Markowitz, 'Expertise in an Age of Polarization: Evaluating Scientists' Political Awareness and Communication Behaviors', *The ANNALS of the American Academy of Political and Social Science* 658(1) (2015): 136–54; Lucas and Warman, 'Disrupting Polarized Discourses'.
31. On policy failure in animal health see Claire A. Dunlop, 'Pathologies of Policy Learning: What Are They and How Do They Contribute to Policy Failure?' *Policy and Politics* 45(1) (January 2017): 19–37; Grant, 'Intractable Policy Failure'.
32. See Sects. 1.1 and 6.1. for further discussion of these expert reviews.

33. On expectations in science-policy see Brown and Beynon-Jones, 'Reflex Regulation'.
34. Bob Hudson, 'Why Policy Failure Is so Common in the UK', *LSE Business Review* (blog), 26 January 2019; Tom Sasse and Emma Norris, 'Moving On', 16 January 2019; Katy Wilkinson, 'Organised Chaos: An Interpretive Approach to Evidence-Based Policy Making in Defra', *Political Studies* 59(4) (December 2011): 959–77; Parker, 'The Rothschild Report (1971) and the Purpose of Government-Funded R&D'; Dunlop, 'Pathologies of Policy Learning'.
35. See Sects. 2.2–2.4, 4.3, and 6.2–6.4.
36. In line with most researchers working in this area, I think it is generally more realistic and useful to think about science–society relations in terms of multiple 'publics' rather than 'the public': Jason Chilvers and Matthew Kearnes, *Remaking Participation: Science, Environment and Emergent Publics* (New York: Routledge, 2015).
37. The most in-depth work to date exploring wider public attitudes to badger culling confines itself to Wales: see Enticott, 'Public Attitudes to Badger Culling to Control Bovine Tuberculosis in Rural Wales'.
38. OPM Group, 'Defra Bovine TB Citizen Dialogue'.
39. Claire Marris, 'The Construction of Imaginaries of the Public as a Threat to Synthetic Biology', *Science as Culture* 24(1) (2015): 83–98; J. Barnett et al., 'Imagined Publics and Engagement around Renewable Energy Technologies in the UK', *Public Understanding of Science* 21(1) (2012): 36–50; Bickerstaff, Simmons and Pidgeon, 'Situating Local Experience of Risk'.
40. Lester and Hutchins, 'The Power of the Unseen'; Maye et al., '"Present Realities" and the Need for a "Lived Experience" Perspective in Brexit Agri-Food Governance'; Jennings and Lodge, 'Brexit, the Tides and Canute'; Lodge and Matus, 'Science, Badgers, Politics'.
41. Enticott, 'Market Instruments, Biosecurity and Place-Based Understandings of Animal Disease'; Robinson, 'A History of Bovine Tuberculosis Eradication Policy in Northern Ireland'; Philip A. Robinson, 'Farmers and Bovine Tuberculosis: Contextualising Statutory Disease Control within Everyday Farming Lives', *Journal of Rural Studies* 55(Supplement) C (1 October 2017): 168–80; Maye, 'Geography Matters'.
42. Philip A. Robinson, 'A History of Bovine Tuberculosis Eradication Policy in Northern Ireland', *Epidemiology and Infection* 143(15) (2015): 3182–95.
43. Angela Cassidy, 'The UK's Bovine TB Strategy: A Prospective View from History', Submission to Defra, Bovine TB Strategy review 2018: call for evidence (Exeter: University of Exeter, 2018).

44. See also Prentice Jamie C. et al., 'When to Kill a Cull: Factors Affecting the Success of Culling Wildlife for Disease Control', *Journal of The Royal Society Interface* 16(152) (6 March 2019): 20180901.
45. Olmstead and Rhodes, *Arresting Contagion*; Atkins, *A History of Uncertainty*; Waddington, *The Bovine Scourge.*
46. Susan Boonman-Berson, Clemens Driessen and Esther Turnhout, 'Managing Wild Minds: From Control by Numbers to a Multinatural Approach in Wild Boar Management in the Veluwe, the Netherlands', *Transactions of the Institute of British Geographers* 44(2) (2019): 2–15.
47. Simon Pooley et al., 'An Interdisciplinary Review of Current and Future Approaches to Improving Human–Predator Relations', *Conservation Biology* 31(3) (2017): 513–23; Hill, 'Perspectives of "Conflict" at the Wildlife–Agriculture Boundary'.
48. Boonman-Berson, Driessen and Turnhout, 'Managing Wild Minds'; Sarah L. Crowley, Steve Hinchliffe and Robbie A McDonald, 'Nonhuman Citizens on Trial: The Ecological Politics of a Beaver Reintroduction', *Environment and Planning A* 49(8) (1 August 2017): 1846–66; Crowley, Hinchliffe and McDonald, 'Conflict in Invasive Species Management'.
49. Price et al., 'From Contradiction to Contrast in a Countryside Conflict'; Saunders and Keenan, 'Conflict Framing in the Control of Bovine Tuberculosis'; Sandover, Kinsley and Hinchliffe, 'A Very Public Cull'.
50. Christl A. Donnelly et al., 'Four Principles to Make Evidence Synthesis More Useful for Policy', *Nature* 558(7710) (June 2018): 361; Andy Stirling and Clive Mitchell, 'Evaluate Power and Bias in Synthesizing Evidence for Policy', *Nature* 563 (5 September 2018): 33.
51. Lisa Rosner, *The Technological Fix: How People Use Technology to Create and Solve Problems* (New York: Routledge, 2013).
52. See Godfray et al., 'A Strategy for Achieving Bovine Tuberculosis Free Status for England', 2, 107–8; Boyd, 'Making Science Count in Government'.
53. See Sects. 5.4 and 7.3.
54. Warren Pearce et al., 'Beyond Counting Climate Consensus', *Environmental Communication* 11(6) (23 July 2017): 723–30; K. M. Centellas, R. E. Smardon and S. Fifield, 'Calibrating Translational Cancer Research: Collaboration without Consensus in Interdisciplinary Laboratory Meetings', *Science, Technology & Human Values* 39(3) (October 2013): 311–35.
55. For excellent practical examples, see the work of *History & Policy* (http://www.historyandpolicy.org/) and e.g. Virginia Berridge, 'Thinking in Time: Does Health Policy Need History as Evidence?' *The Lancet* 375(9717) (2010): 798–99; Abigail Woods, 'The Lowe Report and Its Echoes from History', *The Veterinary Record* 169(17) (October 2011):

434–36; Pat Thane, *Unequal Britain: Equalities in Britain since 1945* (London: Bloomsbury Publishing, 2010); Hugh Pemberton, 'Policy Networks and Policy Learning UK Economic Policy in the 1960s and 1970s', *Public Administration* 78(4) (1 January 2000): 771–92.

56. Price et al., 'From Contradiction to Contrast in a Countryside Conflict'.

BIBLIOGRAPHY

Mass Media Sources

Unless listed below, mass media references can be sourced from the following digital archives:

BBC Genome—online archive of British Broadcasting Corporation *Radio Times* magazine listings

Gale NewsVault: *The Independent* Digital Archive

Gale NewsVault: *Daily Mail* Historical Archive

Gale NewsVault: *The Telegraph* Historical Archive

Gale NewsVault: *The Times* Digital Archive

ProQuest Historical Newspapers: *The Guardian* and *The Observer*

UKPressOnline: *Daily Mirror* archive

Nexis-UK, news media database published by LexisNexis Legal and Professional

Ashby, Eric. 'At Home with Badgers: Wildlife on One'. *The Radio Times*. BBC Television, 13 April 1978. https://genome.ch.bbc.co.uk/77ba3e9e375249eb884d18f966e72d00.

Bale, Peter. 'Badger Watch'. *The Radio Times*. BBC Television, 5 May 1977. https://genome.ch.bbc.co.uk/1d86acdee53343378e43723bcc639ade.

Bateson, Patrick. 'Culling Badgers Could Increase the Problem of TB in Cattle|Letters'. *The Observer*, 14 October 2012, sec. Global. https://www.theguardian.com/theobserver/2012/oct/14/letters-observer.

BBC. 'Anger after Badger Found Shot in Gut'. *BBC News Online*, 23 September 2014, sec. Somerset. https://www.bbc.com/news/uk-england-somerset-29315243.

———. 'Badgers "moved Goalposts" in Cull'. *BBC News*, 9 October 2013, sec. England. https://www.bbc.co.uk/news/uk-england-24459424.

———. 'Benn Confirms TB Cull Rejection'. *BBC News Online*, 7 July 2008. http://news.bbc.co.uk/1/hi/sci/tech/7493846.stm.

———. 'Farmers' Union Backs Staying in EU'. *BBC News Online*, 18 April 2016a, sec. UK. https://www.bbc.com/news/uk-36078112.

———. 'Obituary: Richard Adams'. *BBC News Online*, 27 December 2016b, sec. UK. https://www.bbc.com/news/uk-10788325.

Carrington, Damian, and Jamie Doward. 'Badger Cull "Mindless", Say Scientists'. *The Observer*, 13 October 2012, sec. Environment. http://www.theguardian.com/environment/2012/oct/13/badger-cull-mindless.

Clarke, Philip. 'Farmer Support for Brexit as Strong as Ever, FW Poll Reveals'. *Farmers Weekly*, 22 December 2017. https://www.fwi.co.uk/news/farmer-support-brexit-strong-ever-fw-poll-reveals.

Duncan, Amy. 'Channel 5 Horrifies Viewers by Showing Watership Down on Easter Sunday (Again)'. *Metro*, 16 April 2017. https://metro.co.uk/2017/04/16/channel-5-showed-watership-down-on-easter-sunday-and-its-scarred-viewers-for-life-6578101/.

Flood, Alison. 'Watership Down Author Richard Adams: I Just Can't Do Humans'. *The Guardian*, 4 January 2015, sec. Books. https://www.theguardian.com/books/2015/jan/04/richard-adams-watership-down-interview.

Hart-Davis, Duff. 'Country Matters: Guardians of the Haunted House'. *The Independent*, 11 June 1994. http://www.independent.co.uk/voices/country-matters-guardians-of-the-haunted-house-1421781.html.

Hattenstone, Simon, and Patrick Barkham. 'Michael Eavis Throws Support behind Badger Cull'. *The Guardian*, 21 June 2013. https://www.theguardian.com/environment/2013/jun/21/michael-eavis-badger-cull-glastonbury-festival.

Linley, Mike. 'Survival: Badger Woman'. Norwich: Anglia Television, 9 February 1995.

Lowe, David. 'Princess Anne: Gas Is Much Nicer Way of Culling Badgers'. *Countryfile*. BBC Television, 8 April 2014. https://www.bbc.com/news/av/entertainment-arts-26894760/princess-anne-gas-is-much-nicer-way-of-culling-badgers.

Mance, Henry. 'Britain Has Had Enough of Experts, Says Gove'. *Financial Times*, 3 June 2016. https://www.ft.com/content/3be49734-29cb-11e6-83e4-abc22d5d108c.

May, Brian. 'This Cruel Badger Cull Is Pointless—and I Can Prove It, Says Queen Guitarist Brian May'. *Mail Online*, 20 October 2012a. https://www.dailymail.

co.uk/news/article-2220734/This-cruel-badger-cull-pointless%2D%2DI-prove-says-Queen-guitarist-Brian-May.html.

———. 'Vegetarian Rock Stars Don't Vote Tory. I Did. But I'll Never Vote for Cameron after His Bloody Badger Cull'. *Mail Online*, 25 August 2012b. https://www.dailymail.co.uk/debate/article-2193595/Brian-May-I-voted-Tory-But-Ill-vote-Cameron-bloody-badger-cull.html.

Meikle, James. 'English Badgers Earn a Reprieve, as Government Rejects Mass Cull'. *The Guardian*, 4 July 2008, sec. UK news. https://www.theguardian.com/environment/2008/jul/04/wildlife.conservation.

Rosen, Martin. *Watership Down*. Film. United Kingdom: Nepenthe Productions Ltd, 1978.

Scott, Peter, and Desmond Hawkins. 'Badgers'. *The Radio Times*. BBC Television, 12 November 1954. https://genome.ch.bbc.co.uk/c28140ea6560458696f962560142258c.

Tasker, Johann. 'In the Hot Seat: Tim Farron of the Lib Dems'. *Farmers Weekly*, 14 September 2009. https://www.fwi.co.uk/livestock/health-welfare/livestock-diseases/bovine-tb/in-the-hot-seat-tim-farron-of-the-lib-dems.

Wildscreen. 'WildFilmHistory—Badger Watch (1977)'. WildFilmHistory, 2008. http://web.archive.org/web/20170304143202/http://www.wildfilmhistory.org/film/288/Badger+Watch.html.

Wright, Liz. 'Obituary: Miriam Kelly'. *The Guardian*, 28 August 2008. http://www.theguardian.com/theguardian/2008/aug/29/2.

(All URLs last accessed 6 March 2019)

Primary Sources

Adams, Richard. *Watership Down*. London: Rex Collings Ltd, 1972.

Advisory Committee on Pesticides. 'Pesticide Poisoning of Animals in 2004: Investigations of Suspected Incidents in the United Kingdom'. London: Defra, 2005. http://www.hse.gov.uk/pesticides/resources/Other/53947_PSD_BrochureFINALVERSION(1).pdf.

Agriculture Committee. 'Badgers and Bovine TB, Vol.II: Fifth Report of Session 1998–1999(HC 233-II)'. Agriculture Committee Reports. London: House of Commons: HMSO, 20 April 1999. https://publications.parliament.uk/pa/cm199899/cmselect/cmagric/233/23302.htm.

Allen, A. R., R. A. Skuce and A. W. Byrne. 'Bovine Tuberculosis in Britain and Ireland—A Perfect Storm? The Confluence of Potential Ecological and Epidemiological Impediments to Controlling a Chronic Infectious Disease'. *Frontiers in Veterinary Science* 5 (2018): 109. https://doi.org/10.3389/fvets.2018.00109.

Amlaner, Charles J. and David W. MacDonald, eds. *A Handbook on Biotelemetry and Radio Tracking: Proceedings of an International Conference on Telemetry and Radio Tracking in Biology and Medicine, Oxford, 20–22 March 1979.* Oxford: Pergamon Press, 1980.

Anderson, R. M., Helen C. Jackson, Robert M. May and Anthony M. Smith. 'Population Dynamics of Fox Rabies in Europe'. *Nature* 289(5800) (26 February 1981): 765–71.

Anderson, R. M., and Robert M. May. 'Population Biology of Infectious Diseases: Part I'. *Nature* 280(5721) (2 August 1979): 361–67.

Anderson, R. M., and W. Trewhella. 'Population Dynamics of the Badger (Meles Meles) and the Epidemiology of Bovine Tuberculosis (Mycobacterium Bovis)'. *Philosophical Transactions of the Royal Society B: Biological Sciences* 310(1145) (1985): 327–81.

Anon. 'The Mammal Society of the British Isles'. *Nature* 173 (22 May 1954): 980.

Backhouse, K. M., and H. V. Thompson. 'Myxomatosis'. *Nature* 176(4494) (1955): 1155–56.

Badgers Act (1973). http://www.legislation.gov.uk/ukpga/1973/57/enacted.

Baker, Simon J. 'Escaped Exotic Mammals in Britain'. *Mammal Review* 20(2–3) (1 June 1990): 75–96.

Barasona, J. A., J. Vicente, I. Díez-Delgado, J. Aznar, C. Gortázar and M. J. Torres. 'Environmental Presence of Mycobacterium Tuberculosis Complex in Aggregation Points at the Wildlife/Livestock Interface'. *Transboundary and Emerging Diseases* 64(4) (2 July 2017): 1148–58.

Barkham, Patrick. *Badgerlands: The Twilight World of Britain's Most Enigmatic Animal.* London: Granta Books, 2014.

Barrow, P. A. 'Aspects of the Epidemiology of Bovine Tuberculosis in Badgers and Cattle. II. The Development and Use of a Typing System for Mycobacterium Bovis'. *The Journal of Hygiene* 86(3) (1981): 247–57.

Barrow, P. A., and J. Gallagher. 'Aspects of the Epidemiology of Bovine Tuberculosis in Badgers and Cattle. I. The Prevalence of Infection in Two Wild Animal Populations in South-West England'. *The Journal of Hygiene* 86(3) (1981): 237–45.

Bielby, Jon, Flavie Vial, Rosie Woodroffe and Christl A. Donnelly. 'Localised Badger Culling Increases Risk of Herd Breakdown on Nearby, Not Focal, Land'. Ed. Emmanuel Serrano Ferron. *PLoS ONE* 11(10) (October 2016): e0164618–e0164618. http://dx.plos.org/10.1371/journal.pone.0164618.

Bourne, John, Christl A. Donnelly, David R. Cox, George Gettinby, John P. McInerney, W. Ivan Morrison and Rosie Woodroffe. 'An Epidemiological Investigation into Bovine Tuberculosis: Towards a Science Based Control Strategy'. Independent Scientific Group on Cattle TB. London: Defra, December 2004.

———. 'Bovine TB: Second Report of the Independent Scientific Group on Cattle TB'. Independent Scientific Group on Cattle TB. London: Defra, December 1999.

———. 'Bovine TB: The Scientific Evidence, Final Report of the Independent Scientific Group on Cattle TB'. Independent Scientific Group on Cattle TB. London: Defra, 2007.

———. 'Bovine TB: Towards a Sustainable Policy to Control TB in Cattle'. Independent Scientific Group on Cattle TB. London: Defra, July 1998.

———. 'Independent Scientific Group on Cattle TB: Report of the Work of the Group & Its Published Findings in 2005'. Independent Scientific Group on Cattle TB. London: Defra, 2005.

Boyd, I. 'Making Science Count in Government'. *ELife* 2 (July 2013): e01061–e01061. http://elife.elifesciences.org/lookup/doi/10.7554/eLife.01061.

Broughan, J. M., J. Judge, E. Ely, R. J. Delahay, G. Wilson, R. S. Clifton-Hadley, A. V. Goodchild, H. Bishop, J. E. Parry and S. H. Downs. 'A Review of Risk Factors for Bovine Tuberculosis Infection in Cattle in the UK and Ireland'. *Epidemiology & Infection* 144(14) (October 2016): 2899–2926.

Broughan, J. M., D. Maye, P. Carmody, L. A. Brunton, A. Ashton, W. Wint, N. Alexander et al. 'Farm Characteristics and Farmer Perceptions Associated with Bovine Tuberculosis Incidents in Areas of Emerging Endemic Spread'. *Preventive Veterinary Medicine* 129 (1 July 2016): 88–98.

Brown, A. C. L. 'Animal Health 1972: Report of the Chief Veterinary Officer'. London: Ministry of Agriculture, Fisheries and Food, 1972.

———. 'Animal Health 1973: Report of the Chief Veterinary Officer'. London: Ministry of Agriculture, Fisheries and Food, 1973.

———. 'Animal Health 1974: Report of the Chief Veterinary Officer'. London: Ministry of Agriculture, Fisheries and Food, 1975.

———. 'Animal Health 1977: Report of the Chief Veterinary Officer'. London: Ministry of Agriculture, Fisheries and Food, 1977.

Brown, J. A., C. L. Cheeseman and S. Harris. 'Studies on the Spread of Bovine Tuberculosis from Badgers to Cattle'. *Journal of Zoology* 227(4) (August 1992): 694–96.

Brunton, Lucy A., Christl A. Donnelly, Heather O'Connor, Alison Prosser, Stuart Ashfield, Adam Ashton, Paul Upton et al. 'Assessing the Effects of the First 2 Years of Industry-Led Badger Culling in England on the Incidence of Bovine Tuberculosis in Cattle in 2013–2015'. *Ecology and Evolution* 7(18) (1 September 2017): 7213–30.

Buesching, Christina D., J. R. Clarke, Stephen A. Ellwood, C. M. King, C. Newman and D. W. Macdonald. 'The Mammals of Wytham Woods'. In *Wytham Woods: Oxford's Ecological Laboratory*. Oxford: Oxford University Press, 2010.

Burke, Norah. *King Todd: The True Story of a Wild Badger; and of the Deer, Foxes, and Other Animals in the Forest Where He Lived/Illustrated by D. J. Watkins-Pitchford*. London: Putnam, 1963.

Burns, Lord, Victoria Edwards, John Marsh, Lord Soulsby and Michael Winter. 'Report of Committee of Inquiry into Hunting with Dogs in England & Wales'. London: HMSO, 9 June 2000. http://webarchive.nationalarchives.gov.uk/20080727002638/http://www.huntinginquiry.gov.uk/mainsections/report.pdf.

Byrne, Andrew W., D. Paddy Sleeman, James O'Keeffe and John Davenport. 'The Ecology of the European Badger (Meles Meles) in Ireland: A Review'. *Biology & Environment: Proceedings of the Royal Irish Academy* 112(1) (January 2012): 105–32.

Cabinet Office. 'Modernising Government'. London: HMSO, 1999. http://webarchive.nationalarchives.gov.uk/20131205101137/http://www.archive.official-documents.co.uk/document/cm43/4310/4310.htm.

———. 'Prince of Wales Correspondence with the Prime Minister'. GOV.UK, 13 May 2015. https://www.gov.uk/government/publications/prince-of-wales-correspondence-with-the-prime-minister.

———. 'The Coalition: Our Programme for Government'. London: HMSO, 2010. https://assets.publishing.service.gov.uk/government/uploads/system/uploads/attachment_data/file/78977/coalition_programme_for_government.pdf.

CBAG. 'A History Lesson of Direct Action & Badger Culls. | Badger Killers'. Badger Killers—Coalition of Badger Action Groups, 14 April 2014. https://web.archive.org/web/20140606040738/http://badger-killers.co.uk/a-history-lesson-of-direct-action-badger-culls/.

Centres for Disease Control and Prevention. 'CDC—The Emergency Response Safety and Health Database: Systemic Agent: SODIUM CYANIDE—NIOSH'. CDC—The Emergency Response Safety and Health Database, 27 September 2018. https://www.cdc.gov/niosh/ershdb/emergencyresponsecard_29750036.html.

Chambers, M., S. Gordon, F. Olea-Popelka and P. Barrow. *Bovine Tuberculosis*. Wallingford, Oxfordshire: CABI, 2018.

Charity Commission. 'Charity Details: Badger Trust'. Registered Charities in England and Wales, 2016. http://beta.charitycommission.gov.uk/charity-details/?regid=1111440&subid=0.

———. 'Charity Details: National Federation Of Badger Groups'. Registered Charities in England and Wales, 2006. http://beta.charitycommission.gov.uk/charity-details/?regid=1041772&subid=0.

———. 'Charity Details: The Save Me Trust'. 2017. http://beta.charitycommission.gov.uk/charity-details/?regid=1082568&subid=0.

Cheeseman, C. L. 'Why a Badger Cull Won't Work'. *Badgergate*, 9 June 2013. https://www.badgergate.org/guest-articles/why-a-badger-cull-wont-work/.

Cheeseman, C. L., W. J. Cresswell, S. Harris and P. J. Mallinson. 'Comparison of Dispersal and Other Movements in Two Badger (*Meles Meles*) Populations'. *Mammal Review* 18, no. 1 (1 March 1988): 51–59.

Cheeseman, C. L., and Stephen Harris. 'Methods of Marking Badgers (*Meles Meles*), Notes from the Mammal Society—No. 44'. *Journal of Zoology* 197(2) (1 June 1982): 289–91.

Cheeseman, C. L., G. W. Jones, J. Gallagher and P. J. Mallinson. 'The Population Structure, Density and Prevalence of Tuberculosis (*Mycobacterium Bovis*) in Badgers (*Meles Meles*) from Four Areas in South-West England'. *Journal of Applied Ecology* 18(3) (1981): 795–804.

Cheeseman, C. L., and P. J. Mallinson. 'Behaviour of Badgers (*Meles Meles*) Infected with Bovine Tuberculosis'. *Journal of Zoology* 194(2) (1 June 1981): 284–89.

———. 'Radio Tracking in the Study of Bovine Tuberculosis in Badgers'. In *A Handbook on Biotelemetry and Radio Tracking*, 649–56. Oxford: Pergamon, 1980.

Cheeseman, C. L., J. W. Wilesmith and F. A. Stuart. 'Tuberculosis—The Disease and Its Epidemiology in the Badger, A Review'. *Epidemiology and Infection* 103(1) (August 1989): 113–25.

Cheeseman, C. L., J. W. Wilesmith, F. A. Stuart and P. J. Mallinson. 'Dynamics of Tuberculosis in a Naturally Infected Badger Population'. *Mammal Review* 18(1) (1988): 61–72.

Clark, Michael. *Badgers/Michael Clark; with Illustrations by the Author.* London: Whittet, 1988.

Clements, E. D., Ernest G. Neal and D. W. Yalden. 'The National Badger Sett Survey'. *Mammal Review* 18(1) (1 March 1988): 1–9.

Clifton-Hadley, R. S., J. W. Wilesmith, M. S. Richards, P. Upton and S. Johnston. 'The Occurrence of Mycobacterium Bovis Infection in Cattle in and around an Area Subject to Extensive Badger (Meles Meles) Control'. *Epidemiology and Infection* 114 (1995): 179–93.

Clifton-Hadley, R. S., J. W. Wilesmith and F. A. Stuart. 'Mycobacterium-Bovis in the European Badger (Meles Meles)—Epidemiologic Findings in Tuberculous Badgers from a Naturally Infected Population'. *Epidemiology and Infection* 111(1) (August 1993): 9–19.

Conlan, Andrew James Kerr, Martin Vordermeier, Mart C. M. de Jong and James L. N. Wood. 'The Intractable Challenge of Evaluating Cattle Vaccination as a Control for Bovine Tuberculosis'. *ELife* 7 (5 June 2018): e27694. https://doi.org/10.7554/eLife.27694.

Cressey, Daniel. 'Scientists Track Badger–Cow Encounters to Understand Cattle TB'. *Nature News*, 5 August 2016.

Crowcroft, Peter. *Elton's Ecologists: A History of the Bureau of Animal Population*. Chicago: University of Chicago Press, 1991.

Cruelty to Animals Act: 1835: 5 & 6 William 4 c.59: (1835). http://statutes.org.uk/site/the-statutes/nineteenth-century/1835-5-6-william-4-c-59-cruelty-to-animals-act/.

Davidson, Jennifer A., Miranda G. Loutet, Catherine O'Connor, Cathriona Kearns, Robert M. M. Smith, Maeve K. Lalor, H. Lucy Thomas, Ibrahim Abubakar and Dominik Zenner. 'Epidemiology of *Mycobacterium Bovis* Disease in Humans in England, Wales, and Northern Ireland, 2002–2014'. *Emerging Infectious Diseases* 23(3) (March 2017): 377–86.

Defra. 'A Strategy for Achieving Officially Bovine Tuberculosis Free Status for England'. London: HMSO, 3 April 2014a. https://www.gov.uk/government/publications/a-strategy-for-achieving-officially-bovine-tuberculosis-free-status-for-england.

———. 'Badger Culling Pilots: Independent Expert Panel'. GOV.UK, 2013. https://www.gov.uk/government/groups/badger-culling-pilots-independent-expert-panel.

———. 'Bovine Tuberculosis (BTB) Strategy Review 2018: Terms of Reference'. GOV.UK, 15 March 2018a. https://www.gov.uk/government/publications/a-strategy-for-achieving-bovine-tuberculosis-free-status-for-england-2018-review/bovine-tuberculosis-btb-strategy-review-2018-terms-of-reference.

———. 'Bovine Tuberculosis: The Government's Approach to Tackling the Disease and Consultation on a Badger Control Policy'. London: Department of Environment and Rural Affairs, 2010. http://archive.defra.gov.uk/corporate/consult/tb-control-measures/100915-tb-control-measures-condoc.pdf.

———. 'Cage-Trapping and Dispatch of Badgers under Licence to Prevent the Spread of Bovine TB in Cattle'. 26 August 2014b. https://www.gov.uk/government/publications/cage-trapping-and-dispatch-of-badgers-under-licence-to-prevent-the-spread-of-bovine-tb-in-cattle.

———. 'Press Release: Landmark Agriculture Bill to Deliver a Green Brexit'. GOV.UK, 12 September 2018b. https://www.gov.uk/government/news/landmark-agriculture-bill-to-deliver-a-green-brexit.

———. 'Public Consultation on Controlling the Spread of Bovine Tuberculosis in Cattle in High Incidence Areas in England: Badger Culling Summary of Responses'. London: Defra, July 2006. http://webarchive.nationalarchives.gov.uk/20061027120000/http://www.defra.gov.uk/corporate/consult/badgers-tbcontrols/index.htm.

———. 'The Government's Policy on Bovine TB and Badger Control in England'. London: HMSO, 2011a.

———. 'Total Cost of The Randomised Badger Culling Trial—A Freedom of Information Request to Department for Environment, Food and Rural Affairs'. *WhatDoTheyKnow*, 5 September 2011b. https://www.whatdotheyknow.com/request/total_cost_of_the_randomised_bad.

Defra TB Advisory Group. 'TB Advisory Group Letter to Jeff Rooker'. 16 October 2007. https://web.archive.org/web/20080726222053/http://www.defra.gov.uk/animalh/tb/pdf/rooker-161007.pdf.

Delahay, R. J., J. Davison, D. W. Poole, A. J. Matthews, C. J. Wilson, M. J. Heydon and T. J. Roper. 'Managing Conflict between Humans and Wildlife: Trends in Licensed Operations to Resolve Problems with Badgers Meles Meles in England'. *Mammal Review* 39, no. 1 (January 2009): 53–66.

Donnelly, Christl A., Ian Boyd, Philip Campbell, Claire Craig, Patrick Vallance, Mark Walport, Christopher J. M. Whitty, Emma Woods and Chris Wormald. 'Four Principles to Make Evidence Synthesis More Useful for Policy'. *Nature* 558(7710) (June 2018): 361.

Donnelly, Christl A., Rosie Woodroffe, D. R. Cox, John Bourne, George Gettinby, Andrea M. Le Fevre, John P. McInerney and W. Ivan Morrison. 'Impact of Localized Badger Culling on Tuberculosis Incidence in British Cattle'. *Nature* 426(6968) (December 2003): 834–37.

Downs, Sara H., Jessica E. Parry, Paul A. Upton, Jennifer M. Broughan, Anthony V. Goodchild, Javier Nuñez-Garcia, Matthias Greiner et al. 'Methodology and Preliminary Results of a Systematic Literature Review of Ante-Mortem and Post-Mortem Diagnostic Tests for Bovine Tuberculosis'. *Preventive Veterinary Medicine* 153 (1 May 2018): 117–26.

Drabble, Phil. *No Badgers in My Wood; Illustrations by Eileen A. Soper.* London: Joseph, 1979.

Dunnet, George M., David M. Jones and John P. McInerney. 'Badgers and Bovine Tuberculosis: Review of Policy'. London: HMSO, 1986.

Dyer, Dominic. *Badgered to Death: The People and Politics of the Badger Cull.* Kingston Upon Thames: Canbury Press, 2016.

Edginton, J., and R. Lynch. 'THE TOXICITY OF HYDROGEN CYANIDE BY INHALATION TO FERRETS AND BADGERS'. Salisbury: Chemical Defense Establishment, Porton Down, 1982. https://www.gov.uk/government/publications/investigations-into-gassing-badgers-as-a-culling-option.

Eustace, George. 'Bovine TB: Written Statement—HCWS720'. House of Commons, 24 May 2018. https://www.parliament.uk/business/publications/written-questions-answers-statements/written-statement/Commons/2018-05-24/HCWS720/.

Farm Crisis Network. 'Stress and Loss: A Report on the Impact of Bovine TB on Farming Families'. 2009. http://www.tbfreeengland.co.uk/assets/4200.

Fenner, Frank. *Nature, Nurture and Chance: The Lives of Frank and Charles Fenner*. Canberra: ANU E Press, 2006.

Fitter, Richard, and Jacqui Morris. 'The Fauna and Flora Preservation Society—Conserving Wildlife for 90 Years'. *Journal of Biological Education* 27(2) (1 June 1993): 103–6.

Fitzgerald, S. D., and J. B. Kaneene. 'Wildlife Reservoirs of Bovine Tuberculosis Worldwide: Hosts, Pathology, Surveillance, and Control'. *Veterinary Pathology* 50(3) (May 2013): 488–99.

Flowerdew, John R. 'Advances in the Conservation of British Mammals, 1954–2004: 50 Years of Progress with the Mammal Society'. *Mammal Review* 34(3) (July 2004): 169–210.

Food and Environment Research Agency. Central Science Laboratory: Our History (graphic). 16 September 2009, hosted by Wikipedia at: https://en.wikipedia.org/w/index.php?title=File:CSL_timeline.PNG&oldid=468477845.

Freeman, J. A. 'Research in Progress at the Pest Infestation Control Laboratory'. *EPPO Bulletin* 4(3) (1 September 1974): 291–94.

Gallagher, J., I. Macadam, J. Sayer and L. P. Van Lavieren. 'Pulmonary Tuberculosis in Free-Living Lechwe Antelope in Zambia'. *Tropical Animal Health and Production* 4(4) (December 1972): 204–13.

Gallagher, J., R. H. Muirhead and K. J. Burn. 'Tuberculosis in Wild Badger (*Meles Meles*) in Gloucestershire—Pathology'. *Veterinary Record* 98(1) (1976): 9–14.

Gallagher, J., and J. Nelson. 'Cause of Ill Health and Natural Death in Badgers in Gloucestershire'. *The Veterinary Record* 105(24) (15 December 1979): 546–51.

Giesler, Rebecca, and Elena Ares. 'Badger Culling in England'. *House of Commons Library Briefing Paper*, House of Commons Library Briefing Paper, 6837 (12 April 2018). https://researchbriefings.parliament.uk/ResearchBriefing/Summary/SN06837#fullreport.

Godfray, H. Charles J., Robert N. Curnow, Christopher Dye, Dirk U. Pfeiffer, William J. Sutherland and Mark E. J. Woolhouse. 'Independent Scientific Review of the Randomised Badger Culling Trial and Associated Epidemiological Research'. CSL, 4 March 2004. https://web.archive.org/web/20041205044107/http://www.defra.gov.uk:80/science/publications/2004/GodfreyReport_BovineTBEpidemiology.pdf.

Godfray, H. Charles J., Christl A. Donnelly, R. Glyn Hewinson, Michael Winter and James L. N. Wood. 'Bovine TB Strategy Review: Report to Rt Hon Michael Gove MP, Secretary of State, Defra'. London: Defra, 2018. https://assets.publishing.service.gov.uk/government/uploads/system/uploads/attachment_data/file/756942/tb-review-final-report-corrected.pdf.

Godfray, H. Charles J., Christl A. Donnelly, Rowland R. Kao, David W. Macdonald, Robbie A. McDonald, Gillian Petrokofsky, James L. N. Wood et al. 'A Restatement of the Natural Science Evidence Base Relevant to the Control of Bovine Tuberculosis in Great Britain'. *Proceedings of the Royal Society B: Biological Sciences* 280(1768) (2013): 1–18.

Gormley, Eamonn, Deirdre N. Bhuachalla, James O'Keeffe, Denise Murphy, Frank E. Aldwell, Tara Fitzsimons, Paul Stanley et al. 'Oral Vaccination of Free-Living Badgers (*Meles Meles*) with Bacille Calmette Guerin (BCG) Vaccine Confers Protection against Tuberculosis'. *PLoS ONE* 12(1) (January 2017): e0168851–e0168851. http://dx.plos.org/10.1371/journal.pone.0168851.

Gortázar, C., J. F. Ruiz-Fons and U. Höfle. 'Infections Shared with Wildlife: An Updated Perspective'. *European Journal of Wildlife Research* 62(5) (1 October 2016): 511–25.

Gortázar, Christian, Iratxe Diez-Delgado, Jose Angel Barasona, Joaquin Vicente, Jose De La Fuente and Mariana Boadella. 'The Wild Side of Disease Control at the Wildlife–Livestock–Human Interface: A Review'. *Frontiers in Veterinary Science* 1(January) (2015): 1–12.

Gosling, L. M., and S. J. Baker. 'The Eradication of Muskrat and Coypus from Britain'. *Biological Journal of the Linnean Society* 38 (1989): 39–51.

Grace, Delia. 'Zoonoses of Poverty: Measuring and Managing the Multiple Burdens of Zoonoses and Poverty'. In *Zoonoses—Infections Affecting Humans and Animals: Focus on Public Health Aspects*, 1127–37. Dordrecht: Springer Netherlands, 2015.

Griffiths, H. I., David H. Thomas and Council of Europe. 'The Conservation and Management of the European Badger (*Meles Meles*)'. Strasbourg: Council of Europe Publishing, 1997.

Harris, Stephen. 'Badgers and TB'. *Nature* 288 (11 December 1980): 532.

Judge, Johanna, Robbie A. McDonald, Neil Walker and Richard J. Delahay. 'Effectiveness of Biosecurity Measures in Preventing Badger Visits to Farm Buildings'. *PLoS ONE* 6(12) (December 2011): e28941–e28941. http://dx.plos.org/10.1371/journal.pone.0028941.

Judge, Johanna, Gavin J. Wilson, Roy Macarthur, Robbie A. McDonald and Richard J. Delahay. 'Abundance of Badgers (*Meles Meles*) in England and Wales'. *Scientific Reports* 7(1) (2017): 276.

Kidner, Pauline. *Tribute to Eunice Overend by Pauline Kidner, Secret World Wildlife Rescue—Badger Trust Conference*. 2016. https://www.youtube.com/watch?v=X3LBxYjcbdw.

King, David, Timothy J. Roper, Douglas B. Young, Mark E. J. Woolhouse and Dan Collins. 'Bovine Tuberculosis in Cattle and Badgers'. London: Defra, 30 July 2007. https://web.archive.org/web/20080726221416/http://www.defra.gov.uk/animalh/tb/pdf/badgersreport-king.pdf.

King, Elaine. 'Elaine King | LinkedIn'. 2018. https://www.linkedin.com/in/elainejking/?trk=public-profile-join-page.

King, R. J. 'The Badger Gate'. *Quarterly Journal of Forestry* 58(4) (1964): 311–19.

Krebs, J. R., R. M. Anderson, T. Clutton-Brock, I. Morrison, D. Young and C. A. Donnelly. 'Bovine Tuberculosis in Cattle and Badgers: Report by the Independent Scientific Review Group'. London: Ministry of Agriculture, Fisheries and Food, 1997.

Kruuk, Hans. *The Spotted Hyena: A Study of Predation and Social Behavior*. Chicago: Chicago: University of Chicago Press, 1972.

Lancashire Badger Group. 'Badger Trust's New CEO Is Leading Anti-Cull Spokesman'. *Lancashire Badger Group* (blog), 24 February 2014. http://

www.lancashirebadgergroup.org.uk/2014/02/24/badger-trusts-new-ceo-leading-anti-cull-spokesman/.

Lancum, F. Howard. *Wild Birds and the Land.* MAFF Bulletin 140. London: Ministry of Agriculture, Fisheries & Food: HMSO, 1948.

———. *Wild Mammals and the Land.* MAFF Bulletin 150. London: Ministry of Agriculture, Fisheries & Food: HMSO, 1951.

Lane, Julie M., and Robbie A. McDonald. 'Welfare and "Best Practice" in Field Studies of Wildlife'. In *The UFAW Handbook on the Care and Management of Laboratory and Other Research Animals*, ed. Robert Hubrecht and James Kirkwood, 92–106. Chichester, UK: Wiley-Blackwell, 2010.

Little, T. W., K. J. Burn and P. Stuart. 'Virulence for Calves of Tubercle Bacilli Isolated from Badgers'. *Veterinary Record* 96(24) (1975): 533.

Little, T. W., P. F. Naylor and J. W. Wilesmith. 'Laboratory Study of *Mycobacterium Bovis* Infection in Badgers and Calves'. *The Veterinary Record* 111(24) (1982): 550–57.

Loya, Y. 'Recolonisation of Red Sea Corals Affected by Natural Catastrophes and Man-Made Perturbations'. *Ecology* 57(2) (1976): 278–89.

MacDonald, David W. *Rabies and Wildlife: A Biologist's Perspective.* Oxford: Oxford University Press, 1980.

———. 'Radio-Tracking: Some Applications and Limitations'. In *Animal Marking*, 192–204. London: Palgrave, 1978.

Macrae, W. D. 'The Eradication of Bovine Tuberculosis in Great Britain'. *J Roy Agric Soc Engl* 122 (1961): 64–71.

MAFF. 'Bovine Tuberculosis in Badgers. Eighth Report by the Ministry of Agriculture, Fisheries and Food'. London: Ministry of Agriculture, Fisheries & Food: HMSO, August 1984.

———. 'Bovine Tuberculosis in Badgers. Eleventh Report by the Ministry of Agriculture, Fisheries and Food'. London: Ministry of Agriculture, Fisheries & Food: HMSO, August 1987.

———. 'Bovine Tuberculosis in Badgers. Fifteenth Report by the Ministry of Agriculture, Fisheries and Food'. London: Ministry of Agriculture, Fisheries & Food: HMSO, 1991.

———. 'Bovine Tuberculosis in Badgers. Fourteenth Report by the Ministry of Agriculture, Fisheries and Food'. London: Ministry of Agriculture, Fisheries & Food: HMSO, July 1990.

———. 'Bovine Tuberculosis in Badgers. Report by the Ministry of Agriculture, Fisheries and Food'. London: Ministry of Agriculture, Fisheries & Food: HMSO, November 1976.

———. 'Bovine Tuberculosis in Badgers. Second Report by the Ministry of Agriculture, Fisheries and Food'. London: Ministry of Agriculture, Fisheries & Food: HMSO, December 1977.

———. 'Bovine Tuberculosis in Badgers. Seventeenth Report by the Ministry of Agriculture, Fisheries and Food'. London: Ministry of Agriculture, Fisheries & Food: HMSO, 1994.

———. 'Bovine Tuberculosis in Badgers. Seventh Report by the Ministry of Agriculture, Fisheries and Food'. London: Ministry of Agriculture, Fisheries & Food: HMSO, August 1983.

———. 'Bovine Tuberculosis in Badgers. Sixth Report by the Ministry of Agriculture, Fisheries and Food'. London: Ministry of Agriculture, Fisheries & Food: HMSO, August 1982.

———. 'Bovine Tuberculosis in Badgers. Third Report by the Ministry of Agriculture, Fisheries and Food'. London: Ministry of Agriculture, Fisheries & Food: HMSO, July 1979.

———. 'Pest Infestation Control-Combining the Report of the Infestation Control Laboratory 1968–70 and Pest Infestation Research 1970'. London: Ministry of Agriculture, Fisheries & Food: HMSO, 1973.

Malins, Wickham. *Bully & the Badger: The Remarkable Story of a Badger Cub Fostered by a Bull Terrier and Eventually Returned to the Wild. With Drawings by Eileen A. Soper; Foreword by Ernest G. Neal.* London: Robert Yeatman, 1974.

Mary Gillham Archive Project. '"A Dedicated Naturalist": The Mary Gillham Archive Project'. Peoples Collection Wales, 19 June 2017. https://www.peoplescollection.wales/users/17069.

McCallan, L., C. Brooks, C. Couzens, F. Young, J. McNair and A. W. Byrne. 'Assessment of Serological Tests for Diagnosis of Bovine Tuberculosis'. *Veterinary Record* 181(4) (22 July 2017): 90–90.

McDonald, Robbie A. 'Animal Health: How to Control Bovine Tuberculosis'. *Nature* 511(7508) (July 2014): 158–59.

McGinness, Stephen. 'Bovine Tuberculosis'. *House of Commons Library Research Paper* 63 (1998): 29. https://researchbriefings.parliament.uk/ResearchBriefing/Summary/RP98-63.

Melchett, Peter Robert Henry Mond, and Louise Brodie. *Peter Melchett Interviewed by Louise Brodie.* British Library Oral Histories. London: British Library, 2010.

Meyer, Richard. *The Fate of The Badger Second Edition. New 30th Anniversary Edition 1986–2016.* 2nd edition. Cornwall: Fire-raven Writing, 2016.

More, Simon J. 'What Is Needed to Eradicate Bovine Tuberculosis Successfully: An Ireland Perspective'. *Vet J* 180(3) (June 2009): 275–78.

More, Simon J., Erik Houtsma, Liam Doyle, Guy McGrath, Tracy A. Clegg, Ricardo de la Rua-Domenech, Anthony Duignan et al. 'Further Description of Bovine Tuberculosis Trends in the United Kingdom and the Republic of Ireland, 2003–2015'. *Veterinary Record* 183(23) (15 December 2018): 717.

Muirhead, R. H. 'Bovine Tuberculosis in Wild Badgers in South Gloucestershire'. *State Veterinary Journal* 27(1) (1972): 197–205.

Muirhead, R. H., J. Gallagher and K. J. Burn. 'Tuberculosis in Wild Badgers in Gloucestershire: Epidemiology'. *Vet Rec.* 95(24) (1974): 552–55.

Munro, Ranald, Tim Coulson, Neville Gregory, Timothy J. Roper, Peter Watson and Piran C. L. White. 'Pilot Badger Culls in Somerset and Gloucestershire Report by the Independent Expert Panel'. London: Defra, 5 March 2014. https://www.gov.uk/government/groups/badger-culling-pilots-independent-expert-panel.

Murray, Ruth R. 'Live Trapping of Badgers, Their Removal, Release and Rehabilitation in a New Area'. *Mammal Review* 1(3) (1 September 1970): 86–92.

Nature, and S. L. Zuckerman. 'The Great Badger Debate'. *Nature* 289(5799) (19 February 1981): 628–30.

Neal, Ernest G. *The Badger*. New Naturalists Monographs 1. London: Collins, 1948.

———. *The Badger Man*. Ely: Providence Press, 1994.

———. 'The National Badger Survey'. *Mammal Review* 2(2) (1972): 55–64.

Neal, Ernest G., and Chris Cheeseman. *Badgers*. London: A&D Poyser, 1996.

Newell, D. G., and R. Glyn Hewinson. 'Control of Bovine Tuberculosis by Vaccination'. *Veterinary Record* 136(18) (6 May 1995): 459–63.

O'Connor, Catherine M., Daniel T. Haydon, Rowland R. Kao and Catherine M. O'Connor. 'An Ecological and Comparative Perspective on the Control of Bovine Tuberculosis in Great Britain and the Republic of Ireland'. *Preventive Veterinary Medicine* 104(3–4) (May 2012): 185–97.

Olea-Popelka, Francisco, Adrian Muwonge, Alejandro Perera, Anna S. Dean, Elizabeth Mumford, Elisabeth Erlacher-Vindel, Simona Forcella et al. 'Zoonotic Tuberculosis in Human Beings Caused by *Mycobacterium Bovis*—A Call for Action'. *The Lancet. Infectious Diseases*, September 2016.

OPM Group. 'Defra Bovine TB Citizen Dialogue. Cross-Cutting Summary'. London: Defra, April 2015. https://assets.publishing.service.gov.uk/government/uploads/system/uploads/attachment_data/file/300420/pb14154-bovine-tb-citizen-dialogue-summary.pdf.

Overend, Eunice D. TB in British Badgers. *Oryx* 13(3) (1976): 240–2.

Overend, Eunice D. 'Badgers and TB—Does Gassing Spread the Disease?' *Oryx* 15(4) (August 1980): 338–40.

———. *Oral History Recording of an Interview with Eunice Overend*. Oral history recording. Home in Frome. Taunton, 2012. ADQP/1/2/45. Somerset Heritage Centre. http://somerset-cat.swheritage.org.uk/records/A/DQP/1/2/45.

Overy, Caroline, and E. M. Tansey. *A History of Bovine TB c.1965–c. 2000*. Vol. 55. Wellcome Witnesses to Twentieth Century Medicine. London: Queen Mary University of London, 2015. https://archive.org/details/W55LoRes.

Paice, Jim. 'New Measures to Control Bovine TB in Badgers'. GOV.UK, 15 September 2010. https://www.gov.uk/government/news/new-measures-to-control-bovine-tb-in-badgers.

PBD Biotech. 'APHA Grants Access to New Actiphage Technology for Chronic TB Breakdowns | PBD Biotech'. 21 May 2018. http://www.pbdbio.com/news/apha-protocol-grants-access-to-new-actiphage-technology-for-chronic-tb-breakdowns/.

Pearce, J. W. R., L. P. Pugh and Sir John Ritchie. *Animal Health: A Centenary, 1865–1965: A Century of Endeavour to Control Diseases of Animals*. London: Ministry of Agriculture, Fisheries & Food: HMSO, 1965.

Pease, Alfred E. *The Badger—A Monograph*. London: Lawrence and Bullen Ltd, 1898.

Pest Infestation Control Laboratory. 'Pest Infestation Control Laboratory Report, 1971–73'. London: HMSO, 1975a.

———. 'Pest Infestation Control Laboratory Report, 1974–76'. London: HMSO, 1978.

———. 'Pest Infestation Control Laboratory Report, 1977–79'. London: HMSO, 1981.

———. 'Pest Infestation Control Leaflet'. London: HMSO, c. 1975.

Phillips, N. A., J. Bridgeman and M. Ferguson-Smith. 'The Inquiry into BSE and Variant CJD in the United Kingdom'. London: HMSO, 2000. http://webarchive.nationalarchives.gov.uk/20060525120000/http://www.bseinquiry.gov.uk/index.htm.

Pitt, Frances. *Diana, My Badger: Being the Story of Diana the Badger, her sister Jemima, and Squire Brock Whom Diana Met in the Woods*. [The Library of Animal Friends. vol. 10.]. London: Arrowsmith, 1929.

———. 'The Badger—A Creature of the Night'. In *Woodland Creatures: Being Some Wild Life Studies*, 11–35. London, G. Allen & Unwin Ltd, 1922. http://archive.org/details/woodlandcreature00pittrich.

Political Scrapbook. 'Best of the Badger: The 5 Funniest Responses to Paterson's Own Goal'. *Political Scrapbook*, 10 October 2013. https://politicalscrapbook.net/2013/10/5-funniest-responses-to-badger-goalposts-gaffe/.

Power, A. P., B. G. A. Watts and MAFF. *The Badger Control Policy: An Economic Assessment*. London: Ministry of Agriculture, Fisheries & Food: HMSO, 1987.

Prentice Jamie C., Naomi J. Fox, Michael R. Hutchings, C. L. White Piran, S. Davidson Ross and Marion Glenn. 'When to Kill a Cull: Factors Affecting the Success of Culling Wildlife for Disease Control'. *Journal of The Royal Society Interface* 16(152) (6 March 2019): 20180901.

Prospect. 'The State of Natural England 2018–19'. London: Prospect: The Trade Union for Professionals, 2018. https://www.prospect.org.uk/campaigns/natural-england.

Proud, Andrew J. 'Some Lessons from the History of the Eradication of Bovine Tuberculosis in Great Britain'. *Government Veterinary Journal* 16 (2006): 11–18.

Ransome, Roger. *Natural History of Hibernating Bats*. London: Christopher Helm Ltd/Mammal Society, 1990.

Ratcliffe, Edna Jane. *Through the Badger Gate. The Story of Badgers, Their Persecution and Protection, and of a Cub Reared and Returned to the Wild*. London: Bell, 1974.

Rees, H. W. 'Animal Health 1980: Report of the Chief Veterinary Officer'. London: Ministry of Agriculture, Fisheries and Food, 1980.

———. 'Animal Health 1984: Report of the Chief Veterinary Officer'. London: Ministry of Agriculture, Fisheries and Food, 1984.

———. 'Animal Health 1985: Report of the Chief Veterinary Officer'. London: Ministry of Agriculture, Fisheries and Food, 1985.

———. 'Animal Health 1986: Report of the Chief Veterinary Officer'. London: Ministry of Agriculture, Fisheries and Food, 1986.

———. 'Animal Health 1987: Report of the Chief Veterinary Officer'. London: Ministry of Agriculture, Fisheries and Food, 1987.

Richards, R. A., W. A. Watson, E. Boughton and K. Meldrum. 'Inquiry into Bovine TB in West Cornwall'. London: Ministry of Agriculture, Fisheries and Food, 1972.

Robertson, Andrew. 'TB Knowledge Exchange'. TB Knowledge Exchange, 2018. http://www.tbknowledgeexchange.co.uk.

Rodriguez-Campos, Sabrina, Noel H. Smith, Maria B. Boniotti and Alicia Aranaz. 'Overview and Phylogeny of *Mycobacterium Tuberculosis* Complex Organisms: Implications for Diagnostics and Legislation of Bovine Tuberculosis'. *Research in Veterinary Science* 97(S) (2014): S5–19.

Roper, Timothy J. *Badger*. London: Collins, 2010.

Rozins, Carly, Matthew J. Silk, Darren P. Croft, Richard J. Delahay, Dave J. Hodgson, Robbie A. McDonald, Nicola Weber and Mike Boots. 'Social Structure Contains Epidemics and Regulates Individual Roles in Disease Transmission in a Group-Living Mammal'. *Ecology and Evolution* 8(23) (2018): 12044–55.

RSPCA Wild Animals Advisory Committee. 'Badgers and Bovine Tuberculosis: The Case for Further Investigation'. Horsham: Royal Society for the Prevention of Cruelty to Animals, 1979.

Sainsbury, R. M. Q., and J. Gallagher. 'TB Controls'. *Veterinary Record* 161(4) (28 July 2007): 143.

Sanchez-Hidalgo, Andrea, Andrés Obregón-Henao, William H. Wheat, Mary Jackson and Mercedes Gonzalez-Juarrero. 'Mycobacterium Bovis Hosted by Free-Living-Amoebae Permits Their Long-Term Persistence Survival Outside of Host Mammalian Cells and Remain Capable of Transmitting Disease to Mice'. *Environmental Microbiology* 19(10) (October 2017): 4010–21.

Sandoval Barron, Elsa, Ben Swift, Julian Chantrey, Robert Christley, Richard Gardner, Chris Jewell, Ian McGrath et al. 'A Study of Tuberculosis in Road Traffic-Killed Badgers on the Edge of the British Bovine TB Epidemic Area'. *Scientific Reports* 8(1) (6 December 2018): 17206.

Save Me Trust. 'Bovine TB Symposium 2017—Save Me Trust'. Dr Brian May's Save Me Trust: Giving Animals a Voice, 28 March 2017. http://www.save-me.org.uk/bovine-tb-symposium-2017.

Saved and Safe Ltd. 'BeatbTB'. 2014. http://www.beatbtb.com/.

Scott Henderson, J. 'Report of the Committee on Cruelty to Wild Animals. Cmd 8266, June 1951'. London: Home Office/Scottish Home Department, June 1951.

Select Committee on Agriculture. 'House of Commons—Agriculture—Fifth Report'. London: House of Commons, 27 April 1999. https://publications.parliament.uk/pa/cm199899/cmselect/cmagric/233/23305.htm#n80.

Silk, Matthew J., Darren P. Croft, Richard J. Delahay, David J. Hodgson, Mike Boots, Nicola Weber and Robbie A. McDonald. 'Using Social Network Measures in Wildlife Disease Ecology, Epidemiology, and Management'. *BioScience* 67(3) (1 March 2017): 245–57.

Soper, Eileen Alice. *When Badgers Wake/Written and Illustrated by Eileen A. Soper.* London: Routledge & Kegan Paul, 1955.

Soper, Eileen Alice. *Eileen Soper's Book of Badgers.* London: Constable and Robinson, 1992.

Stuart, F. A., and J. W. Wilesmith. 'Tuberculosis in Badgers: A Review'. *Rev. Sci. Tech. Off. Int. Epiz.* 7(4) (1988): 929–35.

Swan, George J. F., Steve M. Redpath, Stuart Bearhop and Robbie A. McDonald. 'Ecology of Problem Individuals and the Efficacy of Selective Wildlife Management'. *Trends in Ecology & Evolution* 32(7) (July 2017): 518–30.

Swift, Benjamin M. C., Thomas W. Convery and Catherine E. D. Rees. 'Evidence of *Mycobacterium Tuberculosis* Complex Bacteraemia in Intradermal Skin Test Positive Cattle Detected Using Phage-RPA'. *Virulence* 7(7) (2 October 2016): 779–88.

Swinton, J., F. Tuyttens, D. MacDonald, D. J. Nokes, C. L. Cheeseman and R. Clifton-Hadley. 'A Comparison of Fertility Control and Lethal Control of Bovine Tuberculosis in Badgers: The Impact of Perturbation Induced Transmission'. *Philosophical Transactions of the Royal Society of London. Series B, Biological Sciences* 352(1353) (May 1997): 619–31.

Symes, R. G. 'Badger Damage: Fact or Fiction?' In *Mammals as Pests*, ed. Rory Putman, 196–206. London: Chapman and Hall, 1989.

Thoen, Charles O., James H. Steele and John B. Kaneene. *Zoonotic Tuberculosis: Mycobacterium Bovis and Other Pathogenic Mycobacteria.* Malden, MA: John Wiley & Sons, 2014.

Thompson, H. V. 'Animal Welfare and the Control of Vertebrates'. In *Proceedings of the Fourteenth Vertebrate Pest Conference*, 5–8. Sacramento, California, 1990. http://digitalcommons.unl.edu/vpc14.

———. 'The Rabbit Disease—Myxomatosis'. *Annals of Applied Biology* 41, no. 2 (1954): 358–66.

Thompson, H. V., and Carolyn M. King, eds. *The European Rabbit: History and Biology of a Successful Colonizer*. Oxford: Oxford University Press, 1994.

Thompson, H. V., and A. N. Worden. *The Rabbit*. New Naturalists Monographs 13. London: Collins, 1956.

Tinbergen, N., G. J. Broekhuysen, F. Feekes, J. C. W. Houghton, Hans Kruuk and E. Szulc. 'Egg Shell Removal by the Black-Headed Gull, *Larus Ridibundus*.: A Behaviour Component of Camouflage'. *Behaviour* 19(1/2) (1962): 74–117.

Topsell, Edward, Conrad Gessner, Thomas Moffett and John Rowland. *The History of Four-Footed Beasts and Serpents*. London: Printed by E. Cotes, for G. Sawbridge [etc.], 1658. http://archive.org/details/historyoffourfoo 00tops.

Tuyttens, F. A. M., D. W. Macdonald and B. Long. 'Spatial Perturbation Caused by a Badger (Meles Meles) Culling Operation: Implications for the Function of Territoriality and the Control of Bovine Tuberculosis (Mycobacterium Bovis)'. *Journal of Animal Ecology* 69 (2000): 815–28.

Universities Federation for Animal Welfare. 'UFAW Annual Report, 1973–1974'. South Mimms: Universities Federation for Animal Welfare, 1974.

———. 'UFAW Annual Report, 1974–1975'. South Mimms: Universities Federation for Animal Welfare, 1975.

———. 'Obituaries: Harry V. Thompson'. *Universities Federation for Animal Welfare News-Sheet*, 2004. https://www.ufaw.org.uk/downloads/news-sheets/ufaw-spring-news-2004.pdf.

Veterinary Record. 'Combining Plant and Animal Health'. *Veterinary Record* 175(8) (August 2014): 182.

WHO. 'WHO | Roadmap for Zoonotic Tuberculosis'. 2017. http://www.who.int/tb/publications/2017/zoonotic_TB/en/.

WHO, and FAO. 'JOINT WHO/FAO Expert Group on Zoonoses; Report on the First Session'. *World Health Organization Technical Report Series* 40 (May 1951): 1–47.

Who's Who. 'Krebs, Baron, (John Richard Krebs) (Born 11 April 1945)'. In *WHO'S WHO & WHO WAS WHO*. Oxford: Oxford University Press, 2018. http://www.ukwhoswho.com/view/10.1093/ww/9780199540884.001.0001/ww-9780199540884-e-23438.

Wilesmith, J. W., G. A. Wells, M. P. Cranwell and J. B. Ryan. 'Bovine Spongiform Encephalopathy: Epidemiological Studies'. *The Veterinary Record* 123(25) (December 1988): 638–44.

Worden, A. N., ed. *The UFAW Handbook on the Care and Management of Laboratory Animals: With an Appendix on Statistical Analysis.* Baltimore: Williams and Wilkins, 1947.

Yalden, D. W., and R. F. Shore. 'Yellow-Necked Mice *Apodemus Flavicollis* at Woodchester Park, 1968–1989'. *Journal of Zoology* 224(2) (1 June 1991): 329–32.

ZSL. 'Eradicating TB from Cattle and Badgers—A Review of Evidence'. London: Zoological Society of London, September 2018. https://www.zsl.org/sites/default/files/media/2018-09/ZSL_Eradicating_TB_Report_final_24Sep18.pdf.

Zuckerman, S. L. 'Badgers, Cattle and Tuberculosis'. London: HMSO, 1980.

(All URLs last accessed 6 March 2019)

Secondary Literature

Agar, Jon. *The Government Machine: A Revolutionary History of the Computer.* Cambridge, MA: MIT Press, 2003.

———. 'Transition: Sea Change in the Long 1960s'. In *Science in the 20th Century and Beyond*, 403–32. Cambridge: Polity, 2012.

———. 'What Happened in the Sixties?' *The British Journal for the History of Science* 41(4) (2008): 567–600.

———. 'Future Forecast—Changeable and Probably Getting Worse': The UK Government's Early Response to Anthropogenic Climate Change. *Twentieth Century British History* 26(4) (2015): 602–28.

Alcayna-Stevens, Lys. 'Habituating Field Scientists'. *Social Studies of Science* 46(6) (2016): 833–53.

Allen, Daniel, Charles Watkins and David Matless. '"An Incredibly Vile Sport": Campaigns against Otter Hunting in Britain, 1900–39'. *Rural History* 27(1) (April 2016): 79–101.

Anderson, A. *Media, Environment and the Network Society.* Cham, Switzerland: Springer, 2014.

Anderson, Warwick. 'Natural Histories of Infectious Disease: Ecological Vision in Twentieth-Century Biomedical Science'. *Osiris* 19 (2004): 39–61.

———. 'Nowhere to Run, Rabbit: The Cold-War Calculus of Disease Ecology'. *History and Philosophy of the Life Sciences* 39(2) (2017): 13.

Arluke, Arnold B., Lynda Birke and Mike Michael. *The Sacrifice: How Scientific Experiments Transform Animals and People.* West Lafayette, IN: Perdue University Press, 2007.

Asdal, Kristin. '"Interested Methods" and "Versions of Pragmatism"'. *Science, Technology, & Human Values* 43(4) (7 May 2018): 748–55.

Ashall, Vanessa, Kate M. Millar and Pru Hobson-West. 'Informed Consent in Veterinary Medicine: Ethical Implications for the Profession and the Animal "Patient"'. *Food Ethics* 1(3) (1 March 2018): 247–58.

Atkins, Peter J. *A History of Uncertainty: Bovine Tuberculosis in Britain, 1850 to the Present*. Winchester: Winchester University Press, 2016.

———. *Liquid Materialities: A History of Milk, Science and the Law*. Farnham: Ashgate Publishing, Ltd, 2010a.

———. 'Lobbying and Resistance with Regard to Policy on Bovine Tuberculosis in Britain, 1900—1939: An Inside/Outside Model'. In *Tuberculosis Then and Now: Perspectives on the History of an Infectious Disease*, 197–220. Montreal: McGill-Queen's University Press, 2010b.

Atkins, Peter J., and Philip A. Robinson. 'Bovine Tuberculosis and Badgers in Britain: Relevance of the Past'. *Epidemiology and Infection* 141(7) (January 2013): 1437–44.

Ayres, Sarah, Mark Sandford and Tessa Coombes. 'Policy-Making "Front" and "Back" Stage: Assessing the Implications for Effectiveness and Democracy'. *The British Journal of Politics and International Relations* 19(4) (1 November 2017): 861–76.

Baldwin, Claudia, Tanzi Smith and Chris Jacobson. 'Love of the Land: Social–Ecological Connectivity of Rural Landholders'. *Journal of Rural Studies* 51 (2017): 37–52.

Barkham, Patrick. *Badgerlands: The Twilight World of Britain's Most Enigmatic Animal*. London: Granta Books, 2014.

Barnes, Barry, David Bloor and John Henry. *Scientific Knowledge: A Sociological Analysis*. Chicago: University of Chicago Press, 1996.

Barnett, J., K. Burningham, G. Walker and N. Cass. 'Imagined Publics and Engagement around Renewable Energy Technologies in the UK'. *Public Understanding of Science* 21(1) (2012): 36–50.

Barry, Andrew. 'Political Situations: Knowledge Controversies in Transnational Governance'. *Critical Policy Studies* 6(3) (October 2012): 324–36.

Bartrip, Peter W. J. *Myxomatosis: A History of Pest Control and the Rabbit*. London: I.B.Tauris, 2008a.

———. 'Myxomatosis in 1950s Britain'. *Twentieth Century British History* 19(1) (2008b): 83–105.

Bashford, Alison. *Global Population: History, Geopolitics, and Life on Earth*. New York: Columbia University Press, 2014.

Baym, Nancy K., and danah boyd. 'Socially Mediated Publicness: An Introduction'. *Journal of Broadcasting & Electronic Media* 56(3) (1 July 2012): 320–29.

Bea, Sara. 'The Good, the Bad and the Difficult: Sharpening STS Tools to Navigate Conflicting Normativities in the Medical Practice of Deceased Organ Donation'. In *EASST2018: Meetings—Making Science, Technology and Society Together*. University of Lancaster, 2018. https://nomadit.co.uk/easst/easst2018/conferencesuite.php/panels/6224.

Beale, Graeme Robert. 'Tinbergian Practice, Themes and Variations : The Field and Laboratory Methods and Practice of the Animal Behaviour Research

Group under Nikolaas Tinbergen at Oxford University'. PhD, University of Edinburgh, 2008. https://www.era.lib.ed.ac.uk/handle/1842/4103.

Beierl, Barbara Hardy. 'The Sympathetic Imagination and the Human–Animal Bond: Fostering Empathy through Reading Imaginative Literature'. *Anthrozoös* 21(3) (1 September 2008): 213–20.

Beinart, William, and Karen Brown. *African Local Knowledge & Livestock Health: Diseases & Treatments in South Africa*. Woodbridge: Boydell & Brewer Ltd, 2013.

Bell, M., and John Sheail. 'Experts, Publics and the Environment in the UK: Twentieth-Century Translations'. *Journal of Historical Geography* 31(3) (2005): 496–512.

Bell, Michael M., Sarah E. Lloyd and Christine Vatovec. 'Activating the Countryside: Rural Power, the Power of the Rural and the Making of Rural Politics'. *Sociologia Ruralis* 50(3) (June 2010): 205–24.

Bennett, R. M. 'The Political Economy of Bovine Tuberculosis in Great Britain'. *Revue Scientifique et Technique de l'OIE* 36(1) (1 January 2017): 105–14.

Benson, Etienne. 'Animal Writes: Historiography, Disciplinarity, and the Animal Trace'. In *Making Animal Meaning*, ed. Linda Kalof and Georgina M. Montgomery, 3–16. East Lansing: Michigan State University Press, 2011.

———. *Wired Wilderness: Technologies of Tracking and the Making of Modern Wildlife*. Baltimore: Johns Hopkins University Press, 2010.

Berridge, Virginia. 'Thinking in Time: Does Health Policy Need History as Evidence?' *The Lancet* 375(9717) (2010): 798–99.

Berry, Dominic. 'The Resisted Rise of Randomisation in Experimental Design: British Agricultural Science, c.1910–1930'. *History and Philosophy of the Life Sciences* 37(3) (2015): 242–60.

Bickerstaff, K., and P. Simmons. 'The Right Tool for the Job? Modeling, Spatial Relationships, and Styles of Scientific Practice in the UK Foot and Mouth Crisis'. *Environment and Planning D: Society and Space* 22 (2004): 393–412.

Bickerstaff, K., P. Simmons and N. Pidgeon. 'Situating Local Experience of Risk: Peripherality, Marginality and Place Identity in the UK Foot and Mouth Disease Crisis'. *Geoforum* 37(5) (2006): 844–58.

Bishop, Patrick. 'Badgers and Bovine Tuberculosis: The Relationship between Law, Policy and Science Badger Trust v Welsh Ministers [2010] EWCA Civ 807'. *Journal of Environmental Law* 24(1) (1 March 2012): 145–54.

Black, Lawrence, Hugh Pemberton and Pat Thane, eds. *Reassessing 1970s Britain*. Manchester: Manchester University Press, 2013.

Bloor, David. *Knowledge and Social Imagery* (2nd edition). 1976. Reprint, Chicago: University of Chicago Press, 1991.

Blue, G. 'Food, Publics, Science'. *Public Understanding of Science* 19(2) (April 2009): 147–54.

Bocking, Stephen. *Ecologists and Environmental Politics: A History of Contemporary Ecology*. New Haven: Yale University Press, 1997.

———. 'Nature on the Home Front: British Ecologists' Advocacy for Science and Conservation'. *Environment and History* 18(2) (May 2012): 261–81.

Bonney, Rick, Jennifer L. Shirk, Tina B. Phillips, Andrea Wiggins, Heidi L. Ballard, Abraham J. Miller-Rushing and Julia K. Parrish. 'Next Steps for Citizen Science'. *Science* 343(6178) (2014): 1436–37.

Boonman-Berson, Susan, Clemens Driessen and Esther Turnhout. 'Managing Wild Minds: From Control by Numbers to a Multinatural Approach in Wild Boar Management in the Veluwe, the Netherlands'. *Transactions of the Institute of British Geographers* 44(2) (2019): 2–15.

Brassley, Paul. 'Murrains to Mad Cows: A Very Short History of Governments, People and Animal Diseases'. In *Contested Countryside: Rural Politics and Land Controversy in Modern Britain*, ed. Jeremy Burchardt and Philip Conford, 145–67. London: I.B.Tauris, 2008.

———. 'Wartime Productivity and Innovation, 1939–45'. In *The Front Line of Freedom: British Farming in the Second World War*. edited by Brian Short, Charles Watkins, and John Martin, 44–54, Exeter: British Agricultural History Society, 2006.

Bresalier, Michael. 'From Healthy Cows to Healthy Humans: Integrated Approaches to World Hunger, c.1930–1965'. In *Animals and the Shaping of Modern Medicine: One Health and Its Histories*, ed. Abigail Woods, Michael Bresalier, Angela Cassidy and Rachel Mason Dentinger, 119–60. Cham, Switzerland: Palgrave Macmillan, 2018.

———. 'Neutralizing Flu: "Immunological Devices" and the Making of a Virus Disease'. In *Crafting Immunity: Working Histories of Clinical Immunology*, ed. Kenton Kroker, Jennifer Keelan and Pauline Mazumdar, 107–45. Farnham: Ashgate, 2008.

Bresalier, Michael, Angela Cassidy and Abigail Woods. 'One Health in History'. In *One Health: The Theory and Practice of Integrated Health Approaches*, ed. Jakob Zinsstag, Esther Schelling, Maxine Whittaker, Marcel Tanner and David Waltner-Toews, 1–15. Wallingford, Oxfordshire: CABI, 2015. https://www.cabi.org/openresources/43410/.

Broto, V. C. 'Environmental Conflicts, Research Projects and the Generation of Collective Expectations: A Case Study of a Land Regeneration Project in Tuzla, Bosnia and Herzegovina'. *Public Understanding of Science* 21(4) (November 2010): 432–46.

Brown, Karen. 'Environmental and Veterinary History—Some Themes and Suggested Ways Forward'. *Environment and History* 20(4) (November 2014): 547–59.

Brown, Mark B. 'Politicizing Science: Conceptions of Politics in Science and Technology Studies'. *Social Studies of Science* 45(1) (December 2015): 3–30.

Brown, Nik, and Siân M. Beynon-Jones. '"Reflex Regulation": An Anatomy of Promissory Science Governance'. *Health, Risk & Society* 14(3) (2012): 223–40.

Brown, Nik, and Mike Michael. 'A Sociology of Expectations: Retrospecting Prospects and Prospecting Retrospects'. *Technology Analysis & Strategic Management* 15(1) (March 2003): 3–18.

Bucchi, Massimiano. *Science and the Media: Alternative Routes to Scientific Communications.* New York: Routledge, 1998.

Buller, Henry, and Emma Roe. *Food and Animal Welfare.* London: Bloomsbury, 2016.

Burchardt, Jeremy. *Paradise Lost: Rural Idyll and Social Change in England since 1800.* London: I.B.Tauris, 2002.

Burkhardt, Richard W. 'Ethology, Natural History, the Life Sciences, and the Problem of Place'. *Journal of the History of Biology* 32(3) (1999): 489–508.

———. *Patterns of Behavior: Konrad Lorenz, Niko Tinbergen, and the Founding of Ethology.* Chicago: University of Chicago Press, 2005.

Burnett, D. Graham. *The Sounding of the Whale: Science and Cetaceans in the Twentieth Century.* Chicago: University of Chicago Press, 2012.

Burt, Jonathan. 'Solly Zuckerman: The Making of a Primatological Career in Britain, 1925–1945'. *Studies in History and Philosophy of Biological and Biomedical Sciences* 37(2) (June 2006): 295–310.

Bynum, Helen. *Spitting Blood: The History of Tuberculosis.* Oxford: Oxford University Press, 2012.

Cairney, Paul. 'The UK Government's Imaginative Use of Evidence to Make Policy'. *British Politics*, 5 January 2018.

Carter, Neil. 'Greening the Mainstream: Party Politics and the Environment'. *Environmental Politics* 22(1) (1 February 2013): 73–94.

Carter, Neil, and Ben Clements. 'From "Greenest Government Ever" to "Get Rid of All the Green Crap": David Cameron, the Conservatives and the Environment'. *British Politics* 10(2) (1 June 2015): 204–25.

Cassidy, Angela. 'Badger–Human Conflict: An Overlooked Historical Context for Bovine TB Debates in the UK'. In *Understanding Conflicts about Wildlife: A Biosocial Approach*, ed. Catherine M. Hill, Amanda D. Webber and Nancy E. C. Priston. Oxford: Berghahn Books, 2017.

———. '"Big Science" in the Field: Experimenting with Badgers and Bovine TB, 1995–2015'. *History and Philosophy of the Life Sciences* 37(3) (2015): 305.

———. 'Communicating the Social Sciences: A Specific Challenge?' In *Handbook of Public Communication of Science and Technology*, 2nd edition, ed. Massimiano Bucchi and Brian Trench, 186–98. New York: Routledge, 2014.

———. 'Evolutionary Psychology as Public Science and Boundary Work'. *Public Understanding of Science* 15(2) (April 2006): 175–205.

———. 'One Health? Building an Interdisciplinary Bandwagon at the Interfaces of Animal Health, Human Health and the Environment'. In *Investigating*

Interdisciplinary Collaboration: Theory and Practice Across Disciplines, ed. Scott Frickel, Mathieu Albert and Barbara Prainsack. New Brunswick, NJ: Rutgers University Press, 2016. https://www.ncbi.nlm.nih.gov/books/NBK395883/.

———. 'The (Sexual) Politics of Evolution: Popular Controversy in the Late 20th-Century United Kingdom'. *History of Psychology* 10(2) (May 2007): 199–226.

———. 'The UK's Bovine TB Strategy: A Prospective View from History'. Submission to Defra, Bovine TB Strategy Review 2018: Call for Evidence. Exeter: University of Exeter, 2018.

———. 'Vermin, Victims and Disease: UK Framings of Badgers in and beyond the Bovine TB Controversy'. *Sociologia Ruralis* 52(2) (April 2012): 192–204.

Cassidy, Angela, Rachel Mason Dentinger, Kathryn Schoefert and Abigail Woods. 'Animal Roles and Traces in the History of Medicine, c.1880–1980'. *BJHS Themes* 2 (January 2017): 11–33. https://doi.org/10.1017/bjt.2017.3.

Cassidy, Angela, Simon J. Lock and Georgina Voss. 'Sexual Nature? (Re)Presenting Sexuality and Science in the Museum'. *Science as Culture* 25(2) (2016): 214–38.

Centellas, K. M., R. E. Smardon and S. Fifield. 'Calibrating Translational Cancer Research: Collaboration without Consensus in Interdisciplinary Laboratory Meetings'. *Science, Technology & Human Values* 39(3) (October 2013): 311–35.

Chew, Matthew K. 'A Picture Worth Forty-One Words: Charles Elton, Introduced Species and the 1936 Admiralty Map of British Empire Shipping'. *The Journal of Transport History* 35(2) (2014): 225–35.

Chew, Matthew K., and Andrew L. Hamilton. 'The Rise and Fall of Biotic Nativeness: A Historical Perspective'. *Fifty Years of Invasion Ecology: The Legacy of Charles Elton*, edited by David M. Richardson, 35–47. Chichester, Sussex: John Wiley & Sons, Ltd, 2010.

Chilvers, Jason, and Matthew Kearnes. *Remaking Participation: Science, Environment and Emergent Publics*. New York: Routledge, 2015.

Christianson, Scott. *Fatal Airs: The Deadly History and Apocalyptic Future of Lethal Gases That Threaten Our World*. Santa Barbara: ABC-CLIO, 2010.

Clark, J. F. M. 'Pesticides, Pollution and the UK's Silent Spring, 1963–64: Poison in the Garden of England'. *Notes and Records: The Royal Society Journal of the History of Science* 3 (15 February 2017): 297–327.

Coates, Peter, David Moon and Paul Warde, eds. *Local Places, Global Processes: Histories of Environmental Change in Britain and Beyond*. Oxford: Windgather Press, 2016.

Cole, Lucinda. 'Of Mice and Moisture: Rats, Witches, Miasma and Early Modern Theories of Contagion'. *Journal for Early Modern Cultural Studies* 10(2) (2014): 65–84.

Collins, H. M. 'In Praise of Futile Gestures: How Scientific Is the Sociology of Scientific Knowledge?' *Social Studies of Science* 26(2) (1996): 224–29.

Collins, H. M., and R. Evans. 'The Third Wave of Science Studies: Studies of Expertise and Experience'. *Social Studies of Science* 32(2) (2002): 235–96.

Convery, Ian, Cathy Bailey, Maggie Mort and Josephine Baxter. 'Death in the Wrong Place? Emotional Geographies of the UK 2001 Foot and Mouth Disease Epidemic'. *Journal of Rural Studies* 21(1) (January 2005): 99–109.

Cooper, Timothy, and Anna Green. 'The "Torrey Canyon" Disaster, Everyday Life, and the "Greening" of Britain'. *Environmental History* 22(1) (January 2017): 101–26.

Convery, Ian, Maggie Mort, Cathy Bailey and Josephine Baxter. *Animal Disease and Human Trauma*. Basingstoke: Palgrave Macmillan, 2008.

Cosslett, Tess. *Talking Animals in British Children's Fiction, 1786–1914*. Aldershot: Ashgate, 2006.

Cronin, J. Keri. *Art for Animals: Visual Culture and Animal Advocacy, 1870–1914*. Pennsylvania: Pennsylvania State University Press, 2018.

Crowcroft, Peter. *Elton's Ecologists: A History of the Bureau of Animal Population*. Chicago: University of Chicago Press, 1991.

Crowley, Sarah L., Steve Hinchliffe and Robbie A. McDonald. 'Conflict in Invasive Species Management'. *Frontiers in Ecology and the Environment* 15(3) (2017a): 133–41.

———. 'Nonhuman Citizens on Trial: The Ecological Politics of a Beaver Reintroduction'. *Environment and Planning A* 49(8) (1 August 2017b): 1846–66.

———. 'Killing Squirrels: Exploring Motivations and Practices of Lethal Wildlife Management'. *Environment and Planning E: Nature and Space* 1(1–2) (2018): 120–43.

Dale, Corinne. *The Natural World in the Exeter Book Riddles*. Woodbridge: Boydell & Brewer, 2017.

Dam, Mie S., and Mette N. Svendsen. 'Treating Pigs: Balancing Standardisation and Individual Treatments in Translational Neonatology Research'. *BioSocieties* 13(2) (2018): 349–67.

Davies, Gail. 'Networks of Nature: Stories of Natural History Film-Making at the BBC'. PhD, London: University of London, 1998. http://discovery.ucl.ac.uk/5188/.

———. 'Science, Observation and Entertainment: Competing Visions of Postwar British Natural History Television, 1946–1967'. *Cultural Geographies* 7(4) (2000): 432.

Davies, Gail, Beth Greenhough, Pru Hobson-West and Robert G. W. Kirk. 'Science, Culture, and Care in Laboratory Animal Research: Interdisciplinary Perspectives on the History and Future of the 3Rs'. *Science, Technology, & Human Values* 43(4) (2018): 603–21.

Davis, Aeron. 'New Media and Fat Democracy: The Paradox of Online Participation'. *New Media & Society* 12(5) (November 2009): 745–61.

Denzin, Norman K., and Yvonna S. Lincoln, eds. *The SAGE Handbook of Qualitative Research*. Fifth edition. Thousand Oaks, CA: SAGE Publications, 2017.

Djerf-Pierre, M. 'When Attention Drives Attention: Issue Dynamics in Environmental News Reporting over Five Decades'. *European Journal of Communication* 27(3) (September 2012): 291–304.

van Dooren, Thom. 'A Day with Crows—Rarity, Nativity and the Violent-Care of Conservation'. *Animal Studies Journal* 4(2) (2015): 1–28.

———. 'Care: Living Lexicon for the Environmental Humanities'. *Environmental Humanities* 5(2) (2014): 291–94.

Döring, Martin, and Brigitte Nerlich. *The Social and Cultural Impact of Foot and Mouth Disease in the UK in 2001: Experiences and Analyses.* Manchester: Manchester University Press, 2009.

Druglitrø, Tone. '"Skilled Care" and the Making of Good Science'. *Science, Technology, & Human Values* 43(4) (2018): 649–70.

Druglitrø, Tone, and Robert G. W. Kirk. 'Building Transnational Bodies: Norway and the International Development of Laboratory Animal Science, ca. 1956–1980'. *Science in Context* 27(2) (April 2014): 333–57.

Duffy, Michael P. 'The Rothschild Experience: Health Science Policy and Society in Britain'. *Science, Technology & Human Values* 11(1) (1986): 68–78.

Dunlop, Claire A. 'Contestation and Contingency in Advisory Governance'. In *Rethinking Governance*, ed. Mark Bevir and R. A. W. Rhodes, 15. New York: Routledge, 2016a.

———. 'Epistemic Communities'. In *Routledge Handbook of Public Policy*, ed. Eduardo Araral, Scott Fritzen, Michael Howlett, M. Ramesh and Xun Wu, 229–44. New York: Routledge, 2012.

———. 'Knowledge, Epistemic Communities and Agenda-Setting'. In *Handbook of Public Policy Agenda-Setting*, ed. N. Zahariadis, 273–96. Cheltenham: Edward Elgar, 2016b.

———. 'Pathologies of Policy Learning: What Are They and How Do They Contribute to Policy Failure?' *Policy & Politics* 45(1) (17 January 2017a): 19–37.

———. 'Policy Learning and Policy Failure: Definitions, Dimensions and Intersections'. *Policy & Politics* 45(1) (17 January 2017b): 3–18.

Edgerton, David. *Britain's War Machine: Weapons, Resources, and Experts in the Second World War.* Oxford: Oxford University Press, 2011.

———. *Warfare State: Britain, 1920–1970.* Cambridge: Cambridge University Press, 2005.

Edwards, Martin. *Control and the Therapeutic Trial: Rhetoric and Experimentation in Britain, 1918–48.* Leiden: Brill, 2007.

Ellis, Colter. 'Boundary Labor and the Production of Emotionless Commodities: The Case of Beef Production'. *Sociological Quarterly* 55(1) (January 2014): 92–118.

———. 'The Symbiotic Ideology: Stewardship, Husbandry, and Dominion in Beef Production'. *Rural Sociology* 78(4) (1 December 2013): 429–49.

Engelmann, Lukas, and Janina Kehr. 'Double Trouble: Towards an Epistemology of Co-Infection'. *Medicine Anthropology Theory* 2(1) (2015): 1–31.

Enticott, G. 'Market Instruments, Biosecurity and Place-Based Understandings of Animal Disease'. *Journal of Rural Studies* 45 (2016a): 312–19.

———. 'Navigating Veterinary Borderlands: "Heiferlumps", Epidemiological Boundaries and the Control of Animal Disease in New Zealand'. *Transactions of the Institute of British Geographers* 42(2) (November 2016b): 153–65.

———. 'Public Attitudes to Badger Culling to Control Bovine Tuberculosis in Rural Wales'. *European Journal of Wildlife Research* 61 (2015): 387.

———. 'Relational Distance, Neoliberalism and the Regulation of Animal Health'. *Geoforum* 52 (March 2014): 42–50.

———. 'Techniques of Neutralising Wildlife Crime in Rural England and Wales'. *Journal of Rural Studies* 27(2) (April 2011a): 200–8.

———. 'The Local Universality of Veterinary Expertise and the Geography of Animal Disease'. *Transactions of the Institute of British Geographers* 37(1) (June 2011b): 75–88.

Enticott, G., Andrew Donaldson, Philip Lowe, Megan Power, Amy Proctor and Katy Wilkinson. 'The Changing Role of Veterinary Expertise in the Food Chain'. *Philosophical Transactions of the Royal Society of London. Series B, Biological Sciences* 366(1573) (July 2011): 1955–65.

Enticott, G., Alex Franklin and Steven Van Winden. 'Biosecurity and Food Security: Spatial Strategies for Combating Bovine Tuberculosis in the UK'. *The Geographical Journal* 178(4) (December 2012): 327–37.

Enticott, G., D. Maye, P. Carmody, R. Naylor, K. Ward, S. Hinchliffe, W. Wint et al. 'Farming on the Edge: Farmer Attitudes to Bovine Tuberculosis in Newly Endemic Areas'. *Veterinary Record* 177(17) (2015): 439.

Enticott, G., and F. Vanclay. 'Scripts, Animal Health and Biosecurity: The Moral Accountability of Farmers' Talk about Animal Health Risks'. *Health, Risk & Society* 13(4) (June 2011): 293–309.

Epstein, S. 'The Construction of Lay Expertise: AIDS Activism and the Forging of Credibility in the Reform of Clinical Trials'. *Science, Technology & Human Values* 20(4) (October 1995): 408–37.

Evans, David. *A History of Nature Conservation in Britain*. London: Routledge, 1997.

Fish, Rob, Matt Lobley and Michael Winter. 'A License to Produce? Farmer Interpretations of the New Food Security Agenda'. *Journal of Rural Studies* 29 (March 2012): 40–49.

Fisher, Rhiannon. '"A Gentleman's Handshake": The Role of Social Capital and Trust in Transforming Information into Usable Knowledge'. *Journal of Rural Studies* 31 (July 2013): 13–22.

Fissell, M. 'Imagining Vermin in Early Modern England'. *History Workshop Journal* 47(47) (March 1999): 1–29.

Flack, Andrew J. P. 'Lions Loose on a Gentleman's Lawn: Animality, Authenticity and Automobility in the Emergence of the English Safari Park'. *Journal of Historical Geography* 54 (2016): 38–49.

Friedman, Raymond Alan. *Front Stage, Backstage: The Dramatic Structure of Labor Negotiations*. Cambridge, MA: MIT Press, 1994.

Gaarder, Emily. *Women and the Animal Rights Movement*. New Brunswick, NJ: Rutgers University Press, 2011.

Gardiner, Andrew. 'The Animal as Surgical Patient: A Historical Perspective in the 20th Century'. *History and Philosophy of the Life Sciences* 31(3–4) (2009): 355–76.

Garforth, Lisa. *Green Utopias: Environmental Hope Before and After Nature*. Cambridge: Polity Press, 2017.

Garner, Robert. *Animals, Politics and Morality*. Manchester: Manchester University Press, 2005.

Gay, Hannah. *The Silwood Circle: A History of Ecology and the Making of Scientific Careers in Late Twentieth-Century Britain*. London: Imperial College Press, 2013.

Gieryn, T. F. 'Boundaries of Science'. In *The Handbook of Science and Technology Studies*, ed. S Jasanoff, 393–456. Thousand Oaks, CA: SAGE, 1995.

Giraud, E., and G. Hollin. 'Care, Laboratory Beagles and Affective Utopia'. *Theory, Culture and Society* 33(4) (July 2016): 27–49.

Goedeke, T. L. L., and S. Rikoon. 'Otters as Actors: Scientific Controversy, Dynamism of Networks, and the Implications of Power in Ecological Restoration'. *Social Studies of Science* 38(1) (February 2008): 111–32.

Goffman, Erving. *The Presentation of Self in Everyday Life*. Garden City, NY: Doubleday, 1959.

Goldman, Mara J., Joana Roque de Pinho and Jennifer Perry. 'Beyond Ritual and Economics: Maasai Lion Hunting and Conservation Politics'. *Oryx* 47(4) (October 2013): 490–500.

Gorman, Richard. 'Therapeutic Landscapes and Non-Human Animals: The Roles and Contested Positions of Animals within Care Farming Assemblages'. *Social & Cultural Geography* 18(3) (May 2016): 315–35.

Gouyon, Jean-Baptiste. 'From Kearton to Attenborough: Fashioning the Telenaturalist's Identity'. *History of Science* 49.1(162) (2011a): 39–74.

———. *The BBC Natural History Unit: Instituting Natural History Film-Making in Britain. History of Science* 49(4) (2011): 425–51.

———. 'Science and Film-Making'. *Public Understanding of Science* 25(1) (1 January 2016): 17–30.

Gradmann, Christoph. *Laboratory Disease: Robert Koch's Medical Bacteriology*. Baltimore: Johns Hopkins University Press, 2009.

———. 'Robert Koch and the Invention of the Carrier State: Tropical Medicine, Veterinary Infections and Epidemiology around 1900'. *Studies in History and*

Philosophy of Biological and Biomedical Sciences 41(3) (September 2010): 232–40.

Grant, Wyn. 'Intractable Policy Failure: The Case of Bovine TB and Badgers'. *The British Journal of Politics & International Relations* 11(4) (2009): 557–73.

———. *Pressure Groups and British Politics*. Basingstoke: Macmillan Education UK, 2000.

Greenhough, Beth, and Emma Roe. 'Exploring the Role of Animal Technologists in Implementing the 3Rs: An Ethnographic Investigation of the UK University Sector'. *Science, Technology, & Human Values* 43(4) (2018): 694–722.

Griffin, Emma. *Blood Sport: Hunting in Britain since 1066*. New Haven: Yale University Press, 2007.

Griggs, Steven, and David Howarth. 'Protest Movements, Environmental Activism and Environmentalism in the United Kingdom'. In *The SAGE Handbook of Environment and Society*, 314–24. London: SAGE Publications Ltd, 2007.

Haas, Peter M. 'Introduction: Epistemic Communities and International Policy Coordination'. *International Organization* 46(1) (1992): 1–35.

Hamblin, Jacob Darwin. *Arming Mother Nature: The Birth of Catastrophic Environmentalism*. Oxford: Oxford University Press, 2013.

Hamilton, Lindsay. 'Bridging the Divide between Theory and Practice: Taking a Co-Productive Approach to Vet–Farmer Relationships'. *Food Ethics* 1(3) (1 March 2018): 221–33.

Hamilton, Lindsay, Nick Evans and James Allcock. '"I Don't Go to Meetings": Understanding Farmer Perspectives on Bovine TB and Biosecurity Training'. *Veterinary Record* Online First (7 January 2019).

Hancock, Helen. 'BBC Trust Impartiality Review: BBC Coverage of Rural Areas in the UK'. A BBC Trust report, June 2014. http://downloads.bbc.co.uk/bbctrust/assets/files/pdf/our_work/rural_impartiality/rural_impartiality.pdf.

Hansen, Anders. 'Communication, Media and the Social Construction of the Environment'. In *The Routledge Handbook of Environment and Communication*, ed. Anders Hansen and Robert Cox, 26–38. New York: Routledge, 2015.

Haraway, Donna J. *Primate Visions: Gender, Race, and Nature in the World of Modern Science*. London: Routledge, 1989.

———. 'The Promises of Monsters: A Regenerative Politics for Inappropriate/d Others'. In *Cultural Studies*, ed. Lawrence Grossberg, Cary Nelson and Paula A. Treichler, 295–337. London: Routledge, 1992.

———. *When Species Meet*. Minneapolis: University of Minnesota Press, 2007.

Harcup, Tony, and Deirdre O'Neill. 'What Is News? News Values Revisited (Again)'. *Journalism Studies* 18(12) (2 December 2017): 1470–88.

von Hardenberg, Wilko Graf, Matthew Kelly, Claudia Leal and Emily Wakild, eds. *The Nature State: Rethinking the History of Conservation*. Abingdon: Routledge, 2017.

Hardy, A. 'Professional Advantage and Public Health: British Veterinarians and State Veterinary Services, 1865–1939'. *Twentieth Century British History* 14(1) (2003): 1–23.

Hardy, Anne. 'John Bull's Beef: Meat Hygiene and Veterinary Public Health in England in the Twentieth Century'. *Review of Agricultural and Environmental Studies—Revue d'Etudes en Agriculture et Environnement* 91(4) (2010): 369–92.

Hardy, Peter. *A Lifetime of Badgers.* Newton Abbot: David and Charles, 1975.

Healy, S. 'Deadly Dingoes: "Wild" or Simply Requiring "Due Process"'. *Social Studies of Science* 37(3) (2007): 443–71.

Henderson, W. 'Continued Growth'. In *Agricultural Research 1931–1981: A History of the Agricultural Research Council and a Review of Developments in Agricultural Science during the Last Fifty Years.* London: Agricultural Research Council, 1981.

Henke, C R. 'Making a Place for Science: The Field Trial'. *Social Studies of Science* 30(4) (2000): 483–511.

Herzog, Hal. *Some We Love, Some We Hate, Some We Eat: Why It's So Hard to Think Straight about Animals.* New York: Harper Collins, 2010.

Hilgartner, Stephen. *Science on Stage: Expert Advice as Public Drama.* Stanford, CA: Stanford University Press, 2000.

Hilgartner, Stephen, and C. L. Bosk. 'The Rise and Fall of Social-Problems—A Public Arenas Model'. *American Journal of Sociology* 94(1) (1988): 53–78.

Hill, Catherine M. 'Perspectives of "Conflict" at the Wildlife–Agriculture Boundary: 10 Years On'. *Human Dimensions of Wildlife* 20(4) (2015): 1–6.

Hilton, Matthew, James McKay, Jean-Francois Mouhot and James Crowson. *The Politics of Expertise: How NGOs Shaped Modern Britain.* Oxford: Oxford University Press, 2013.

Hipperson, Julie. 'Professional Entrepreneurs: Women Veterinary Surgeons as Small Business Owners in Interwar Britain'. *Social History of Medicine* 31(1) (1 February 2018): 122–39.

Holloway, Lewis, and Christopher Bear. 'Bovine and Human Becomings in Histories of Dairy Technologies: Robotic Milking Systems and Remaking Animal and Human Subjectivity'. *BJHS Themes* 2 (January 2017): 215–34. https://doi.org/10.1017/bjt.2017.2.

Honigsbaum, Mark. '"Tipping the Balance": Karl Friedrich Meyer, Latent Infections, and the Birth of Modern Ideas of Disease Ecology'. *Journal of the History of Biology* (December 1935) (November 2015).

Horton, John. 'Producing Postman Pat: The Popular Cultural Construction of Idyllic Rurality'. *Journal of Rural Studies* 24(4) (1 October 2008): 389–98.

Howard, Robert W., and Eunice D. Overend. *Badgers without Bias: An Objective Look at the Controversy about Tuberculosis in Badgers and Cattle/by Robert W. Howard; with Decorations by Eunice D. Overend.* Bristol: Abson/Avon Wildlife Trust, 1981.

Hudson, Bob. 'Why Policy Failure Is so Common in the UK'. *LSE Business Review* (blog), 26 January 2019. https://blogs.lse.ac.uk/businessreview/2019/01/26/why-policy-failure-is-so-common-in-the-uk/.

Huxley, Elspeth. *Peter Scott: Painter and Naturalist.* London: Faber and Faber, 1993.

Hytten, Karen F. 'Dingo Dualisms: Exploring the Ambiguous Identity of Australian Dingoes'. *Australian Zoologist* 35(1) (January 2009): 18–27.

Ibrahim, Yasmin, and Anita Howarth. 'Contamination, Deception and "Othering": The Media Framing of the Horsemeat Scandal'. *Social Identities* 23(2) (March 2017): 212–31.

Inglis, D. 'What Is Worth Defending in Sociology Today? Presentism, Historical Vision and the Uses of Sociology'. *Cultural Sociology* 8(1) (March 2013): 99–118.

Ingram, Paul. 'THE UNITED KINGDOM EXPERIENCE IN THE PRIVATIZATION OF EXTENSION'. In *Public and Private Roles in Agricultural Development: Proceedings of the Twelfth Agricultural Sector Symposium*, ed. J. R. Anderson and C. de Haan. Washington, DC: World Bank Publications, 1988.

Jasanoff, Sheila. *Designs on Nature: Science and Democracy in Europe and the United States.* Princeton: Princeton University Press, 2005.

Jennings, Will, and Martin Lodge. 'Brexit, the Tides and Canute: The Fracturing Politics of the British State'. *Journal of European Public Policy* 26(5) (31 May 2018): 1–18.

Jerolmack, Colin. *The Global Pigeon*. Chicago: University of Chicago Press, 2013.

Jones, Susan D. 'Mapping a Zoonotic Disease: Anglo-American Efforts to Control Bovine Tuberculosis before World War I'. *Osiris* 19 (January 2004): 133–48.

———. 'Population Cycles, Disease, and Networks of Ecological Knowledge'. *Journal of the History of Biology* 70(2) (2017): 357–91.

Jørgensen, Dolly. 'A Blueprint for Destruction: Eco-Activism in Doctor Who during the 1970s'. *Ecozon@: European Journal of Literature, Culture and Environment* 3(2) (2012): 11–26.

Kahan, Dan M., Ellen Peters, Maggie Wittlin, Paul Slovic, Lisa Larrimore Ouellette, Donald Braman and Gregory Mandel. 'The Polarizing Impact of Science Literacy and Numeracy on Perceived Climate Change Risks'. *Nature Climate Change* 2 (May 2012): 732–35.

Kean, Hilda. 'The "Smooth Cool Men of Science": The Feminist and Socialist Response to Vivisection'. *History Workshop Journal* 40 (1995): 16–38.

———. *Animal Rights: Political and Social Change in Britain Since 1800.* Islington: Reaktion Books, 1998.

Keck, Frédéric. 'Feeding Sentinels: Logics of Care and Biosecurity in Farms and Labs'. *BioSocieties* 10(2) (2015): 162–76.

Kelly, Matthew. 'Conventional Thinking and the Fragile Birth of the Nature State in Post-War Britain'. In *The Nature State: Rethinking the History of Conservation*, ed. Wilko Graf von Hardenberg, Matthew Kelly, Claudia Leal and Emily Wakild, 114–34. Abingdon: Routledge, 2017.

Kerr, Anne, and Lisa Garforth. 'Affective Practices, Care and Bioscience: A Study of Two Laboratories'. *The Sociological Review* 64(1) (1 February 2016): 3–20.

Kim, Kiheung. *The Social Construction of Disease: From Scrapie to Prion*. New York: Routledge, 2006.

Kirk, Robert G. W. 'A Brave New Animal for a Brave New World: The British Laboratory Animals Bureau and the Constitution of International Standards of Laboratory Animal Production and Use, circa 1947–1968'. *Isis: An International Review Devoted to the History of Science and Its Cultural Influences* 101(1) (March 2010): 62–94.

———. 'Between the Clinic and the Laboratory: Ethology and Pharmacology in the Work of Michael Robin Alexander Chance, c.1946–1964'. *Medical History* 53(4) (October 2009): 513–36.

———. 'Recovering the Principles of Humane Experimental Technique: The 3Rs and the Human Essence of Animal Research'. *Science, Technology, & Human Values* 43(4) (2018): 622–48.

———. 'The Invention of the "Stressed Animal" and the Development of a Science of Animal Welfare, 1947–86'. *Animal Welfare* 1947 (2014): 86.

Knight, John. 'Introduction'. In *Natural Enemies: People–Wildlife Conflicts in Anthropological Perspective*, ed. John Knight, 1–36. New York: Routledge, 2000.

Koch, Tom. *Disease Maps: Epidemics on the Ground*. Chicago: University of Chicago Press, 2011.

Koch, Tom, and Kenneth Denike. 'Certainty, Uncertainty, and the Spatiality of Disease: A West Nile Virus Example'. *Stochastic Environmental Research and Risk Assessment* 21(5) (August 2007): 523–31.

Kohler, Robert E. *Landscapes and Labscapes: Exploring the Lab–Field Border in Biology*. Chicago: University of Chicago Press, 2002.

Krohn, P. L. 'Solly Zuckerman Baron Zuckerman, of Burnham Thorpe, O.M., K.C.B.' *Biogr. Mems Fell. R. Soc.* 41 (1995): 576–98.

Kroll, G. 'The "Silent Springs" of Rachel Carson: Mass Media and the Origins of Modern Environmentalism'. *Public Understanding of Science* 10 (2001): 403–20.

Kuhn, Raymond. *Politics and the Media in Britain*. Basingstoke: Palgrave Macmillan, 2007.

Kuhn, Thomas S. *The Structure of Scientific Revolutions: 50th Anniversary Edition*. Chicago: University of Chicago Press, 2012.

Lambert, Robert A. 'The Grey Seal in Britain: A Twentieth Century History of a Nature Conservation Success'. *Environment and History* 8(4) (2002): 449–74.

Latour, Bruno. *Science in Action: How to Follow Scientists and Engineers through Society*. Cambridge, MA: Harvard University Press, 1987.

Law, J. 'Disaster in Agriculture: Or Foot and Mouth Mobilities'. *Environment and Planning A* 38(2) (2006): 227–39.

Law, J. 'Care and Killing: Tensions in Veterinary Practice'. In *Care in Practice: On Tinkering in Clinics, Homes and Farms*, ed. A. Mol, I. Moser and J. Pols, 57–69. Bielefeld: Transcript, 2010.

Law, J., and A. Mol. 'The Actor Enacted: Cumbrian Sheep in 2001'. In *Material Agency: Towards a Non-Anthropocentric Approach*, 57–77. Dordrecht: Springer International Publishing, 2008.

Law, J., and I. Moser. 'Contexts and Culling'. *Science, Technology & Human Values* 37(4) (December 2011): 332–54.

Lean, Tom. *Electronic Dreams: How 1980s Britain Learned to Love the Computer*. New York: Bloomsbury Academic, 2016.

Lee, J. H. 'News Values, Media Coverage, and Audience Attention: An Analysis of Direct and Mediated Causal Relationships'. *Journalism & Mass Communication Quarterly* 86(1) (March 2009): 175–90.

Lester, Libby, and Brett Hutchins. 'The Power of the Unseen: Environmental Conflict, the Media and Invisibility'. *Media Culture and Society* 34(7) (October 2012): 847–63.

Lewenstein, B. V. 'From Fax to Facts—Communication in the Cold-Fusion Saga'. *Social Studies of Science* 25(3) (1995): 403–36.

Lobley, Matt, Michael Winter and Rebecca Wheeler. *The Changing World of Farming in Brexit UK*. New York: Routledge, 2018.

Lodge, Martin, and Kira Matus. 'Science, Badgers, Politics: Advocacy Coalitions and Policy Change in Bovine Tuberculosis Policy in Britain'. *Policy Studies Journal* 42(3) (August 2014): 367–90.

Lorimer, J. 'Counting Corncrakes: The Affective Science of the UK Corncrake Census'. *Social Studies of Science* 38(3) (2008): 377–405.

———. 'Nonhuman Charisma'. *Environment and Planning D: Society and Space* 25 (2007): 911–32.

Lovegrove, Roger. *Silent Fields: The Long Decline of a Nation's Wildlife*. Oxford: Oxford University Press, 2007.

Lowe, Philip, Jeremy Phillipson, Amy Proctor and Menelaos Gkartzios. 'Expertise in Rural Development: A Conceptual and Empirical Analysis'. *World Development* 116 (1 April 2019): 28–37.

Lucas, Chloe, and Russell Warman. 'Disrupting Polarized Discourses: Can We Get out of the Ruts of Environmental Conflicts?' *Environment and Planning C: Politics and Space* 36(6) (16 May 2018): 987–1005.

Macdonald, Sharon. *Behind the Scenes at the Science Museum*. Oxford: Berg, 2002.

Magnan, André. 'Food Regimes'. In *The Oxford Handbook of Food History*, edited by Jeffrey M. Pilcher, 370–88. Oxford: Oxford University Press, 2012.

Mahony, Nick, Janet Newman and Clive Barnett. *Rethinking the Public: Innovations in Research, Theory and Politics*. Bristol: Policy Press, 2010.

Maier, Michaela, Jutta Milde, Senja Post, Lars Günther, Georg Ruhrmann and Berend Barkela. 'Communicating Scientific Evidence: Scientists', Journalists' and Audiences' Expectations and Evaluations regarding the Representation of Scientific Uncertainty'. *Communications* 41(3) (2016): 239–64.

Maloney, William A., Grant Jordan and Andrew M. McLaughlin. 'Interest Groups and Public Policy: The Insider/Outsider Model Revisited'. *Journal of Public Policy* 14(1) (1994): 17–38.

Man, Lam Yee. 'Is Risk a Drive for Change? Pollution and Risk Displacement in 1970s to 1980s Hong Kong'. *Nature and Culture* 11(2) (1 June 2016): 165–95.

Marren, Peter. *The New Naturalists: Half a Century of British Natural History*. New York: HarperCollins, 1995.

Marris, Claire. 'The Construction of Imaginaries of the Public as a Threat to Synthetic Biology'. *Science as Culture* 24, no. 1 (2015): 83–98.

Marsh, David, David Toke, Claes Belfrage, Daniela Tepe and Sean McGough. 'Policy Networks and the Distinction between Insider and Outsider Groups: The Case of the Countryside Alliance'. *Public Administration* 87(3) (27 July 2009): 621–38.

Martin, A., N. Myers and A. Viseu. 'The Politics of Care in Technoscience'. *Social Studies of Science* 45(5) (October 2015): 625–41.

Martin, John. *The Development of Modern Agriculture: British Farming since 1931*. Basingstoke: Palgrave Macmillan, 2000.

———. 'The Wild Rabbit: Plague, Polices and Pestilence in England and Wales, 1931–1955'. *Agricultural History Review* 58(2) (2010): 255–76.

Marvin, Garry. *Bullfight*. Champaign, IL: University of Illinois Press, 1994.

———. 'English Foxhunting: A Prohibited Practice'. *International Journal of Cultural Property* 14(3) (2007): 339.

Marvin, Garry, and Susan McHugh. 'In It Together: An Introduction to Human–Animal Studies'. In *Routledge Handbook of Human–Animal Studies*, ed. Garry Marvin and Susan McHugh, 1–9. New York: Routledge, 2014.

———. 'INTERVIEWEE: GARRY MARVIN; INTERVIEWER: SUSAN MCHUGH'. *Antennae: The Journal of Nature in Visual Culture* 39 (2017): 7–20.

Mason Dentinger, Rachel. 'Patterns of Infection and Patterns of Evolution: How a Malaria Parasite Brought "Monkeys and Man" Closer Together in the 1960s'. *Journal of the History of Biology* 49(2) (April 2016): 359–95.

Matless, David. *Landscape and Englishness*. Islington: Reaktion Books, 1998.

Maye, Damian. 'Geography Matters: Farmer Perceptions of a Voluntary TB Risk-Based Trading System'. *The Veterinary Record* 180(6) (February 2017): 146–47.

Maye, Damian, Hannah Chiswell, Mauro Vigani and James Kirwan. '"Present Realities" and the Need for a "Lived Experience" Perspective in Brexit Agri-Food Governance'. *Space and Polity* 22(2) (4 May 2018): 270–86.

Maye, Damian, G. Enticott and Rhiannon Naylor. 'Using Scenario-Based Influence Mapping to Examine Farmers' Biosecurity Behaviour'. *Land Use Policy* 66 (October 2017): 265–77.

Maye, Damian, G. Enticott, Rhiannon Naylor, Brian Ilbery and James Kirwan. 'Animal Disease and Narratives of Nature: Farmers' Reactions to the Neoliberal Governance of Bovine Tuberculosis'. *Journal of Rural Studies* 32 (August 2014): 401–10.

McCulloch, Steven P., and Michael J. Reiss. 'Bovine Tuberculosis and Badger Control in Britain: Science, Policy and Politics'. *Journal of Agricultural and Environmental Ethics* 30(4) (1 August 2017): 469–84.

McLeod, Kari S. 'Our Sense of Snow: The Myth of John Snow in Medical Geography'. *Social Science & Medicine* 50(7–8) (April 2000): 923–35.

McMillen, Christian W. *Discovering Tuberculosis: A Global History, 1900 to the Present*. New Haven: Yale University Press, 2015.

Mehmet, Mehmet, and Peter Simmons. 'Kangaroo Court? An Analysis of Social Media Justifications for Attitudes to Culling'. *Environmental Communication* 12(3) (September 2016): 370–86.

Mellon, Jonathan, and Christopher Prosser. 'Twitter and Facebook Are Not Representative of the General Population: Political Attitudes and Demographics of British Social Media Users'. *Research & Politics* 4(3) (1 July 2017).

Méthot, Pierre-Olivier, and Rachel Mason Dentinger. 'Ecology and Infection: Studying Host–Parasite Interactions at the Interface of Biology and Medicine'. *Journal of the History of Biology* 49(2) (April 2016): 231–40.

Meyer, Morgan. 'Caring for Weak Ties—The Natural History Museum as a Place of Encounter between Amateur and Professional Science'. *Sociological Research Online* 15(2) (2010a): 9.

———. 'The Rise of the Knowledge Broker'. *Science Communication* 32(1) (March 2010b): 118–27.

Meyer, Morgan, and Susan Molyneux-Hodgson. 'Introduction: The Dynamics of Epistemic Communities'. *Sociological Research Online* 15(2) (2010): 1–7.

Miller, David. 'Risk, Science and Policy: Definitional Struggles, Information Management, the Media and BSE'. *Social Science & Medicine* 49(9) (November 1999): 1239–55.

Mills, Brett. *Animals on Television: The Cultural Making of the Non-Human*. London: Palgrave Macmillan, 2017.

———. 'Towards a Theory of Documentary Representation for Animals'. *Screen* 56(1) (1 March 2015): 102–7.

Mitman, Gregg. *Reel Nature: America's Romance with Wildlife on Film.* Cambridge, MA: Harvard University Press, 1999.

Mitsuda, Tatsuya. 'Entangled Histories: German Veterinary Medicine, c.1770–1900'. *Medical History* 61(1) (January 2017): 25–47.

Mokyr, Joel. *The Gifts of Athena: Historical Origins of the Knowledge Economy.* Princeton: Princeton University Press, 2002.

Mol, Annemarie. *The Logic of Care: Health and the Problem of Patient Choice.* New York: Routledge, 2008.

Mol, Annemarie, Ingunn Moser and Jeannette Pols, eds. *Care in Practice: On Tinkering in Clinics, Homes and Farms.* Bielefeld: Transcript Verlag, 2010.

Morel, Thomas, Giuditta Parolini and Cesare Pastorino, eds. *The Making of Useful Knowledge.* Berlin: Max Planck Institute for the History of Science, 2016.

Morris, Patricia. 'Introduction: Euthanasia in Veterinary Medicine'. In *Blue Juice: Euthanasia in Veterinary Medicine*, 1–18. Philadelphia: Temple University Press, 2012.

Mort, M., I. Convery, C. Bailey and J. Baxter. 'The Health and Social Consequences of the 2001 Foot & Mouth Disease Epidemic in North Cumbria'. (2004): 1–153.

Mort, Maggie, Ian Convery, Josephine Baxter and Cathy Bailey. 'Animal Disease and Human Trauma: The Psychosocial Implications of the 2001 UK Foot and Mouth Disease Disaster'. *Journal of Applied Animal Welfare Science* 11(2) (28 May 2008): 133–48.

Motta, Matthew. 'The Polarizing Effect of the March for Science on Attitudes toward Scientists'. *PS: Political Science & Politics* 51 (4) (October 2018): 782–788.

Motta, Renata. 'Social Disputes over GMOs: An Overview'. *Sociology Compass* 8(12) (2014): 1360–76.

Nading, Alex M. 'Humans, Animals, and Health: From Ecology to Entanglement'. *Environment and Society: Advances in Research* 4(1) (December 2013): 60–78.

Naylor, Rhiannon, Alice Hamilton-Webb, Ruth Little and Damian Maye. 'The "Good Farmer": Farmer Identities and the Control of Exotic Livestock Disease in England'. *Sociologia Ruralis* 58(1) (2016): 3–19.

Naylor, Rhiannon, Will Manley, Damian Maye, G. Enticott, Brian Ilbery and Alice Hamilton-Webb. 'The Framing of Public Knowledge Controversies in the Media: A Comparative Analysis of the Portrayal of Badger Vaccination in the English National, Regional and Farming Press'. *Sociologia Ruralis* 57(1) (2017): 3–22.

Nelson, Marie. 'Old English Riddle No. 15: The "Badger": An Early Example of Mock Heroic'. *Neophilologus* 59(3) (1975): 447–50.

Nerlich, B. 'War on Foot and Mouth Disease in the UK, 2001: Towards a Cultural Understanding of Agriculture'. *Agriculture and Human Values* 21(1) (2004): 15–25.

Neustadt, Richard E., and Ernest R. May. *Thinking in Time: The Use of History for Decision Makers.* New York: Simon and Schuster, 1986.

Nisbet, M. C., and E. M. Markowitz. 'Expertise in an Age of Polarization: Evaluating Scientists' Political Awareness and Communication Behaviors'. *The ANNALS of the American Academy of Political and Social Science* 658(1) (2015): 136–54.

Nisbet, M. C. 'Framing Science: A New Paradigm in Public Engagement'. In *Understanding Science: New Agendas in Science*, ed. LeeAnn Kahlor and Patricia A. Stout, 40–67. New York: Routledge, 2009.

Nixon, Sean. 'Trouble at the National Trust: Post-War Recreation, the Benson Report and the Rebuilding of a Conservation Organization in the 1960s'. *Twentieth Century British History* 26(4) (October 2015): 529–50.

Nyhart, Lynn K. *Modern Nature: The Rise of the Biological Perspective in Germany.* Chicago: University of Chicago Press, 2009.

Olmstead, Alan L., and Paul Rhodes. *Arresting Contagion: Science, Policy, and Conflicts over Animal Disease Control.* Cambridge, MA: Harvard University Press, 2015.

Palladino, Paolo. 'Ecological Theory and Pest Control Practice: A Study of the Institutional and Conceptual Dimensions of a Scientific Debate'. *Social Studies of Science* 20, no. 2 (May 1990): 255–81.

———. *Entomology, Ecology and Agriculture: The Making of Science Careers in North America, 1885–1985.* New York: Routledge, 2013.

Parker, Miles. 'The Rothschild Report (1971) and the Purpose of Government-Funded R&D—A Personal Account'. *Palgrave Communications* 2 (August 2016): 16053. https://doi.org/10.1057/palcomms.2016.53.

Parolini, Giuditta. 'Charting the History of Agricultural Experiments'. *History and Philosophy of the Life Sciences* 37(3) (2015): 231–41.

Pearce, Warren, Reiner Grundmann, Mike Hulme, Sujatha Raman, Eleanor Hadley Kershaw and Judith Tsouvalis. 'Beyond Counting Climate Consensus'. *Environmental Communication* 11(6) (23 July 2017): 723–30.

Pearce, Warren, Anna Wesselink and Hal Colebatch. 'Evidence and Meaning in Policy Making'. *Evidence & Policy: A Journal of Research, Debate and Practice* 10(2) (May 2014): 161–65.

Pemberton, Hugh. 'Policy Networks and Policy Learning UK Economic Policy in the 1960s and 1970s'. *Public Administration* 78(4) (1 January 2000): 771–92.

Pemberton, Neil, and Michael Worboys. *Mad Dogs and Englishmen: Rabies in Britain, 1830–2000.* Basingstoke: Palgrave Macmillan UK, 2007.

Perkins, David. *Romanticism and Animal Rights.* Cambridge: Cambridge University Press, 2003.

Petersen, I., H. Heinrichs and H. P. Peters. 'Mass-Mediated Expertise as Informal Policy Advice'. *Science, Technology & Human Values* 35(6) (August 2010): 865–87.

Phoenix, Jessica. 'Local Understandings of Bovine Tuberculosis (Working Title)'. PhD, University of Lancaster, in prep.

Pile, Steve. '"A Load of Bloody Idiots". Somerset Dairy Farmers' View of Their Political World'. *Political Geography Quarterly* 10(4) (October 1991): 405–21.

Pinch, Trevor J., and Wiebe E. Bijker. 'The Social Construction of Facts and Artefacts: Or How the Sociology of Science and the Sociology of Technology Might Benefit Each Other'. *Social Studies of Science* 14(3) (1 August 1984): 399–441.

Poole, Kristopher. 'Foxes and Badgers in Anglo-Saxon Life and Landscape'. *Archaeological Journal* (April 2015): 1–34.

Pooley, S., M. Barua, W. Beinart, A. Dickman, G. Holmes, J. Lorimer, A. J. Loveridge et al. 'An Interdisciplinary Review of Current and Future Approaches to Improving Human–Predator Relations'. *Conservation Biology* 31(3) (2016): 513–23.

Pooley, Simon, M. Barua, W. Beinart, A. Dickman, G. Holmes, J. Lorimer, A. J. Loveridge, D. W. Macdonald, G. Marvin and S. Redpath. 'An Interdisciplinary Review of Current and Future Approaches to Improving Human–Predator Relations'. *Conservation Biology* 31(3) (2017): 513–23.

Potter, Beatrix. *The Tale of Mr. Tod*. London: Frederick Warne & Co., 1908.

Potts, Annie. 'Kiwis against Possums: A Critical Analysis of Anti-Possum Rhetoric in Aotearoa New Zealand'. *Society & Animals* 17(1) (February 2009): 1–20.

Price, Stephan. *Thinking through Badgers: Researching the Controversy Over Bovine Tuberculosis and the Culling of Badgers*. Wilmington, DE: Vernon Press, 2017.

Price, Stephan, Clare Saunders, Stephen Hinchliffe and Robbie A McDonald. 'From Contradiction to Contrast in a Countryside Conflict: Using Q Methodology to Reveal a Diplomatic Space for Doing TB Differently'. *Environment and Planning A* 49(11) (23 August 2017): 2578–94.

Public Domain Review. 'The History of Four-Footed Beasts and Serpents (1658)'. *The Public Domain Review*, 2015. https://publicdomainreview.org/collections/the-history-of-four-footed-beasts-and-serpents-1658/.

Reed, Matthew. '"This Loopy Idea": An Analysis of UKIP's Social Media Discourse in Relation to Rurality and Climate Change'. *Space and Polity* 20(2) (May 2016): 1–16.

Rees, Amanda. 'Animal Agents? Historiography, Theory and the History of Science in the Anthropocene'. *BJHS Themes* 2 (January 2017): 1–10. https://doi.org/10.1017/bjt.2017.11.

———. *The Infanticide Controversy: Primatology and the Art of Field Science*. Chicago: University of Chicago Press, 2009.

Reynolds, David. 'Case Study: TV History: Probing People's Comfortable Assumptions'. *History and Policy*, 18 August 2016. http://www.historyandpolicy.org/case-studies/case-study/david-reynolds.

Riesch, H. 'Changing News: Re-Adjusting Science Studies to Online Newspapers'. *Public Understanding of Science* 20(6) (August 2010): 771–77.

Riesch, Hauke, and Clive Potter. 'Citizen Science as Seen by Scientists: Methodological, Epistemological and Ethical Dimensions'. *Public Understanding of Science* 23(1) (1 January 2014): 107–20.

Robinson, Emily, Camilla Schofield, Florence Sutcliffe-Braithwaite and Natalie Thomlinson. 'Telling Stories about Post-War Britain: Popular Individualism and the "Crisis" of the 1970s'. *Twentieth Century British History* 28 (2), (June 2017): 268–304.

Robinson, Philip A. 'A History of Bovine Tuberculosis Eradication Policy in Northern Ireland'. *Epidemiology and Infection* 143(15) (2015): 3182–95.

———. 'Farmers and Bovine Tuberculosis: Contextualising Statutory Disease Control within Everyday Farming Lives'. *Journal of Rural Studies* 55(Supplement C) (1 October 2017): 168–80.

———. 'Performativity and a Microbe: Exploring Mycobacterium Bovis and the Political Ecologies of Bovine Tuberculosis'. *BioSocieties*, 6 June 2018.

Romero, Adam M. 'Commercializing Chemical Warfare: Citrus, Cyanide, and an Endless War'. *Agriculture and Human Values* 33(1) (March 2016): 3–26.

Rosenberg, Charles. 'Chapter 15—Toward an Ecology of Knowledge: On Discipline, Context, and History'. In *Rise of the Knowledge Worker*, ed. James W. Cortada, 221–32. Boston: Butterworth-Heinemann, 1998.

Rosenberg, Charles E. 'Disease in History: Frames and Framers'. *The Milbank Quarterly* 67 (1989): 1–15.

Rosenberg, Charles E., and Janet Lynne Golden. *Framing Disease: Studies in Cultural History*. New Brunswick, NJ: Rutgers University Press, 1992.

Rosner, Lisa. *The Technological Fix: How People Use Technology to Create and Solve Problems*. New York: Routledge, 2013.

Russell, Edmund P. '"Speaking of Annihilation": Mobilizing for War against Human and Insect Enemies, 1914–1945'. *The Journal of American History* 82(4) (1996): 1505–29.

———. *War and Nature: Fighting Humans and Insects with Chemicals from World War I to Silent Spring*. Cambridge: Cambridge University Press, 2001.

Sandbrook, Dominic. *State of Emergency: The Way We Were. Britain, 1970–1974*. London: Penguin, 2011.

Sandover, Rebecca, Samuel Kinsley and Stephen Hinchliffe. 'A Very Public Cull—The Anatomy of an Online Issue Public'. *Geoforum* 97 (1 December 2018): 106–18.

Sands, Tim. *Wildlife in Trust: A Hundred Years of Nature Conservation*. London: Elliott & Thompson, 2013.

Sarewitz, Daniel. 'How Science Makes Environmental Controversies Worse'. *Environmental Science & Policy* 7(5) (October 2004): 385–403.

Sasse, Tom, and Emma Norris. 'Moving On'. 16 January 2019. https://www.instituteforgovernment.org.uk/publications/moving-on-staff-turnover-civil-service.

Saunders, Clare, and Caroline Keenan. 'Conflict Framing in the Control of Bovine Tuberculosis'. Environment and Sustainability Institute, University of Exeter, in prep.

Saunders-Jones, Dafydd. 'Bovine TB Eradication Programmes in Europe'. Nuffield Farming Scholarships Trust Report, August 2016. nuffieldinternational.org/live/Report/UK/2015/dafydd-saunders-jones.

Sax, Boria. *Imaginary Animals: The Monstrous, the Wondrous and the Human*. Islington: Reaktion Books, 2013.

Sayer, Karen. 'Animal Machines: The Public Response to Intensification in Great Britain, c. 1960–c. 1973'. *Agricultural History* 87(4) (2013): 473–501.

———. 'Brucellosis in Fact and Fiction: The Story of a Zoonosis'. *Veterinary History* 18 (2016): 165–83.

———. 'The "Modern" Management of Rats: British Agricultural Science in Farm and Field during the Twentieth Century'. *BJHS Themes* (January 2017): 1–29. https://doi.org/10.1017/bjt.2017.7.

Schäfer, Mike S. 'Taking Stock: A Meta-Analysis of Studies on the Media's Coverage of Science'. *Public Understanding of Science* 21(6) (December 2012): 650–63.

Scheu, A. M., A.-M. Volpers, A. Summ and B. Blobaum. 'Medialization of Research Policy: Anticipation of and Adaptation to Journalistic Logic'. *Science Communication* 36(6) (September 2014): 706–34.

Schuurman, Nora. 'Performing Good Death at the Veterinary Clinic: Experiences of Pet Euthanasia in Finland'. *Area* 49(2) (2016): 208–14.

Sellick, Jessica, and Richard Yarwood. 'Placing Livestock in Landscape Studies: Pastures New or Out to Graze?' *Landscape Research* 38(4) (August 2013): 404–20.

Sharman, Amelia, and Richard Perkins. 'Post-Decisional Logics of Inaction: The Influence of Knowledge Controversy in Climate Policy Decision-Making'. *Environment and Planning A: Economy and Space* 49(10) (1 October 2017): 2281–99.

Sheail, John. 'Government and the Management of an Alien Pest Species: A British Perspective'. *Landscape Research* 28(1) (2003): 101–11.

———. *Nature in Trust: The History of Nature Conservation in Britain*. Glasgow: Blackie, 1976.

———. 'Nature Protection, Ecologists and the Farming Context: A U.K. Historical Context'. *Journal of Rural Studies* 11(1) (1995): 79–88.

———. '"One and the Same Historic Landscape": A Physical/Cultural Perspective'. *International Journal of Heritage Studies* 13(4–5) (2007a): 321–34.

———. 'The Grey Squirrel (*Sciurus Carolinensis*)—A UK Historical Perspective on a Vertebrate Pest Species'. *Journal of Environmental Management* 55(3) (March 1999): 145–56.

———. 'The Management of an Animal Population: Changing Attitudes towards the Wild Rabbit in Britain'. *Journal of Environmental Management* 33(2) (1991): 189–203.

———. 'The Management of Wildlife and Amenity: A UK Post-war Perspective'. *Contemporary Record* 7(1) (1993): 44–65.

———. 'The Mink Menace: The Politics of Vertebrate Pest Control'. *Rural History* 15(2) (2004): 207–22.

———. '"Torrey Canyon": The Political Dimension'. *Journal of Contemporary History* 42(3) (2007b): 485–504.

———. 'Wartime Rodent-Control in England and Wales'. In *The Front Line of Freedom: British Farming in the Second World War*, edited by Brian Short, Charles Watkins, and John Martin, 55–66. Exeter: British Agricultural History Society, 2006.

Shortall, Orla, Annmarie Ruston, Martin Green, Marnie Brennan, Wendela Wapenaar and Jasmeet Kaler. 'Broken Biosecurity? Veterinarians' Framing of Biosecurity on Dairy Farms in England'. *Preventive Veterinary Medicine* 132 (2016): 20–31.

Shortall, Orla, Lee-Ann Sutherland, Annmarie Ruston and Jasmeet Kaler. 'True Cowmen and Commercial Farmers: Exploring Vets' and Dairy Farmers' Contrasting Views of "Good Farming" in Relation to Biosecurity'. *Sociologia Ruralis* 58(3) (2018): 583–603.

Shuttleworth, Sally. 'Old Weather: Citizen Scientists in the 19th and 21st Centuries'. *Science Museum Group Journal* 3(3) (March 2015). http://journal.sciencemuseum.org.uk/browse/issue-03/old-weather/.

Silk, Matthew J., Darren P. Croft, Richard J. Delahay, David J. Hodgson, Mike Boots, Nicola Weber and Robbie A. McDonald. 'Using Social Network Measures in Wildlife Disease Ecology, Epidemiology, and Management'. *BioScience* 67(3) (1 March 2017): 245–57.

Silverman, Chloe. *Understanding Autism: Parents, Doctors, and the History of a Disorder*. Princeton: Princeton University Press, 2012.

Simberloff, Daniel. 'Charles Elton: Pioneer Conservation Biologist'. *Environment and History* 18(2) (2012): 183–202.

Sismondo, Sergio. *An Introduction to Science and Technology Studies.* Chichester, UK: Wiley-Blackwell, 2010.

van Sittert, Lance. 'Routinising Genocide: The Politics and Practice of Vermin Extermination in the Cape Province c.1889–1994'. *Journal of Contemporary African Studies* 34(1) (2 January 2016): 111–28.

Sluga, Glenda. *Internationalism in the Age of Nationalism*. Pennsylvania: University of Pennsylvania Press, 2013.

Smallman, Melanie. 'Science to the Rescue or Contingent Progress? Comparing 10 Years of Public, Expert and Policy Discourses on New and Emerging Science and Technology in the United Kingdom'. *Public Understanding of Science* 27(6) (1 August 2018): 655–73.

Smocovitis, Vassiliki Betty. *Unifying Biology: The Evolutionary Synthesis and Evolutionary Biology*. Princeton: Princeton University Press, 1996.

Sorensen, Andre. 'Taking Path Dependence Seriously: An Historical Institutionalist Research Agenda in Planning History'. *Planning Perspectives* 30(1) (2 January 2015): 17–38.

Spencer, Adam. 'One Body of Evidence, Three Different Policies: Bovine Tuberculosis Policy in Britain'. *Politics* 31(2) (2011): 91–99.

Star, Susan Leigh. 'Power, Technology and the Phenomenology of Conventions: On Being Allergic to Onions'. *The Sociological Review* 38(S1) (1 May 1990): 26–56.

Steere-Williams, Jacob. 'Performing State Medicine During Its "Frustrating" Years: Epidemiology and Bacteriology at the Local Government Board, 1870–1900'. *Social History of Medicine* 28(1) (September 2014a): 82–107.

———. 'The Perfect Food and the Filth Disease: Milk-Borne Typhoid and Epidemiological Practice in Late Victorian Britain'. *Journal of the History of Medicine and Allied Sciences* 65(4) (October 2014b): 514–45.

Stirling, Andy, and Clive Mitchell. 'Evaluate Power and Bias in Synthesizing Evidence for Policy'. *Nature* 563 (5 September 2018): 33.

Strauss, A., and J. Corbin. 'Grounded Theory Methodology: An Overview'. In *Handbook of Qualitative Research*, ed. N. K. Denzin and Y. S. Lincoln, 273–85. Thousand Oaks, CA: Sage, 1994.

Sunderland, Mary E. 'Modernizing Natural History: Berkeley's Museum of Vertebrate Zoology in Transition'. *Journal of the History of Biology* (September 2012).

Sundqvist, Göran, Des Gasper, Asunción Lera St. Clair, Erlend A. T. Hermansen, Steven Yearley, Irene Øvstebø Tvedten and Brian Wynne. 'One World or Two? Science–Policy Interactions in the Climate Field'. *Critical Policy Studies* 12(4) (2018): 448–68.

Svendsen, Mette N., and Lene Koch. 'Potentializing the Research Piglet in Experimental Neonatal Research'. *Current Anthropology* 54(S7) (October 2013): S118–28.

Syse, Karen Victoria Lykke. 'Otters as Symbols in the British Environmental Discourse'. *Landscape Research* 38(4) (August 2013): 540–52.

———. 'Stumbling over Animals in the Landscape: Methodological Accidents and Anecdotes'. *Nordic Journal of Science and Technology Studies* 2(1) (December 2016): 20.

Taylor, Nik, and Richard Twine. *The Rise of Critical Animal Studies: From the Margins to the Centre*. New York: Routledge, 2014.

Thane, Pat. *Unequal Britain: Equalities in Britain since 1945*. London: Bloomsbury Publishing, 2010.

Thirtle, Colin, Paolo Palladino and Jenifer Piesse. 'On the Organisation of Agricultural Research in the United Kingdom, 1945–1994: A Quantitative

Description and Appraisal of Recent Reforms'. *Research Policy* 26(4–5) (December 1997): 557–76.

Tichelar, Michael. '"Putting Animals into Politics": The Labour Party and Hunting in the First Half of the Twentieth Century'. *Rural History* 17(2) (October 2006): 213–34.

———. *The History of Opposition to Blood Sports in Twentieth Century England: Hunting at Bay*. New York: Taylor & Francis, 2016.

Tilley, Helen. *Africa as a Living Laboratory: Empire, Development, and the Problem of Scientific Knowledge, 1870–1950*. Chicago: University of Chicago Press, 2011.

Tucker, Joshua A., Andrew Guess, Pablo Barbera, Cristian Vaccari, Alexandra Siegel, Sergey Sanovich, Denis Stukal and Brendan Nyhan. 'Social Media, Political Polarization, and Political Disinformation: A Review of the Scientific Literature'. SSRN Scholarly Paper. Rochester, NY: Social Science Research Network, 19 March 2018. https://papers.ssrn.com/abstract=3144139.

UlAin, Qurat, and Terry Whiting. 'Is a "Good Death" at the Time of Animal Slaughter an Essentially Contested Concept?' *Animals* 7(12) (14 December 2017): 99.

Van Zwanenberg, Patrick, and Erik Millstone. 'BSE: A Paradigm of Policy Failure'. *The Political Quarterly* 74(1) (January 2003): 27–37.

———. *BSE: Risk, Science and Governance*. Oxford: Oxford University Press, 2005.

Vandeweerd, Jean-Michel, Nathalie Kirschvink, Peter Clegg, Sandrine Vandenput, Pascal Gustin and Claude Saegerman. 'Is Evidence-Based Medicine so Evident in Veterinary Research and Practice? History, Obstacles and Perspectives'. *The Veterinary Journal* 191(1) (January 2012): 28–34.

Vasterman, Peter, ed. *From Media Hype to Twitter Storm: News Explosions and Their Impact on Issues, Crises, and Public Opinion*. Amsterdam: Amsterdam University Press, 2018a.

———. 'Introduction'. In *From Media Hype to Twitter Storm: News Explosions and Their Impact on Issues, Crises, and Public Opinion*, 17–36. Amsterdam: Amsterdam University Press, 2018b.

Waddington, Keir. *The Bovine Scourge: Meat, Tuberculosis and Public Health, 1850–1914*. Woodbridge: Boydell & Brewer, 2006.

———. 'The Science of Cows: Tuberculosis, Research and the State in the United Kingdom, 1890–1914'. *History of Science* 39(3) (September 2001): 355–81.

———. 'To Stamp out "so Terrible a Malady": Bovine Tuberculosis and Tuberculin Testing in Britain, 1890–1939'. *Medical History* 48(1) (January 2004): 29–48.

Wagner-Egger, P., A. Bangerter, I. Gilles, E. Green, D. Rigaud, F. Krings, C. Staerkle and A. Clemence. 'Lay Perceptions of Collectives at the Outbreak of the H1N1 Epidemic: Heroes, Villains and Victims'. *Public Understanding of Science* 20(4) (March 2011): 461–76.

Wallwork, J., and John A. Dixon. 'Foxes, Green Fields and Britishness: On the Rhetorical Construction of Place and National Identity'. *British Journal of Social Psychology* 43(1) (2004): 21–39.
Ward, Neil. 'Rethinking Rural Policy under New Labour'. In *New Labour's Countryside Rural Policy in Britain since 1997*, ed. M. Woods, 29–43. Bristol: The Policy Press, 2008.
Warrier, Maya. 'The Temple Bull Controversy at Skanda Vale and the Construction of Hindu Identity in Britain'. *International Journal of Hindu Studies* 13(3) (2009): 261–78.
Weich, Kerstin, and Herwig Grimm. 'Editorial'. *Food Ethics* 1(3) (1 March 2018): 205–8.
Whatmore, S. J. 'Mapping Knowledge Controversies: Science, Democracy and the Redistribution of Expertise'. *Progress in Human Geography* 33(5) (July 2009): 587–98.
Wihbey, John. 'Journalists' Use of Knowledge in an Online World'. *Journalism Practice* 11(10) (November 2016): 1267–82.
Wilkie, Rhoda. *Livestock/Deadstock: Working with Farm Animals from Birth to Slaughter*. Philadelphia: Temple University Press, 2010.
Wilkinson, Katy. 'Organised Chaos: An Interpretive Approach to Evidence-Based Policy Making in Defra'. *Political Studies* 59(4) (December 2011): 959–77.
Williams, Roger. 'Some Political Aspects of the Rothschild Affair'. *Science Studies* 3(1) (1973): 31–46.
Wilsdon, James. 'The Past, Present and Future of the Chief Scientific Advisor'. *European Journal of Risk Regulation* 5(3) (September 2014): 293–99.
Wilson, Mark. 'The British Environmental Movement: The Development of an Environmental Consciousness and Environmental Activism, 1945–1975'. PhD, Northumbria University Newcastle, 2014. http://nrl.northumbria.ac.uk/21603/.
Winter, M. 'Intersecting Departmental Responsibilities, Administrative Confusion and the Role of Science in Government: The Case of BSE'. *Parliamentary Affairs* 49(4) (October 1996): 550–65.
Woods, Abigail. 'A Historical Synopsis of Farm Animal Disease and Public Policy in Twentieth Century Britain'. *Philosophical Transactions of the Royal Society of London. Series B, Biological Sciences* 366(1573) (July 2011a): 1943–54.
———. *A Manufactured Plague: The History of Foot-and-Mouth Disease in Britain*. London: Earthscan, 2004.
———. 'From Cruelty to Welfare: The Emergence of Farm Animal Welfare in Britain, 1964–71'. *Endeavour* 36(1) (2012): 14–22.
———. 'From Practical Men to Scientific Experts: British Veterinary Surgeons and the Development of Government Scientific Expertise, c. 1878–1919'. *History of Science* (2013): 457–80.

———. 'Patterns of Animal Disease'. In *Routledge History of Disease*, ed. Mark Jackson, 147–64. New York: Routledge, 2016.

———. 'The Farm as Clinic: Veterinary Expertise and the Transformation of Dairy Farming, 1930–1950'. *Studies in History and Philosophy of Biological and Biomedical Sciences* 38(2) (June 2007): 462–87.

———. 'The Lowe Report and Its Echoes from History'. *The Veterinary Record* 169(17) (October 2011b): 434–36.

Woods, Abigail, Michael Bresalier, Angela Cassidy and Rachel Mason Dentinger. *Animals and the Shaping of Modern Medicine: One Health and Its Histories.* Cham, Switzerland: Palgrave Macmillan, 2018. https://doi.org/10.1017/bjt.2017.3.

Woods, Abigail, and Stephen Matthews. '"Little, If at All, Removed from the Illiterate Farrier or Cow-Leech": The English Veterinary Surgeon, c.1860–1885, and the Campaign for Veterinary Reform'. *Medical History* 54(1) (January 2010): 29–54.

Worboys, M. 'Germ Theories of Disease and British Veterinary Medicine, 1860–1890'. *Medical History* 35(3) (July 1991): 308–27.

Wynne, Brian. 'Creating Public Alienation: Expert Cultures of Risk and Ethics on GMOs'. *Science as Culture* 10(4) (2001): 445–81.

———. 'Misunderstood Misunderstanding: Social Identities and Public Uptake of Science'. *Public Understanding of Science* 1 (1992): 281–304.

(All URLs last accessed 6 March 2019)

Permissions

All chapters in this book were first published by Springer by Angela Cassidy; hereby published with permission under the Creative Commons Attribution License or equivalent. Every chapter published in this book has been scrutinized by our experts. Their significance has been extensively debated. The topics covered herein carry significant information for a comprehensive understanding. They may even be implemented as practical applications or may be referred to as a beginning point for further studies.

We would like to thank the editorial team for lending their expertise to make the book truly unique. They have played a crucial role in the development of this book. Without their invaluable contributions this book wouldn't have been possible. They have made vital efforts to compile up to date information on the varied aspects of this subject to make this book a valuable addition to the collection of many professionals and students.

This book was conceptualized with the vision of imparting up-to-date and integrated information in this field. To ensure the same, a matchless editorial board was set up. Every individual on the board went through rigorous rounds of assessment to prove their worth. After which they invested a large part of their time researching and compiling the most relevant data for our readers.

The editorial board has been involved in producing this book since its inception. They have spent rigorous hours researching and exploring the diverse topics which have resulted in the successful publishing of this book. They have passed on their knowledge of decades through this book. To expedite this challenging task, the publisher supported the team at every step. A small team of assistant editors was also appointed to further simplify the editing procedure and attain best results for the readers.

Apart from the editorial board, the designing team has also invested a significant amount of their time in understanding the subject and creating the most relevant covers. They scrutinized every image to scout for the most suitable representation of the subject and create an appropriate cover for the book.

The publishing team has been an ardent support to the editorial, designing and production team. Their endless efforts to recruit the best for this project, has resulted in the accomplishment of this book. They are a veteran in the field of academics and their pool of knowledge is as vast as their experience in printing. Their expertise and guidance has proved useful at every step.

Their uncompromising quality standards have made this book an exceptional effort. Their encouragement from time to time has been an inspiration for everyone.

The publisher and the editorial board hope that this book will prove to be a valuable piece of knowledge for students, practitioners and scholars across the globe.

Index

E

G

H

I

L

M

N

P

www.ingramcontent.com/pod-product-compliance
Lightning Source LLC
LaVergne TN
LVHW051049220926
848485LV00001BA/53
* 9 7 8 1 6 4 1 1 6 7 7 8 9 *